VITAMIN K
in Health
and Disease

VITAMIN K
in Health
and Disease

John W. Suttie

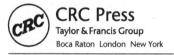

CRC Press
Taylor & Francis Group
Boca Raton London New York

CRC Press is an imprint of the
Taylor & Francis Group, an **informa** business

CRC Press
Taylor & Francis Group
6000 Broken Sound Parkway NW, Suite 300
Boca Raton, FL 33487-2742

ISBN 13: 978-0-3674-5244-5 (pbk)

Library of Congress Cataloging-in-Publication Data

Suttie, J. W. (John Weston), 1934-
    Vitamin K in health and disease / John W. Suttie.
      p. ; cm.
    Includes bibliographical references and index.
    ISBN 978-0-8493-3392-7 (hardcover : alk. paper)
    1. Vitamin K--Health aspects. I. Title.
    [DNLM: 1. Vitamin K. W1 OX626 v.26 2009 / QU 181 S967v 2009]

    QP772.V55S88 2009
    612.3'99--dc22
                                                2009005528

Visit the Taylor & Francis Web site at
http://www.taylorandfrancis.com

and the CRC Press Web site at
http://www.crcpress.com

Contents

Chapter 4

Preface

Research efforts directed toward an understanding of the metabolic role of vitamin K have had a somewhat unusual history. The discovery of this fat-soluble vitamin in the early 1930s was based on the observation of a blood clotting disorder in chicks fed a diet designed to lack cholesterol. It was soon shown that the lack of a previously unknown fat-soluble factor was responsible for the hemorrhagic condition, and it was identified and designated "vitamin K." A decrease in the activity of the plasma procoagulant prothrombin was noted early in these studies, and over the next 20 years, three other plasma procoagulants, factors VII, IX, and X, were found to require vitamin K. These four proteins were collectively called the "vitamin K-dependent clotting factors," and it was another 20 years before other vitamin K-dependent proteins were discovered. An understanding of how vitamin K was involved in the synthesis of these clotting factors was not elucidated during the early phase of vitamin K research as scientists did not know how proteins were synthesized. I became interested in vitamin K research in the mid-1960s and was involved in the efforts of a few small research groups to eventually demonstrate that the biological role of vitamin K is to function as one of the substrates of an enzyme that modifies the biological activity of a small number of proteins by the posttranslational conversion of specific Glu residues to γ-carboxyglutamyl (GLA) residues. A substantial amount of this book deals with the vitamin K-dependent carboxylase, with the vitamin K-epoxide reductase, a closely associated enzyme, and with the identification and function of other vitamin K-dependent proteins and their functions. The book focuses more on the history of the development of our current understanding of vitamin K function than would be found in most extensive reviews, but I feel that the retention of some of the history of any field of research is of value. I have also attempted to keep the discussion of recent advances in this research field as current as a publication schedule will allow, as a number of new and exciting venues of research have opened up in the last few years.

The other major focus of this book is directed toward the nutritional and public health aspects of vitamin K research. The vitamin K requirements of animals and humans were historically based on the amount of vitamin needed for the normal coagulation of blood, and in the case of the healthy adult human, it is essentially impossible to produce a prothrombin time that is out of the "normal" range. The low dietary requirement for the vitamin and the low amounts of vitamin K in most foods prevented the publication of accurate databases to calculate dietary intakes for some time, but these are now available. This book provides what I feel will be helpful tables on food sources, population intakes of vitamin K, and the impact of diet on the circulating levels of vitamin K and of other potential markers which have been used to assess vitamin K status. Much of the public health concerns regarding vitamin K intake has been related to the possible role of vitamin K in the promotion of skeletal health. However, more of the recent efforts are directed toward the possible role of vitamin K in preventing vascular calcification, and there are a number of other public health-related responses that may be associated with vitamin K status that are being currently investigated. These efforts are covered in this book, as well as a discussion of the difficulty in establishing an appropriate dietary reference intake for vitamin K.

As the number of research laboratory leaders involved in vitamin K-related research has always been small, I have had the pleasure of personally knowing most of them as competitors, collaborators, and friends. The open interaction between this group of scientists has aided progress in the field, as have the graduate students, postdocs, and visiting scientists who have worked in my laboratory on vitamin K-related projects: Charles Coven, Dharmishtha Shah, Myrtle Thierry-Palmer, Gary Nelsestuen, David Lorusso, Charles Esmon, Gregory Grant, Johan Stenflo, James Sadowski, Louise Canfield, Jeffrey Finnan, Thomas Carlisle, John McTigue, Reidar Wallin, Donna Whitlon, Megumi Kawai, Lasse Uotila, Ann Larson, Jean Patterson, Takami Ueno, Peter Preusch, Sherwood Lehrman, Tom Brody, Ellen Hildebrandt, Jhan Swanson, Alex Cheung, Richard Pottorf, Angelika Hopfgartner, Kathleen Creedon, Moa Schalin-Karrila, Susumu Funakawa, Gary Wood, Carl Kindberg, James Knobloch, DeAnn Liska, Sharyn Gardill, Yuji Usui, Carol Grossman, Tina Misenheimer, Mark Harbeck, Charlet Keller Reedstrom, Birgit Will-Simmons, Randall Bolger, Pumin Zhang, Cassandra Kight, Margaret Benton, Cynthia Hinck, Alexandra Bach, Richard Moulton, Wei Wu, Robert Davidson, Gwendolyn Alexander, Andrea Garber, Sherri Millis, Anna Sessler, and Zhongjian Lu.

Author

John Suttie is the Katherine Berns Van Donk Steenbock professor emeritus in the Department of Biochemistry and former chair of the Department of Nutritional Sciences at the University of Wisconsin–Madison. He has broad expertise in biochemistry and human nutrition. Dr. Suttie received his B.S., M.S., and Ph.D. degrees from the University of Wisconsin–Madison. He was a National Institutes of Health (NIH) postdoctoral fellow at the National Institute for Medical Research, Mill Hill, England, before joining the University of Wisconsin faculty. His research activities were directed toward the toxicology of inorganic fluorides and the metabolism, mechanism of action, and nutritional significance of vitamin K. He received the Mead Johnson Award, the Osborne & Mendel Award, and the Conrad Elvehjem Award of the American Society for Nutrition (ASN); the Atwater Lectureship from the Agricultural Research Service; the Bristol Myers-Squibb Award for Distinguished Achievement in Nutrition Research; an award for his contributions to hemostasis from the International Society on Thrombosis and Haemostasis; and in 1996 he was elected to the National Academy of Sciences.

Dr. Suttie served as president of the ASN and as their editor-in-chief of the *Journal of Nutrition*. He served as chairman of the Board of Experimental Biology, president of the Federation of American Societies for Experimental Biology (FASEB), and as a member of the National Academy's Board on Agriculture and Natural Resources and the Food and Nutrition Board of the Institute of Medicine. He also served on the Blood Products Advisory Committee of the Food and Drug Administration and the American Heart Association Nutrition Committee, the Public Policy Committees of the ASN and the American Society for Biochemistry and Molecular Biology, the USDA/NAREEE Advisory Board, the International Life Sciences Institute (ILSI) Food, Nutrition and Safety Committee, and on Dietary Guidelines and Dietary Reference Intakes Committees.

1 Historical Background

The dietary essentiality of vitamin K was discovered as the result of a series of experiments carried out by the Danish nutritional biochemist Henrik Dam, working at the University of Copenhagen. Dam was studying the possible essentiality of cholesterol in the diet of the chick and noted [1,2] that chicks ingesting diets that had been extracted with nonpolar solvents to remove the sterols developed subdural or muscular hemorrhages and that blood taken from these animals clotted slowly. As was the case in the discovery of almost all of the vitamins, Dam's observations were not unique. A similar response was subsequently observed by McFarlane and his collaborators [3] at the Ontario Agricultural College in Guelph, Canada, who described a clotting defect seen in experiments designed to assess the nutritive value of different protein sources in purified chick diets. The chicks bled when their wings were banded, and the same response was observed [4] when they fed chicks ether-extracted fish or meat meal in an attempt to establish the vitamin A and D requirements of the chick. Holst and Halbrook [5] in the Division of Poultry Husbandry of the College of Agriculture at the Berkeley campus of the University of California also observed "scurvy-like" symptoms, including internal and external hemorrhages, in chicks fed fish meal and yeast as a protein source. The hemorrhagic condition was cured by the addition of cabbage to the diet, and they concluded from this observation that vitamin C was essential for the chick. It is of interest that, although most North American scientists in the 1930s were capable of reading the German literature, neither the Guelph nor the Berkeley group cited Dam's observations of similar hemorrhagic responses in chicks fed altered diets.

Cribbett and Correll [6] at Kansas State College subsequently failed to reproduce the "scurvy-like" symptoms observed by Holst and Halbrook, and Dam's studies of the hemorrhagic condition as a "new deficiency disease" [7] continued. The observations from Dam's laboratory that lemon juice [2] or ascorbic acid administration [7,8] did not influence the hemorrhagic response provided further evidence against the vitamin C theory, and studies shifted to an attempt to isolate and identify the unknown factor. Progress in elucidating the nature of the hemorrhagic condition was confused to some extent, but not seriously delayed, by the hypothesis of Cook and Scott at the University of California Medical School that the response was caused by the presence of toxic factors in the protein source used [9,10]. Subsequent efforts to identify the new essential factor were initially led by Dam and by Almquist in the Poultry Science Department at Berkeley, who followed up the original observations of Holst and Halbrook.

A series of short, one- to three-page reports by these two groups established the new essential nutrient as being in the nonsterol, nonsaponifiable portion of the lipid extracts of liver and a number of green vegetables [11–13]. In a somewhat more extensive report by Almquist and Stokstad [14] it was noted that Halbrook [15] had found that when fish meal was used as the protein source in the basal (antihemorrhagic factor deficient) ration, the response was variable; and, if the fish meal was kept moistened for some time, the hemorrhagic disease did not develop. The Berkeley group clearly established (Table 1.1) that drying the fish meal slowly, which would have allowed bacterial action, resulted in a protective response that was not obtained when the meal was dried rapidly. These studies also established that the protective action which was developed in wet fish meal could not be explained on the basis of the removal of some water-soluble prohemorrhagic toxic factor in the fish meal. Although these studies pointed out the possibility that bacterial action in the wet fish meal might be involved in developing the antihemorrhagic properties of the product, the authors did not hypothesize that the bacteria were synthesizing the elusive factor. A subsequent report [16] described the demonstration of the presence of the antihemorrhagic factor in an ether extract of the droppings of chicks fed only the basal diet, with the conclusion that "the vitamin was evidently synthesized by bacterial action either after the droppings were voided or within the lower portions of the digestive tract where absorption could not take place readily, or both." These early advances in establishing the nature of the antihemorrhagic factor were made using only rather insensitive whole blood clotting times and the incidence of hemorrhage or mortality as an end point, and it is of interest to review the types of data that were accepted by leading biochemical journals at that time (Tables 1.2 and 1.3). It is apparent the statisticians were not heavily involved in manuscript review during the 1930s. The difficulty in producing a diet that would induce spontaneous hemorrhagic condition in any species other than the chick was not apparent until later, and the fortuitous

TABLE 1.1
Impact of "Slow Drying" on the Antihemorrhagic Factor in Fish Meal Measured by a Chick Bioassay

	% of Chicks	
Diet	Survived	Hemorrhage
Basal diet	0	69
Basal diet with fish meal portion washed with water and rapidly dried at 200°F	6	94
Basal diet with fish meal portion dried by washing with 95% ethanol	19	75
10% of the 65% polished rice in the basal diet replaced with 10% rice bran	37	50
10% of the 65% polished rice in the basal diet replaced with moistened rice bran and the diet slowly dried at room temperature	94	0

Note: Basal diet contained: 20% fish meal (not putrefied), 65% ground polished rice, 12% dried yeast, 1% $CaCO_3$, 1% salt, 1% cod liver oil. White leghorn chicks (15/group) were fed the diets for 6 weeks, while survival rate and incidence of hemorrhagic syndrome were recorded.
Source: Adopted from Almquist and Stokstad [14].

TABLE 1.2
Effect of Liver Fat Fractionation on Antihemorrhagic Activity

Addition to Basal Diet	Whole Blood Clotting Time (min)
None	10, 20, >30, >60, >1000
3% hog liver fat	2, 2, 2, 4, 4
3% fatty acids from fat	5, >30, >30, >30, >60
0.4% nonsaponifiable portion of fat	3, 4, 12, 12, 13
0.4% sterol from fat	15, 60, 75, >60

Note: Basal diet contained: 20% ether extracted dried hog liver, 15% dried yeast, 2.7% salts, 62.3% sucrose with 4% cod liver oil added. White leghorn chicks (5/group) were fed the diets for 30 days.

Source: Adopted from Dam [12].

TABLE 1.3
Effect of Fish Meal and Alfalfa Extracts on Antihemorrhagic Activity

Addition to Basal Diet	Mortality (%)	Hemorrhage (%)
None	87	73
Putrefied fish meal	20	7
Ether extract of putrefied fish meal (2%)	0	0
Dehydrated alfalfa (2%)	0	0
Ether extract of alfalfa, equivalent to 10% alfalfa	7	0
Nonsaponifiable fraction of alfalfa extract	6	0
Saponifiable fraction of alfalfa extract	60	47

Note: Basal diet contained: 20% fish meal (not putrefied), 65% ground polished rice, 12% dried yeast, 1% $CaCO_3$, 1% salt, 1% cod liver oil. White leghorn chicks (15/group) were fed the diets for 6 weeks, while survival rate and incidence of hemorrhagic syndrome were recorded.

Source: Adopted from Almquist and Stokstad [14].

choice of the chick as an experimental animal in the early experiments was essential to the chance discovery of the vitamin.

The term "vitamin K" was first used by Dam in a short note in *Nature* concluding that the factor could not be identical with vitamin A, D, or E; he said "I therefore suggest the term vitamin K for the antihemorrhagic factor" [11]. Although not commented on in the *Nature* article, Dam [17] subsequently pointed out that "the letter K was the first one in the alphabet which had not, with more or less justification, been used to designate other vitamins, and it also happened to be the first letter in the word 'koagulation' according to the Scandinavian and German spellings."

The complex series of enzymatic reactions involved in the coagulation of blood were not well understood in the 1930s, and only prothrombin and fibrinogen were definitely characterized as plasma proteins involved in the formation of a fibrin clot. Dam's group [18] succeeded in preparing a crude plasma prothrombin fraction from chick plasma and demonstrated that its procoagulant activity was decreased when it was obtained from vitamin K-deficient chicks. Quick, at the Marquette University School of Medicine, Milwaukee, who developed the widely used "Quick Prothrombin Time" measurement of plasma procoagulant activity, independently recognized [19] that the clotting defect in chicks fed hemorrhagic diets was due to a decrease in plasma prothrombin. The same report demonstrated that the coagulation defect in sweet clover disease, eventually shown to be due to the presence of Dicumarol™, was also related to a decrease in the prothrombin concentration and that sweet clover disease and the hemorrhagic chick disease were closely related. Although it is now known that the Quick prothrombin time is not specific for prothrombin, at the time of these studies, the other procoagulant vitamin K-dependent proteins had not yet been discovered.

Within a few years of the time that these animal studies were in progress, the hemorrhagic diathesis resulting from obstructive jaundice and the related lack of intestinal bile was shown to be related to a decrease in prothrombin concentration [20–22], and it was realized that this defect was associated with the lack of the same dietary factor responsible for the hemorrhagic disease of chickens that was being studied. Hemorrhagic episodes in patients diagnosed as having hemophilia were, however, not found to have decreased prothrombin concentrations. A short report from the Brinkhous laboratory at the University of Iowa Medical College [20] established that treatment of obstructive jaundice by the administration of bile mixed with a petroleum ether extract of ground alfalfa raised prothrombin levels, as measured by a whole blood clotting time, considerably faster than treatment with bile alone. A very comprehensive review in 1940 by Brinkhous [23] points out the progress made in establishing that hemorrhagic conditions resulting from malabsorption syndromes or starvation and the hemorrhagic disease of the newborn would respond to vitamin K administration. Following these early advances in an understanding of the role of this fat-soluble vitamin, progress in determining the metabolic role of the vitamin was slow. It was not until the early 1950s that the remainder of the classical vitamin K-dependent clotting factors—factors VII, IX, and X—were clearly demonstrated as essential plasma proteins and subsequently shown to require vitamin K for their biosynthesis. It would be over 20 years before the metabolic role of vitamin K as a cofactor in a posttranslational protein modification would be established, and nearly 25 years before any other vitamin K-dependent proteins were discovered.

After the existence of a previously unknown dietary antihemorrhagic factor was demonstrated, an active program to isolate and characterize this factor was begun by a number of research groups. The work was continuously hampered by the tedious nature of the assays used. Early studies by all groups used a "preventative" chick assay where crude fractions of a potentially active compound were added to a hemorrhagic diet that was fed for a number of weeks as the procoagulant ability of blood was monitored. These assays were extremely time consuming, and "curative" assays were subsequently developed. Chicks were first made deficient by feeding a hemorrhagic diet, and the short-term response to the feeding of dietary ingredient, or the administration of a test compound as a tablet was measured. Either whole blood clotting times [12, 24] or crude plasma clotting factor assays [25, 26] were used as a measure of deficiency.

Early studies of dietary components with high vitamin activity demonstrated [13,14,27] that the active compound was lipid soluble and was present in the nonsaponifiable fraction of a lipid extract. Hexane appeared [28] to be the solvent of choice, and large amounts of other pigments were extracted by this procedure. Fractionation proceeded by the bulk methods in use at that time; adsorption and elution from a wide range of inert materials [29], and differential fractionation into various organic solvents. The isolation was aided by the realization [30] that the active fraction was stable to molecular distillation, and low pressure distillation was used extensively as a method of purification. A detailed description of the progress of the various groups involved in the isolation is available in a review of the field in 1941 by Doisy, Binkley, and Thayer [31].

Dam collaborated with Karrer of the University of Zurich in the isolation of the vitamin, and by 1939 they had succeeded [32] in isolating the vitamin as a yellow oil from alfalfa. Although they described some of its chemical properties, they did not recognize it as a quinone derivative. The group led by Almquist and a group at the Squibb Institute for Medical Research led by Ansbacher [33,34] were also isolating the vitamin from alfalfa, and the St. Louis University group led by Doisy was purifying it from both alfalfa and putrefied fish meal. Pure or nearly pure preparations of the vitamin were obtained by the Doisy [35] and Ansbacher [36] groups at nearly the same time as the Dam and Karrer preparation. It was soon recognized [37,38] that the active preparations were quinones. Almquist and Klose [39] had been studying vitamin K activity in bacterial extracts, and discovered the first known chemical compound with vitamin K activity. They demonstrated that phthiocol (2-methyl-3-hydroxy-1,4-naphthoquinone) (Figure 1.1), which had previously been isolated from *Mycobacterium tuberculosis*, had biological activity [40]. This observation led to a number of studies of the structural requirements of compounds with antihemorrhagic activity and the finding that the 2-methyl group of phthiocol, but not the 3-hydroxyl group, was essential for activity. Reports of the biological activity of menadione (2-Me-1,4-naphthoquinone) (Figure 1.1) were published in the July 1939 issue of the *Journal of the American Chemical Society* by the Almquist [41], Fieser [42], Doisy [43], and Ansbacher [44] laboratories. As it could readily be obtained in a pure form and, on a weight basis, had very high biological activity, much of the subsequent animal work in this area utilized the activity of menadione as a reference. Vitamin K_1 (phylloquinone) (Figure 1.1) was characterized as 2-methyl-3-phytyl-1,4-naphthoquinone and synthesized by Doisy's group [45,46], and their identification was confirmed by independent syntheses of this compound by Karrer and collaborators [47], Almquist and Klose [48], and Fieser [49,50].

The Doisy group also isolated a form of the vitamin from putrefied fish meal which in contrast to the oil isolated from alfalfa was a crystalline product. Subsequent studies demonstrated that this compound, called "vitamin K_2," contained an unsaturated side chain, and it was characterized [35] as 2-methyl-3-(*all trans*-farnesylfarnesyl)-1,4-naphthoquinone, the compound now known as menaquinone-6. This structure was assumed to be the correct structure of the first menaquinone isolated for many years. However, Isler et al. [51] later demonstrated that a crystalline form of the vitamin isolated by Doisy's method and shown by mixed melting point determination to be identical to Doisy's compound contained seven, not six, isoprenyl units and was in

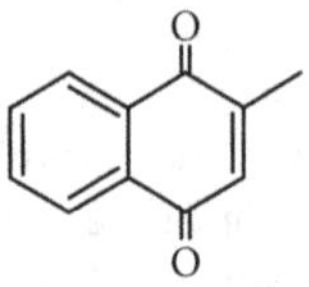

Menadione

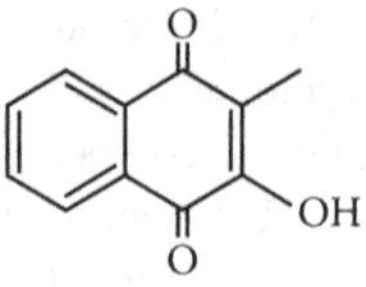

Phthiocol

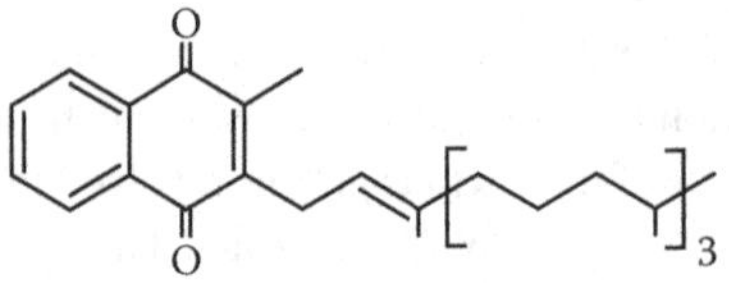

Phylloquinone

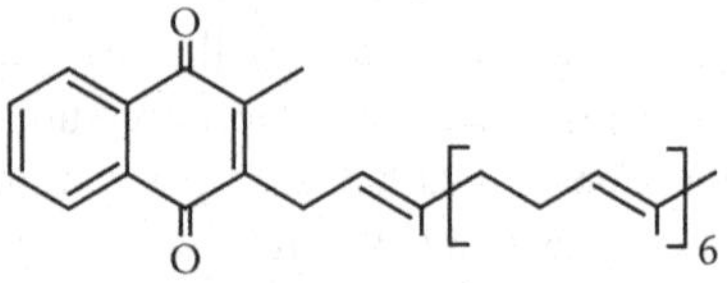

Menaquinone-7 (MK-7)

FIGURE 1.1 Structures of phthiocol, the first chemical compound shown to have antihemorrhagic activity; menadione, the compound used as a standard in most of the early studies involved in isolating the natural antihemorrhagic factor; phylloquinone, the form of the vitamin first isolated from alfalfa; and menaquinone-7, one of a series of compounds with antihemorrhagic properties that were isolated from bacteria.

fact 2-methyl-3-(*all trans*-farnesylgeranylgeranyl)-1,4-naphthoquinone (Figure 1.1) or menaquinone-7, not menaquinone-6. Isler et al. [51] also demonstrated that the crude product obtained from putrefied fish meal did contain some menaquinone-6.

The elucidation of the structure of vitamin K was an extremely competitive research area with a number of large groups involved. Some indication of the effort involved can be gained from an inspection of the large number of papers published in the 1939 issues of the *Journal of the American Chemical Society*, the *Journal of Biological Chemistry*, and *Helvetica Chimica Acta*. Many of these are short notes that appeared within a few weeks of submission, and numerous notes and full papers appeared in various other journals during that year. The result of this concentration of effort in characterization and synthesis was an extremely rapid solution to what was at that time a very difficult problem in organic chemistry. It is not easy at this time to assess the importance of observations made by the different groups involved or to assign priority and credit. A review of the literature from the 1930s does, however, make it difficult to understand why Almquist did not share the Nobel Prize which was awarded to Dam and Doisy in 1943 (Figure 1.2).

Details of the progress in isolation and characterization of vitamin K are available in reviews written by Doisy [31], Almquist [52], and Dam [53] shortly after the characterization of the vitamin. Doisy did not present a lecture upon his receipt of the 1943 Nobel Prize in Physiology and Medicine, but some insights into his progress in the determination of the structure and synthesis of vitamin K are available in an autobiography published in the 1976 issue of the *Annual Review of Biochemistry* [54]. Dam's Nobel lecture [17] contains a number of personal insights into his role in these investigations. Almquist [55,56] has also reviewed his personal involvement in the discovery of vitamin K, and Jukes [57] and Olson [58], both of whom were personally acquainted with the investigators involved, have provided their own insight

In 1943, the Nobel Prize for Physiology or Medicine was awarded to Henrik Carl Peter Dam of the Polytechnic Institute of Copenhagen, Denmark, for his "discovery of vitamin K" and to Edward Adelbert Doisy of the Saint Louis University at St. Louis, Missouri, for his "discovery of the chemical nature of vitamin K." Biographies of each are available at http://nobelprize.org/medicine/laureates/1943/index.html. Herman James Almquist also contributed substantially to the efforts to identify, characterize, and synthesize the natural antihemorrhagic factor but was not included in the award. A biographical sketch of H. Almquist published in 1986 by Jukes (53) indicates that Almquist's publication (13) regarding evidence for the presence of this factor, which followed Dam's publication (11) by 10 weeks, had been held up by the Berkeley administration for a substantial period. The Jukes biography also contains a 1944 letter from Dam to Almquist which suggests that he was not very comfortable with the fact that Almquist had not shared in the prize.

FIGURE 1.2 The discovery of vitamin K led to the award of a Nobel Prize in 1943.

into the race to identify and characterize the antihemorrhagic factor. A biographical sketch of Almquist prepared by Jukes [59] provides additional information on the early studies of this important fat-soluble vitamin.

Additional extensive reviews of the vitamin K field were published prior to the development of an understanding of the biochemical role of the vitamin. Dam [60] and Isler and Wiss [61] surveyed the vitamin K literature in the *Vitamins and Hormones* series. Both the first and second editions of *The Vitamins* [62,63] contain multi-authored sections dealing with various aspects of chemistry and biological activity of vitamin K, and the proceedings of a 1966 symposium held in honor of Professor Dam have been published [64] in *Vitamins and Hormones*.

Very little research that substantially advanced an understanding of the metabolic and nutritional roles of vitamin K was published from the 1940s to the mid-1960s. Three additional plasma procoagulants, factor VII [65,66], factor X [67], and factor IX [68,69] were identified in the early 1950s; and, along with prothrombin (factor II), they came to be known as the "vitamin K-dependent clotting factors." However, the molecular basis for this distinction was not known. In the mid-1950s Martius and Nitz-Litzow [70] and Martius [71] proposed that vitamin K functioned as an electron carrier in the mammalian respiratory chain and that a deficiency of the vitamin would lead to a decrease in ATP production needed for protein synthesis. The apparent rapid turnover rate of prothrombin was postulated to make it a particularly sensitive protein. Studies from a number of laboratories that failed to support this theory have been reviewed by Johnson [72]. In retrospect it is easy to understand that the task of determining how the amount or the activity of a specific protein such as prothrombin could be altered by vitamin K status was impossible if researchers did not know how proteins were synthesized. It is also understandable that the nutritional importance of vitamin K and an understanding of the dietary requirements for the vitamin would be difficult to obtain when the analytical capacity to measure microgram and nanogram amounts of the vitamin in foods and tissues was not yet developed.

Research activity directed toward an understanding of the role of the vitamin K-dependent proteins that had been identified and the function of vitamin K in their synthesis increased in the early 1960s as an understanding of mammalian protein synthesis became available. Researchers whose expertise was in hematology and nutritional biochemistry began to accumulate the data that led to the identification in the mid-1970s of vitamin K as a substrate for a γ-glutamyl carboxylase that drove a posttranslational modification of vitamin K-dependent proteins. Although a large number of investigators contributed to the continual advance in an understanding of the metabolic role of vitamin K in the mid- to late-1960s much of the effort was centered in the laboratories of Connor Johnson at the University of Illinois, Bob Olson at St. Louis University, and John Suttie at the University of Wisconsin. During the same period, Caen Hemker's laboratory at the University of Lieden in the Netherlands identified a circulating, inactive form of prothrombin in the plasma of patients treated with oral anticoagulants. Gary Nelsestuen's group at the University of Minnesota and Johan Stenflo's laboratory at the University of Lund in Sweden provided the characterization of γ-carboxyglutamic acid (Gla) as the missing factor in the "abnormal" prothrombin, and this advance led directly to the demonstration of the vitamin K-dependent carboxylase as the metabolic enzyme with a requirement for the vitamin. Efforts to characterize the properties of this enzyme, detail its mechanism of action, and purify it were actively carried out in a number of laboratories, but initially in the Suttie laboratory, in the laboratory of Barbara and Bruce Furie at Harvard, Paul Dowd at the University of Pittsburgh, Kathy Berkner at the Cleveland Clinic, Cees Vermeer at Maastricht University in The Netherlands, and Darrel Stafford at the University of North Carolina. The products of the vitamin K-dependent carboxylase were Gla residues and the 2,3-epoxide of vitamin K which was shown to be recycled to the reduced form of vitamin K by a vitamin K epoxide reductase (VKOR). Studies from the laboratory of John Matschiner at St. Louis University were key to an understanding of this recycling activity, and the properties of the enzyme were investigated by many of the laboratories working on the carboxylase, and also by Reidar Wallin's group at Wake Forest, and Johannes Oldenburg at the University of Bonn in Germany.

The modification of the primary gene product by the formation of Gla residues gave these proteins their unique biological activity, and the presence of Gla residues in these proteins resulted in the identification of additional vitamin K-dependent proteins by biochemists and molecular biologists which continues to this time. These efforts occurred in the same period of time that the structures of the vitamin K-dependent coagulation factors were being described and the complex process involved in the generation of thrombin from prothrombin was being elucidated. Major efforts in this direction were led by Earl Davie at the University of Washington, Harold Roberts at the University of North Carolina, Craig Jackson at

Washington University, Ken Mann at the University of Vermont, and Chuck Esmon at the Oklahoma Medical Research Foundation. The range of vitamin K-dependent proteins was expanded when Paul Price at the University of California at San Diego and a group led by Paul Gallop and Jane Lian and their collaborators at Harvard found Gla proteins in bone, and Baldomero Olivera at the University of Utah found a large number of Gla-containing peptides in the venom of the *Conus* snail. The availability of analytical techniques suitable for measuring the content of vitamin K in foods, plasma, and tissues was driven by efforts in Martin Shearer's laboratory in London and Jim Sadowski's group at Tufts University, and these efforts have enabled a small number of laboratories to develop the databases of the vitamin K content of foods that are now available. Relationships between vitamin K intake and plasma and tissue concentrations have been determined by these laboratories along with Vermeer's group, while efforts to understand the degradative metabolism of vitamin K have been led by Shearer's laboratory. The metabolic functions of two vitamin K-dependent proteins, osteocalcin and Matrix Gla protein (MGP), are still not well defined, but interest in these proteins has led to epidemiological and controlled population studies that are directed toward an understanding of the possible role of the vitamin in the prevention of chronic disease. These efforts are widespread, but much of it has been initiated by the laboratory of Sarah Booth at Tufts University and by Shearer, Suttie, and Vermeer, as well as a large number of studies in Japan, much of it centered in the Sato and Iwamoto laboratories.

REFERENCES

1. Dam, H. 1929. Cholesterinositoffwechsel in huhnereiern und huhnchen. *Biochem Z* 215:475–492.
2. Dam, H. 1930. Uber die cholesterinsynthese in tierkorper. *Biochem Z* 220:158–163.
3. McFarlane, W.D., W.R. Graham, and G.E. Hall. 1931. Studies in protein nutrition of the chick. I. The influence of different protein concentrates on the growth of baby chicks, when fed as the source of protein in various simplified diets. *J Nutr* 4:331–349.
4. McFarlane, W.D., W.R. Graham, and F. Richardson. 1931. The fat-soluble vitamin requirements of the chick. I. The vitamin A and vitamin D content of fish meal and meat meal. *Biochem J* 25:358–366.
5. Holst, W.F. and E.R. Halbrook. 1933. A "scurvy-like" disease in chicks. *Science* 77:354.
6. Cribbett, R. and J.T. Correll. 1934. On a scurvy-like disease in chicks. *Science* 79:40.
7. Dam, H. 1934. Haemorrhages in chicks reared on artificial diets: A new deficiency disease. *Nature* 133: 909–910.
8. Dam, H. and F. Schonheyder. 1934. A deficiency disease in chicks resembling scurvy. *Biochem J* 28:1355–1359.
9. Cook, S.F. and K.G. Scott. 1935. A bioassay of certain protein supplements when fed to baby chicks. *Proc Soc Exp Biol Med* 33:167–170.
10. Cook, S.F. and K.G. Scott. 1935. Apparent intoxication in poultry due to nitrogenous bases. *Science* 82:465–467.
11. Dam, H. 1935. The antihaemorrhagic vitamin of the chick. Occurrence and chemical nature. *Nature* 135:652–653.
12. Dam, H. 1935. The antihaemorrhagic vitamin of the chick. *Biochem J* 29:1273–1285.

13. Almquist, H.J. and E.L.R. Stokstad. 1935. Dietary haemorrhagic disease in chicks. *Nature* 136:31.
14. Almquist, H.J. and E.L.R. Stokstad. 1935. Haemorrhagic chick disease of dietary origin. *J Biol Chem* 111:105–113.
15. Halbrook, E.R. 1935. Thesis. University of California.
16. Almquist, H.J. and E.L.R. Stokstad. 1936. Factors influencing the incidence of dietary hemorrhagic disease in chicks. *J Nutr* 12:329–335.
17. Dam, H. 1964. The discovery of vitamin K, its biological functions and therapeutical application. In *Nobel Lectures Physiology or Medicine 1942–1962*, 9–26. New York: Elsevier.
18. Dam, H., F. Schonheyder, and E. Tage-Hansen. 1936. Studies on the mode of action of vitamin K. *Biochem J* 30:1075–1079.
19. Quick, A.J. 1937. The coagulation defect in sweet clover disease and in the hemorrhagic chick disease of dietary origin. A consideration of the source of prothrombin. *Am J Physiol* 118:260–271.
20. Warner, E.D., K.M. Brinkhous, and H.P. Smith. 1938. Bleeding tendency of obstructive jaundice: Prothrombin deficiency and dietary factors. *Proc Soc Exp Biol Med* 37:628–630.
21. Butt, C.R., A.M. Snell, and A.E. Osterberg. 1938. The use of vitamin K and bile in treatment of the hemorrhagic diathesis in cases of jaundice. *Mayo Clin Proc* 13:74–80.
22. Dam, H. and J. Glavind. 1938. Vitamin K in human pathology. *Lancet* i:720–721.
23. Brinkhous, K.M. 1940. Plasma prothrombin; vitamin K. *Medicine* 19:329–416.
24. Thayer, S.A., R.W. McKee, S.B. Binkley, D.W. MacCorquodale, and E.A. Doisy. 1939. The assay of vitamins K_1 and K_2. *Proc Soc Exp Biol Med* 41:194–197.
25. Schonheyder, F. 1936. The quantitative determination of vitamin K. I. *Biochem J* 30:890–896.
26. Almquist, H.J. and A.A. Klose. 1939. Determination of the anti-hemorrhagic vitamin. *Biochem J* 33:1055–1060.
27. Almquist, H.J. 1937. The anti-hemorrhagic vitamin. *Poultry Sci* 16:166–172.
28. Almquist, H.J. 1936. Purification of the antihemorrhagic vitamin. *J Biol Chem* 114:241–245.
29. Dam, H. and F. Schonheyder. 1936. The occurrence and chemical nature of vitamin K. *Biochem J* 30:897–901.
30. Almquist, H.J. 1936. Purification of the antihemorrhagic vitamin by distillation. *J Biol Chem* 115:589–591.
31. Doisy, E.A., S.B. Binkley, and S.A. Thayer. 1941. Vitamin K. *Chem Rev* 28:477–517.
32. Dam, H., A. Geiger, J. Glavind, P. Karrer, W. Karrer, E. Rothschild, and H. Salomon. 1939. Isolierung des vitamins K in hochgereinigter form. *Helv Chim Acta* 22:310–313.
33. Ansbacher, S. 1938. New observations on the vitamin K deficiency of the chick. *Science* 88:221.
34. Ansbacher, S. 1939. A quantitative biological assay of vitamin K. *J Nutr* 17:303–315.
35. Binkley, S.B., D.W. MacCorquodale, S.A. Thayer, and E.A. Doisy. 1939. The isolation of vitamin K_1. *J Biol Chem* 130:219–234.
36. Fernholz, E., S. Ansbacher, and M.L. Moore. 1939. On the color reaction for vitamin K. *J Am Chem Soc* 61:1613–1614.
37. Karrer, P. and A. Geiger. 1939. Vitamin K aus alfalfa. *Helv Chim Acta* 22:945–948.
38. McKee, R.W., S.B. Binkley, D.W. MacCorquodale, S.A. Thayer, and E.A. Doisy. 1939. The isolation of vitamins K_1 and K_2. *J Am Chem Soc* 61:1295.
39. Almquist, H.J. and A.A. Klose, Color reactions in vitamin K concentrates. 1939. *J Am Chem Soc* 61:1610–1611.

40. Almquist, H.J. and A.A. Klose. 1939. The anti-hemorrhagic activity of pure synthetic phthiocol. *J Am Chem Soc* 61:1611.
41. Almquist, H.J. and A.A. Klose. 1939. The antihemorrhagic activity of certain naphthoquinones. *J Am Chem Soc* 61:1923–1924.
42. Fieser, L.F., D.M. Bowen, W.P. Campbell, E.M. Fry, and M.D. Gates. 1939. Synthesis of antihemorrhagic compounds. *J Am Chem Soc* 61:1926–1927.
43. Thayer, S.A., L.C. Cheney, S.B. Binkley, D.W. MacCorquodale, and E.A. Doisy. 1939. Vitamin K activity of some quinones. *J Am Chem Soc* 61:1932.
44. Ansbacher, S. and E. Fernholz. 1939. Simple compounds with vitamin K activity. *J Am Chem Soc* 61:1924–1925.
45. Binkley, S.B., L.C. Cheney, W.F. Holcomb, R.W. McKee, S.A. Thayer, D.W. MacCorquodale, and E.A. Doisy. 1939. The constitution and synthesis of vitamin K_1. *J Am Chem Soc* 61:2558–2559.
46. MacCorquodale, D.W., L.C. Cheney, S.B. Binkley, W.F. Holcomb, R.W. McKee, S.A. Thayer, and E.A. Doisy. 1939. The constitution and synthesis of vitamin K_1. *J Biol Chem* 131:357–370.
47. Karrer, P., A. Geiger, R. Legler, A. Ruegger, and H. Salomon. 1939. Uber die isolierung des alpha-phyllochinones (vitamin K aus alfalfa) sowie uber dessen entdeckungsgeschechter. *Helv Chim Acta* 22:1464–1470.
48. Almquist, H.J. and A.A. Klose. 1939. Synthetic and natural antihemorrhagic compounds. *J Am Chem Soc* 61:2557–2558.
49. Fieser, L.F. 1939. Synthesis of 2-methyl-3-phytyl-1,4-naphthoquinone. *J Am Chem Soc* 61:2559–2561.
50. Fieser, L.F. 1939. Identity of synthetic 2-methyl-3-phytyl-1,4-naphthoquinone and vitamin K_1. *J Am Chem Soc* 61:2561.
51. Isler, O., R. Ruegg, L.H. Chapard-dit-Jean, A. Winterstein, and O. Wiss. 1958. Synthese und isolierung von vitamin K_2 und isoprenologen verbindungen. *Helv Chim Acta* 41:786–807.
52. Almquist, H.J. 1941. Vitamin K. *Physiol Rev* 21:194–216.
53. Dam, H. 1942. Vitamin K, its chemistry and physiology. *Adv Enzymol* 2:285–324.
54. Doisy, E.A. 1976. An autobiography. *Annu Rev Biochem* 45:1–9.
55. Almquist, H.J. 1975. The early history of vitamin K. *Am J Clin Nutr* 28:656–659.
56. Almquist, H.J. 1979. Vitamin K: Discovery, identification, synthesis, functions. *Fed Proc* 38:2687–2689.
57. Jukes, T.H. 1980. Vitamin K: A reminiscence. *TIBS* 5:140–141.
58. Olson, R.E. 1979. Discovery of vitamin K. *TIBS* 4:118–120.
59. Jukes, T.H. 1987. Herman James Almquist (1903–): Biographical sketch. *J Nutr* 117:409–415.
60. Dam, H. 1948. Vitamin K. *Vitamins and Hormones* 6:27–53.
61. Isler, O. and O. Wiss. 1959. Chemistry and biochemistry of the K vitamins. *Vitamins and Hormones* 17:53–90.
62. Sebrell, W.H. Jr and R.S. Harris (eds.). 1954. *The Vitamins*, Vol. 2. New York: Academic Press.
63. Sebrell, W.H. and R.S. Harris (eds.). 1971. *The Vitamins*. New York: Academic Press.
64. Harris, R.S., I.G. Wool, J.A. Loraine, G.F. Marian, and K.V. Thiman (eds.). 1966. *Vitamins and Hormones*, Vol. 24. New York: Academic Press.
65. Owen, C.A. Jr, T.B. Magath, and J.L. Bollman. 1951. Prothrombin conversion factors in blood coagulation. *Am J Physiol* 166:1–11.
66. Koller, F., A. Loeliger, and F. Duckert. 1951. Experiments on a new clotting factor (factor VII). *Acta Haematol* 6:1–18.
67. Hougie, C., E.M. Barrow, and J.B. Graham. 1957. Stuart clotting defect. I. Segregation of an hereditary hemorrhagic state from the heterogeneous group heretofore called "stable factor" (SPCA, proconvertin, factor VII) deficiency. *J Clin Invest* 36:485–496.

68. Aggeler, P.M., S.G. White, M.B. Glendening, E.W. Page, T.B. Leake, and G. Bates. 1952. Plasma thromboplastin component (PTC) deficiency: A new disease resembling hemophilia. *Proc Soc Exp Biol Med* 79:692–694.

69. Biggs, R., A.S. Douglas, R.G. MacFarlane, J.V. Dacie, W.R. Pitney, C. Merskey, and J.R. O'Brien. 1952. Christmas disease. A condition previously mistaken for haemophilia. *Brit Med J* ii:1378–1382.

70. Martius, C. and D. Nitz-Litzow. 1954. Oxydative phosphorylierung und vitamin K mangel. *Biochim Biophys Acta* 13:152–153.

71. Martius, C. 1966. Mode of action of vitamin K in animals. *Vitamins and Hormones* 24:441–445.

72. Paolucci, A.M., P.B. RamaRao, and B.C. Johnson. 1963. Vitamin K deficiency and oxidative phosphorylation. *J Nutr* 81:17–22.

2 Active Forms, Antagonists, Physical Properties, and Synthesis of Vitamin K

2.1 NOMENCLATURE AND STRUCTURES OF K VITAMERS

The nomenclature of compounds possessing vitamin K activity has been modified a number of times since the discovery of the vitamin. The designation of phylloquinone as K_1, menadione as K_3, and all menaquinones as K_2 was used for some time, but the nomenclature in general use at the present time (Table 2.1) is that most recently adopted by the IUPAC-IUB Subcommittee on Nomenclature of Quinones [1].

The term *vitamin K* is used as a generic descriptor of 2-methyl-1,4-naphthoquinone (menadione), and any derivatives of this compound that exhibit an antihemorrhagic activity in animals fed a vitamin K-deficient diet (Figure 2.1). The compound 2-methyl-3-phytyl-1,4-naphthoquinone, found in all green plants, should be designated as phylloquinone rather than vitamin K_1. The United States Pharmacopeia (USP) nomenclature for phylloquinone is phytonadione. A number of compounds with antihemorrhagic activity that were first isolated from putrified fish meal and at that time called vitamin K_2 are a series of multiprenyl menaquinones with unsaturated side chains that are found in animal tissues and bacteria. A menaquinone with 7 isoprenoid units, or 35 carbons in the side chain, was once called vitamin $K_{2(35)}$ but is now more appropriately called menaquinone-7 (MK-7). Vitamins of the menaquinone series with up to 13 prenyl groups have been identified, as well as several partially saturated members of this series. At one time, there was an effort by the International Union of Nutritional Sciences (IUNS) to alter the IUPAC nomenclature to refer to menadione as "menaquinone," phylloquinone as "phytylmenaquinone," and a vitamin with an unsaturated side chain as a "prenylmenaquinone." This nomenclature was not thought by many investigators to be useful and is seldom seen in the literature. Inappropriate nomenclature of the different forms of vitamin K is used rather often. The most common deviations from appropriate nomenclature that are currently seen are the use of vitamin K_3 for menadione and references in both the title and text of scientific publications to vitamin K_2 when the study involves a specific menaquinone such as MK-4.

TABLE 2.1

Vitamin K Nomenclature

Structure	Original	IUPAC
2-Methyl-1, 4-naphthoquinone	K_3	Menadione
2-Methyl-3-phytyl-1, 4-naphthoquinone	K_1	Phylloquinone (K)
2-Methyl-3-multiprenyl-1, 4-naphthoquinone (class)	$K_{2(n)}$	Menaquinone-n (MK-n)
2-Methyl-3-farnesylgeranyl-geranyl-1, 4-naphthoquinone	$K_{2(35)}$	Menaquinone-7 (MK-7)
2-Methyl-3-geranyl-geranyl-1,4-naphthoquinone	$K_{2(20)}$	Menaquinone-4 (MK-4)

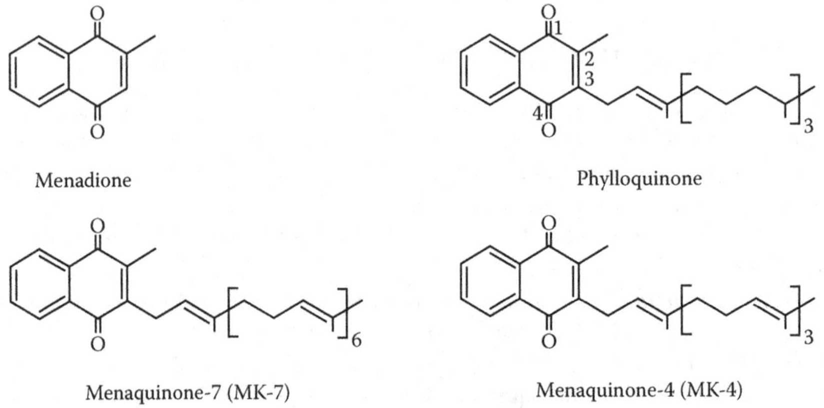

Menadione

Phylloquinone

Menaquinone-7 (MK-7)

Menaquinone-4 (MK-4)

FIGURE 2.1 Common biologically active forms of vitamin K.

2.2 ACTIVE FORMS OF VITAMIN K

After vitamin K was discovered, a large number of chemically related compounds were synthesized and their biological activities compared by the use of some type of chick bioassay. Much of the information related to the biological activity of a large number of compounds synthesized by Fieser and coworkers has been summarized in a single paper [2], and other data relative to these early efforts have been reviewed and summarized elsewhere [3–5]. The data from the earlier studies are somewhat difficult to use in comparing the relative activity of different compounds because of variations in methods of assay, but they did establish the basic structure needed for biological activity.

The first simple compound with antihemorrhagic activity to be discovered was 2-methyl-3-hydroxy-1,4-naphthoquinone, commonly called "phthicol." This compound (see Figure 1.1) had relatively weak activity, and it was soon recognized that menadione was much more active. Most studies of the biological activities of newly synthesized naphthoquinones related the activity of these compounds to that of menadione. The 2-methyl group is usually considered essential for activity, and alterations at this position, such as the 2-ethyl derivative of 1,4-napthoquinone, resulted

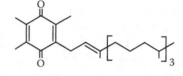

Desmethyl-phylloquinone

2',3'dihydro-phylloquinone

2,3-dimethyl-
1,4-naphthoquinone

2-methyl-3-octadecyl-
1,4-naphthoquinone

2,6-dimethyl-3-phytyl-
1,4-naphthoquinone

2,5,6-Me-3-phytyl-
1,4-benzoquinone

FIGURE 2.2   Structures with partial vitamin K activity, assayed in vitamin K-deficient chicks, see Table 2.2.

TABLE 2.2
Relationship between Vitamin K Activity and Structure[a]

Compound	Effective Dose (µg)
Phylloquinone	1
2',3'-Dihydro-phylloquinone	8
2-Methyl-3-octadecyl-1,4-naphthoquinone	25
2,3-Dimethyl-1,4-naphthoquinone	50
Desmethyl-phylloquinone	50
2,5,6-Methyl-3-phytyl-1,4-benzoquinone	Inactive
2,6-Dimethyl-3-phytyl-1,4-naphthoquinone	Inactive

[a] The data represent a curative assay of vitamin K-deficient chicks and are based on an 18-h response to the administration of the different compounds into the crop in 0.1 ml of peanut oil [2]. An effective dose was that which reduced the whole blood-clotting time from in excess of 60 min to less than 10 min. The largest dose tested was 1,000 µg.

in a marked decrease in activity or in inactive compounds. This was not due to the inability of the 2-ethyl-1,4 naphthoquinone to be alkylated, as 2-ethyl-3-phytyl-1,4-naphthoquinone was also found to lack substantial activity. There is some evidence that the 2-methyl group may not be absolutely essential, as des-Me-phylloquinone did have measurable activity in these early studies. Although there were early suggestions that the 2-methyl-naphthoquinone ring structure itself (menadione) might be a biologically active form of the vitamin, it is now known that it is readily alkylated to menaquinone-4, a highly active form of the vitamin, following ingestion.

The range of compounds that can be utilized by animals is wide, and compounds such as 2-methyl-4-amino-1-naphthol and even 2-methyl-1-naphthol are oxidized to menadione following ingestion and have similar activity. 2-Methyl-4-amino-1-naphthol is a fungistatic and bactericidal agent used as a wine preservative and is referred to as vitamin K_6 in that context. The reduced forms of the substituted 1,4-naphthoquinones, the corresponding hydroquinones, will spontaneously oxidize to the quinone form, but they can be stabilized by esterification. Compounds such as the diphosphate, the disulfate, the diacetate (sometimes referred to as vitamin K_4), and the dibenzoate of reduced vitamin Ks have been prepared and they are also biologically active forms.

The structures of a number of compounds related to natural vitamin K are shown in Figure 2.2, and their biological activity determined by chick bioassay is summarized in Table 2.2. Studies of these 2-methyl-1,4-naphthoquinone variants [2] have revealed that polyisoprenoid side chains are the most effective substituents at the 3-position. The biological activity of phylloquinone is reduced by saturation of the double bond to form 2-methyl-3-(β-γ-dihydrophytyl)-1,4-naphthoquinone. This compound is, however, considerably more active than 2-methyl-3-octadecyl-1,4-naphthoquinone, which has an unbranched alkyl side chain of similar size. Natural phylloquinone isolated from plants is the *trans* isomer, but synthetic phylloquinone contains about 20% of the *cis* isomer which is essentially inactive [6] when studied in a rat model following intracardial injection. The naphthoquinone nucleus cannot be altered appreciably, as methylation to form 2,6-dimethyl-3-phytyl-1,4-naphthoquinone results in loss of activity, and the benzoquinone most closely corresponding to phylloquinone, 2,5,6-trimethyl-3-phytyl-1,4-benzoquinone, is inactive. The data in Table 2.2 were obtained by the use of an 18-h curative test on vitamin K-deficient chickens following oral administration. This type of assay allows sufficient time for metabolic alterations of the administered form to an active form of the vitamin, and response seen would be influenced by bioavailability and metabolism of the compound as well as its activity as a substrate of the vitamin K-dependent carboxylase. Analogs of phylloquinone with differing numbers of saturated isoprenoid groups at the 3-position have been assessed for their relative activity, with phylloquinone being the most active (Table 2.3) in the deficient chick curative assays that were used.

The spectrum of menaquinones produced by a limited number of obligate and facultative anaerobic organisms is broad [7,8], and the distribution of menaquinones produced by various cultured microorganisms has been investigated and used as a taxonomic tool [9]. The data in Table 2.4 illustrate the range

TABLE 2.3
Relative Activity of Vitamin K Isoprenalogs[a]

Number of C atoms in Side Chain	Phylloquinone Series	Menaquinone Series	
	Oral (Chick)	Oral (Chick)	Intracardial (Rat)
10	10	15	<2
15	30	40	–
20	100	100	13
25	80	>120	15
30	50	100	170
35	–	70	1,700
40	–	68	–
45	–	60	2,500
50	–	25	1,700

Note: Relative biological activity (molar) phylloquinone = 100.

[a] Data were obtained by bioassays based on the normalization of clotting times of deficient animals [4,87].

TABLE 2.4
Fecal Menaquinone Concentrations in Germ-Free Rats Inoculated with Single Organisms

Organism	MKs Found	Concentration (ng/g ± SEM)
Bifidobacterium longum	0	–
Clostridium ranosum	0	–
Escherichia coli	7	245 ± 23
	8	6,176 ± 256
Bacteroides vulgatus	3	66 ± 10
	4	77 ± 6
	7	18 ± 2
	8	46 ± 4
	9	338 ± 18
	10	6,657 ± 949
	11	749 ± 81

Note: Germ-free Wistar mature rats (five per group) were housed under germ-free conditions for 10 days following oral inoculations with single organisms. The rats were fed an irradiation sterilized diet, and dried feces were analyzed for the presence of MK-3 through MK-13 (for details, see Kindberg et al. [10]).

of menaquinones produced when four organisms present in the human gut were isolated and administered to germ-free rats [10].

The predominant menaquinones produced by human gut bacteria are from MK-6 to MK-10, and the relative biological activity of these various vitamin K isoprenalogs appears to be dependent on the route of administration. Data obtained by the oral administration of the vitamin to vitamin K-deficient chicks (Table 2.3) show that isoprenalogs with three to five isoprenoid groups in either a menaquinone- or a phylloquinone-type compound have maximum activity. The lack of effectiveness of higher isoprenalogs in this type of assay may be due to the relatively poor absorptions of these compounds. However, when the intracardial injection of vitamin K to deficient rats is used as a criterion, the very high molecular weight isoprenalogs of the menaquinone series are the most active, and maximum activity was observed with MK-9. In addition to the long-chain menaquinones produced by gut bacteria that contribute to the vitamin K status of all individuals, there are bacteria that produce 2-methyl-1,4-naphthoquinones that are substantially modified from these forms. Partial saturations of the isoprenyl side chain of menaquinones are formed by some bacteria, and forms of the vitamin with a completely saturated side chain have been identified [11,12]. Less common alterations such as additional methylation of the naphthoquinone ring [13] or substantial modification of the isoprenyl side chain [14] have been identified in some organisms (Figure 2.3), but the metabolic role of these forms of the vitamin have not been determined.

Once the biochemical role of vitamin K was determined, it became possible to directly assess the activity of various analogs of the vitamin as substrates for the vitamin K-dependent carboxylase (see Chapter 4). The results of some of these studies are shown in Table 2.5 and Figure 2.4. These data indicate that alterations in the structure of the vitamin which lowers their activity appear to be directly related to the compound's ability to function as a substrate for the carboxylase, whereas the animal studies are greatly dependent on bioavailability and cellular transport as well as their biochemical role. The data also suggest that modifications of the

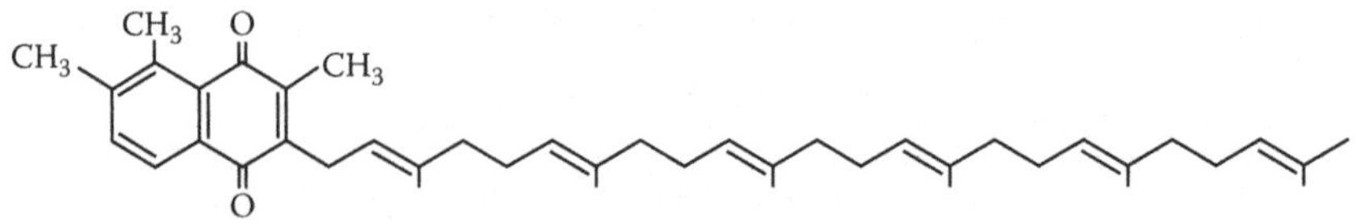

2,7 and 8-trimethyl-3-farnesylfarnesyl-1,4-naphthoquinone

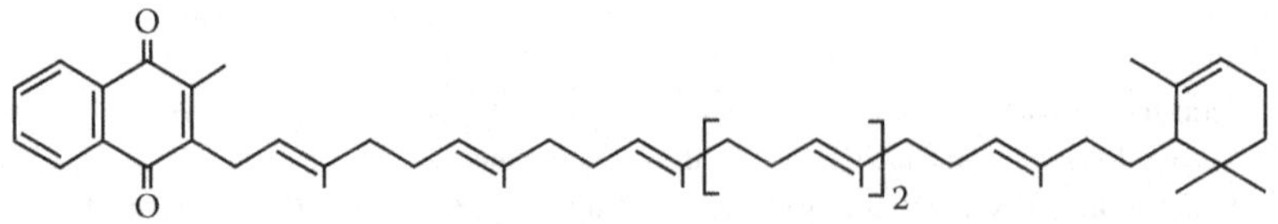

II,III-Tetrahydro-ω-(2,6,6-trimethylcyclohex-2-enylmethyl)-menaquinone-6

FIGURE 2.3   Structures of minor forms of vitamin K found in bacteria.

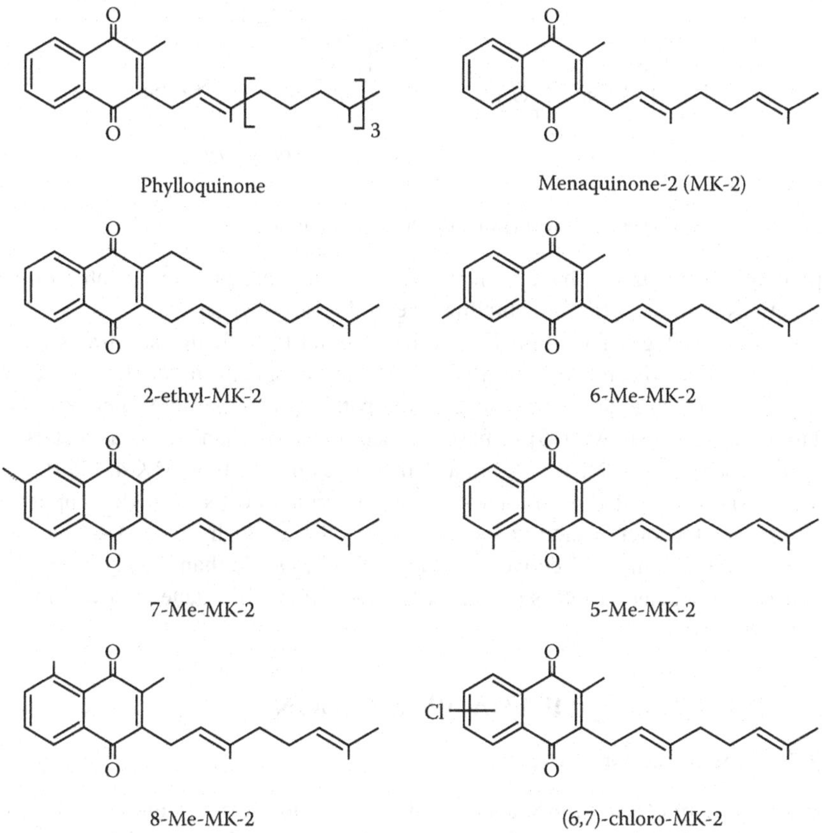

FIGURE 2.4 Structures with partial vitamin K activity, assayed as substrates for the vitamin K-dependent carboxylase, see Table 2.5.

TABLE 2.5

Activity of Vitamin K Analogs as Substrates for the Microsomal Vitamin K-Dependent Carboxylase

Substrate	Carboxylase Activity[a]
Phylloquinone	100
Menaquinone-2	80
2-Ethyl-menaquinone-2	11
6-Me-menaquinone-2	100
7-Me-menaquinone-2	71
5-Me-menaquinone-2	8
8-Me-menaquinone-2	18
(6,7)-Chloro-menaquinone-2	62

[a] Data are expressed as the activity of saturating amounts of the reduced form of each vitamin relative to that of phylloquinone [50,59].

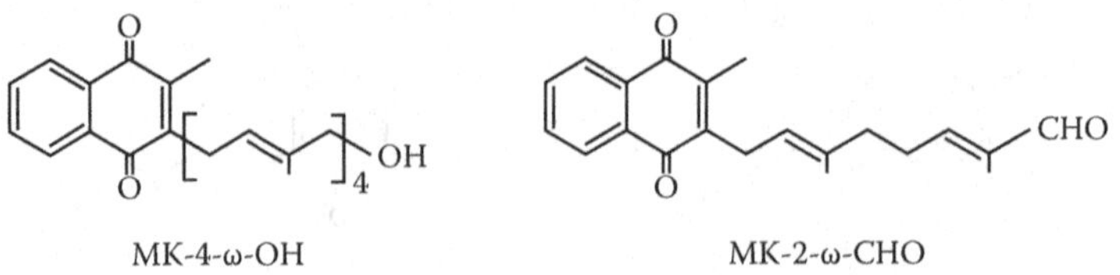

MK-4-ω-OH   MK-2-ω-CHO

FIGURE 2.5 ω-Oxygenated form of short-chain menaquinones.

naphthoquinone ring can have variable effects, which are probably related to their interactions with the vitamin K binding site in the carboxylase.

Very few analogs of vitamin K have been found to be better substrates for the carboxylase than the natural forms of the vitamin, but the ω-aldehyde of MK-4 (Figure 2.5) which is an intermediate in the pathway of vitamin K metabolic degradation, has been shown [15] to have a much lower K_m than MK-4 as a substrate for the carboxylase and a V_{max}/K_m that is five times higher than MK-4. Short-chain menaquinones have also been found to attack malignant cells through an apoptotic response (see Chapter 8), and in some cell types the ω-aldehyde of MK-2 has been shown to be much more effective in inducing this response than MK-2. Whether or not these ω-oxygenated forms of vitamin K are active when generated within cells is not known.

2.3   ANTAGONISTS OF VITAMIN K ACTION

2.3.1   COUMARIN DERIVATIVES

The antagonism of vitamin K action can occur either at the vitamin binding site of the vitamin K-dependent carboxylase or through an inhibition of the vitamin K epoxide reductase that recycles the epoxide product of carboxylase action back to the reduced, metabolically active, form of the vitamin (see Chapter 4). The first vitamin K antagonist discovered was being actively investigated during the same period of time that Dam and Almquist were involved in establishing the essentiality of vitamin K in the diet. The history of the discovery of the anticoagulant action of coumarin derivatives has been well documented [16,17] and has also been discussed by Link in a publication [18] that should be read by anyone with an interest in this subject. A hemorrhagic disease of cattle, which was eventually traced to the consumption of improperly cured sweet clover hay, was prevalent in the Canadian and American Midwest in the 1920s, and was commonly referred to as "sweet clover disease." Early investigators recognized that the disease could be cured by the substitution of good hay for the spoiled hay and that if serious hemorrhages did not develop the animals could be aided by transfusion with whole blood from healthy animals. By the early 1930s, it was established that the cause of the prolonged clotting times was a decrease in the prothrombin activity of blood. The compound present in spoiled sweet clover responsible for this disease was studied by a number of investigators but was finally isolated and characterized by Link's group during the period from 1933 to 1941. As there was no chemical method that could be used to follow the concentration of the active factor during attempts to purify it, a reproducible bioassay was essential for success. The assay used [19] was a modification of the "Quick 1-stage prothrombin time" utilizing rabbit plasma. As the sensitivity of the response to the oral administration of a partially purified preparation of the active factor varied substantially between individual rabbits, each assay was compared to the response seen with administration of a standard dose of spoiled sweet clover hay to the same rabbit. Although the purification assays were time consuming, the active hemorrhagic agent was eventually crystallized [20], characterized as 3,3'-methyl-*bis*-(4-hydroxycoumarin) [21], and given the trade name Dicumarol (Figure 2.6). Dicumarol, the antagonist that was first isolated, was successfully used as a clinical agent to replace heparin for anticoagulant therapy in some early studies. However, questions about the activity and pharmacokinetics of Dicumarol led to the synthesis of a large number of substituted 4-hydroxycoumarins both in Link's laboratory and elsewhere, and the ability of over 100 4-hydroxycoumarins to act as anticoagulants was defined within a few years of the characterization of Dicumarol [22]. The most successful of these, as a clinical drug prescribed for the long-term lowering of the vitamin K-dependent clotting factors, have been warfarin, 3-(α-acetonylbenzyl)-4-hyroxycoumarin or its sodium salt; phenprocoumarol, 3-(1-phenylpropyl)-4-hydroxycoumarin; and acenocoumarol, 3-(α-acetonyl-4-nitrobenzyl)-4-hydroxycoumarin. The various drugs that have been used differ in the degree to which they are absorbed from the intestine and in their plasma turnover rate presumably because of differing rates of metabolism. Their effectiveness as an inhibitor of their target enzyme, the vitamin K epoxide reductase, also varies [23]. As these drugs are synthetic compounds, the clinically used drugs are racemic mixtures, and studies of the two optical isomers of Warfarin have shown that they differ both in their effectiveness as anticoagulants and in the influence of other drugs on their metabolism. These oral anticoagulants, almost exclusively warfarin in the United States, are very widely used and, because of dietary and genetic interactions, the correct dosage for a patient can vary significantly (see Chapter 7).

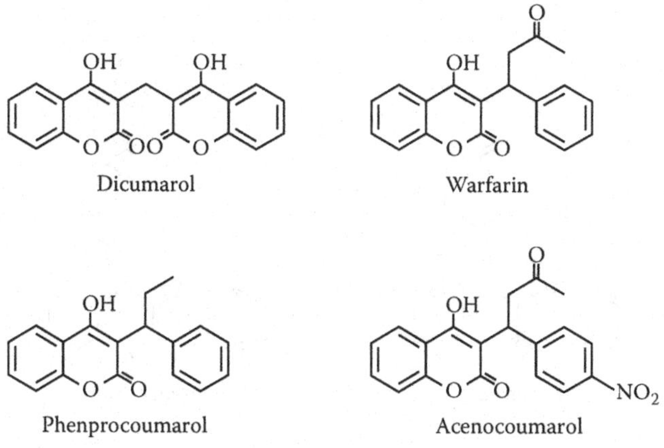

Dicumarol

Warfarin

Phenprocoumarol

Acenocoumarol

FIGURE 2.6   Structures of coumarin-based oral anticoagulants.

In addition to its use as a clinical anticoagulant, warfarin has been widely used as an effective and safe rodenticide. Rats are not easy to poison as they very rapidly become "bait shy," and if they consume a nonlethal amount of a toxic compound, they will refuse to consume more of the bait. The lethal action of warfarin is death from internal hemorrhage which occurs a few days after the lethal dose is consumed, and rats tend to continue to consume bait until death. Warfarin was number 42 in a series of coumarin derivatives synthesized in Link's laboratory in the 1940s, and it was the compound focused on as a potential rodenticide. Rats are much more sensitive to warfarin than rabbits are [24] and as it was less susceptible to being counteracted by varying amounts of vitamin K in the normal food of rodents, it appeared to be a more lethal bait. The Wisconsin Alumni Research Foundation heavily promoted the use of warfarin as a rodenticide, and its name was derived by the combination of the first letters of the organization's name with the "arin" from coumarin. Warfarin was first used as a rodenticide in the late 1940s, and soon became the most widely used rodenticide in the market.

By the early 1960s concern regarding warfarin's effectiveness was expressed because of the identification of anticoagulant-resistant rat populations, first in Northern Europe [25,26] and subsequently in the United States [27]. These rats have an increased resistance to warfarin, a decreased activity of the vitamin K epoxide reductase [28], and an increased requirement for vitamin K [29]; and the resistant rat populations appear to have the same genetic alteration as that observed [30] in some human patients who require large doses of warfarin to reach a targeted degree of anticoagulation. Concern over the spread of the anticoagulant-resistant rat population led to a renewed interest in the synthesis of a number of compounds that not only are effective in the warfarin-resistant rat [31] but also are much more active in normal animals than most compounds synthesized in the past (Figure 2.7). There are some differences in the nature of the warfarin resistance observed in rats obtained from different geographic locations [32], but the underlying basic genetic basis of the resistance is similar in all, an altered vitamin K epoxide reductase [32,33] resulting from at least eight different mutations. Oral anticoagulants that are effective in resistant rodents have kinetic inhibition values for the vitamin K epoxide reductase that

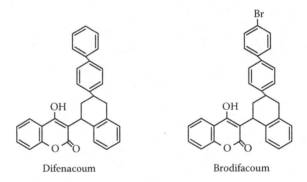

Difenacoum   Brodifacoum

FIGURE 2.7 Structures of coumarin-based anticoagulants that have been effective in warfarin-resistant rats.

are lower than warfarin, which has a K_i of 0.72 μM for the epoxide reductase activity of susceptible rats and 29 μM for resistant rats. In contrast to these values, brodifacoum, one of the more effective replacements for warfarin, has K_is of 0.04 μM and 0.09 μM for susceptible and resistant rats [34]. In addition to an alteration in the epoxide reductase, different strains of resistant rodents may have variations in the absorption, cellular uptake, or metabolism of the anticoagulants [35] and possibly alterations in the expression of the hepatic protein calumenin, which can influence the activity of the vitamin K-dependent carboxylase [36]. As would be expected, resistance to the second generation of anticoagulants has also been observed as they become more widely used [32,37].

At the present time, the readily purchased rat poisons that originally contained warfarin now contain one of these more effective 4-hydroxycoumarin derivatives. These compounds are more hydrophobic [34] and are cleared from the body much more slowly than warfarin. This has raised concerns that these "superwarfarins" can have serious impacts on wild birds and companion animals [38,39] and accidental or intentional ingestion by humans [40–42]. Long-term administration of vitamin K is required to reverse the impact of these compounds [43].

2.3.2 1,3-INDANDIONES

Another class of oral anticoagulants that block vitamin K activity is the 2-substituted 1,3-indandiones [44]. A large number of these compounds have been synthesized, and two of the most studied members of this series have been 2-phenyl-1,3-indandione and 2-pivalyl-1,3-indandione (Figure 2.8). These compounds have had some commercial use as rodenticides and have been studied clinically as possible oral anticoagulants. However, they do carry the potential for hepatic toxicity [45] and are no longer used clinically. The mechanism of action of these compounds has not been studied as extensively as the 4-hydroxycoumarins, but the observations that warfarin-resistant rats are also resistant to the indandiones and the ability of these compounds to inhibit the conversion of the 2,3-epoxide of vitamin K to the vitamin [46] would suggest that the mechanism of action of the indandiones is similar to that of the 4-hydroxycoumarins.

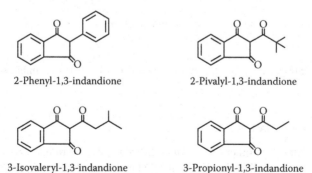

2-Phenyl-1,3-indandione   2-Pivalyl-1,3-indandione

3-Isovaleryl-1,3-indandione   3-Propionyl-1,3-indandione

FIGURE 2.8 Structures of indandiones that antagonize vitamin K action.

2.3.3   2-HALO-3-PHYTYL-1,4-NAPHTHOQUINONES

In the course of a series of investigations into the ability of phylloquinone to overcome the action of warfarin, Lowenthal, MacFarlane, and McDonald [47] found
that the replacement of the 2-methyl group of phylloquinones by a chlorine atom
to form 2-chloro-3-phytyl-1,4-naphthoquinone (Figure 2.9) or its bromine analog
resulted in compounds that were potent antagonists of vitamin K. The most active
of these two compounds was the chloro derivative, commonly called "Chloro-K,"
and in contrast to the coumarin and indandione derivatives, Chloro-K acted as
if it were a true competitive inhibitor of the vitamin at its active site [48]. The
observation [49] that the chlorinated form of a benzoquinone analog of vitamin K,
2-chloro-5,6-dimethyl-1,4-benzoquinone was also an antagonist of vitamin K provided further evidence of a direct action of these compounds. More recent in vitro
studies [50] utilizing the availability of the vitamin K-dependent carboxylase have
shown that reduced Chloro-K is a direct competitive inhibitor of reduced phylloquinone, the substrate for the enzyme. Chloro-K also interferes with enzymes
responsible for metabolizing vitamin K, and significant alterations in the tissue
distribution of radioactive vitamin K were observed [51] when it was administered
at the same time as Chloro-K. Because of its distinctly different mechanism of
action than the commonly used coumarin anticoagulants, Chloro-K has been used
as a probe of the mechanism of action of vitamin K, and as it is an effective anticoagulant in coumarin anticoagulant-resistant rats [52], it has been suggested as a
possible rodenticide [53].

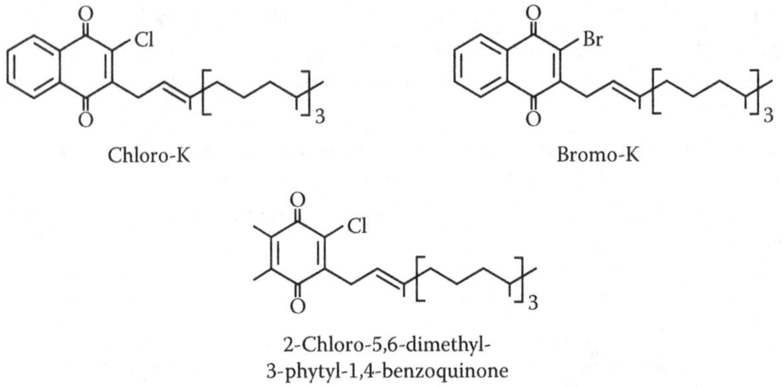

Chloro-K   Bromo-K

2-Chloro-5,6-dimethyl-
3-phytyl-1,4-benzoquinone

FIGURE 2.9   Structures of halogen-modified compounds known to be inhibitors of vitamin K
action.

2.3.4   OTHER ANTAGONISTS

There are a number of other compounds that appear to be rather structurally unrelated to either vitamin K or the coumarins that have been found to have anticoagulant
activity (Figure 2.10). The first of these, 2,3,5,6-tetrachloro-4-pyridinol, was shown
[54] to have anticoagulant activity, and on the basis of its action in warfarin-resistant

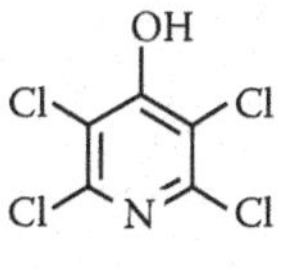

2,3,5,6-Tetrachloro-
4-pyridinol

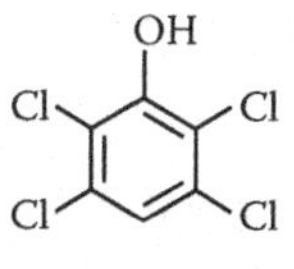

2,3,5,6-Tetrachlorophenol

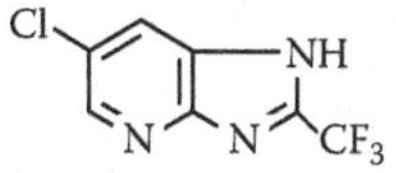

6-Chloro-2-trifluoromethylimidazo-
[4,5-*b*]-pyrimidine

FIGURE 2.10   Structures of inhibitors of vitamin K action with no structural relationship to vitamin K or to coumarin-based antagonists.

rats [46], it would appear that it functions as a direct antagonist of the vitamin. Subsequent studies of this antagonist [55] indicated that although vitamin K would reverse the action of this antagonist in animals, reduced phylloquinone would not reverse its ability to inhibit the vitamin K-dependent carboxylase in an in vitro study. It has also been shown [56] that the inhibitory action of tetrachloropyridinol extends to a large number of polychlorinated phenols and that 2,3,5,6-tetrachlorophenol is as effective an inhibitor of the carboxylase as the initially described antagonist. A number of di- and trichlorophenols also inhibit the carboxylase, but not as effectively as the two shown in Figure 2.10. The molecular action of this inhibitor has not been established, but it does not appear to be a direct competitive inhibitor of the reduced vitamin K-binding site of the carboxylase. A second series of compounds that appear to be structurally unrelated to the vitamin are the 6-substituted imidazole [4,5-*b*]pyrimidines. These compounds have been described [57] as antagonists of the vitamin, and the action of 6-chloro-2-trifluoromethyl-imidazo[4,5-*b*]pyrimidine in warfarin-resistant rats would suggest that they are functioning in the same way as a coumarin or an indandione type of compound. The in vitro action of this compound has not been studied.

2.3.5   INACTIVE FORMS OF VITAMIN K AS INHIBITORS

Early studies of the biological activity of different forms of vitamin K utilized chick bioassays and were capable of demonstrating that some lacked activity but were less effective in identifying compounds that were acting as inhibitors of active vitamers.

Partial purification of the vitamin K-dependent carboxylase made it possible to study the impact of a number of analogs of phylloquinone on the carboxylase, rather than indirectly through their effect on clotting factor levels in animals. The data in Figure 2.11 and Table 2.6 present the results of an in vitro study of the maximal activity of the reduced forms of a number of phylloquinone derivatives as substrates for the carboxylase and their ability to act as an inhibitor of the enzyme when phylloquinone is used as a substrate [58,59]. These compounds differed

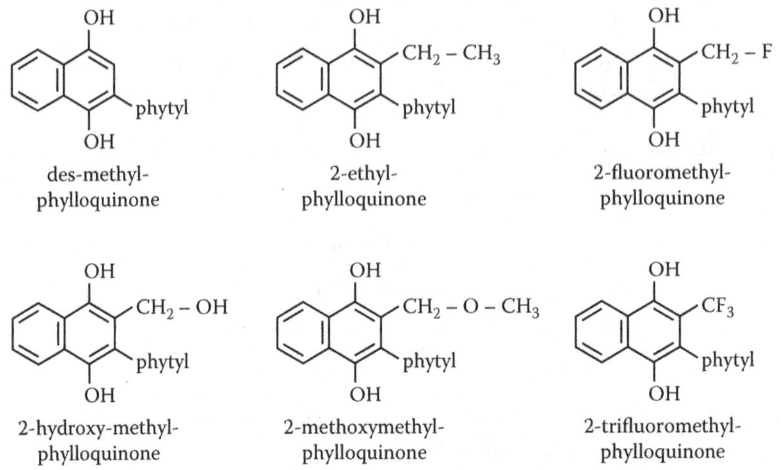

FIGURE 2.11 Structures of phylloquinone analogs modified at the 2-position.

TABLE 2.6

The Effect of Alteration of the Constituent at the 2-Position of the Naphthoquinone Ring on the Activity of Phylloquinone Analogs to Function as Substrates or Inhibitors of the Vitamin K-Dependent Carboxylase

Alteration of Phylloquinone Structure	Substrate Activity V_{max}	Inhibitor Activity K_i (µM)
Phylloquinone	100	–
Des-methyl-phylloquinone	<5	NI
2-Ethyl-phylloquinone	10	NI
2-Fluoromethyl phylloquinone	<2	US
2-Hydroxymethyl phylloquinone	<2	5
2-Methoxymethyl phylloquinone	<2	12
2-Trifluormethyl phylloquinone	<2	60

Note: Phylloquinone analogs were reduced and assayed for carboxylase activity in rat liver microsomes or partially purified carboxylase preparations and activity expressed as percent of V_{max} for phylloquinone. Inhibitor activity of the reduced analogs was assessed with reduced phylloquinone as a substrate. NI = no inhibitor; US = unstable in incubation. For details, see References [50,58,59].

only in the group that was located on the 2-position of the naphthoquinone ring. Deletion of the 2-methyl group, or the substitution of an ethyl group for a methyl group, results in very low substrate activity, but these compounds were not inhibitors. However, the 2-hydroxymethyl analog of phylloquinone, which was not a carboxylase substrate, was found to be a very good inhibitor, and the 2-trifluoromethyl analog which lacked substrate activity was also an inhibitor of the carboxylase. The 2-hydroxymethyl analog of phylloquinone, the most effective compound studied, was not found to be an anticoagulant when administered to rats, but it is not known if this analog of phylloquinone was capable of reaching the active site of the enzyme when ingested.

2.4   USE OF VITAMIN K TO SUPPLEMENT DIETS AND RATIONS

Although the intake of vitamin K within the population is extremely variable and some individuals consume very small amounts, evidence of clinically significant deficiencies are extremely rare (see Chapter 7). Newborn infants are given a vitamin K supplement which is also prescribed for patients with lipid malabsorption problems, and phylloquinone is used to rapidly reverse elevated International Normalized Ratio (INR) values during attempts to manage Warfarin therapy [60]. Vitamin K is increasingly being added to over-the-counter multivitamin supplements and to calcium supplements. At one time, a water-soluble form of menadione, menadiol sodium diphosphate, which was sold as Kappadione or Synkayvite, was widely used, but the danger of hyperbilirubinemia associated with menadione usage led to the use of intramuscular injectable phylloquinone as the desired form of the vitamin. Phylloquinone (USP phytonadione) is marketed as AquaMEPHYTON, Konakion, Mephyton, and Mono-Kay and used in most countries. These products contain detergents such as polysorbate-80 or polyethoxylated castor oil and, although they were not formulated for oral administration, they have been administered to newborn infants in this manner (see Chapter 7). A product containing a mixed micellar preparation of phylloquinone rather than synthetic detergents (Konakion MM) is used in a number of countries and appears to be more effectively absorbed from the gut than the intramuscular preparations. In Japan and other Asian countries, MK-4 rather than phylloquinone is widely used. At the present time enteral feeding products contain varying amounts of vitamin K as phylloquinone, and the U.S. Food and Drug Administration has recently set a requirement [61] for parenteral adult multivitamin products of 150 µg of phylloquinone per day.

The use of over-the-counter vitamin K preparations as dietary supplements does not appear to be as prevalent a practice as the use of many other vitamins. Some, but not all, "multivitamin" preparations contain phylloquinone at a reasonable level of intake. Many calcium supplements contain vitamin D, and some of these now also contain phylloquinone. A popular chewable calcium supplement also contains both vitamin D and phylloquinone. Dietary supplements containing only vitamin K do not appear to be commonly found in drugstores, and only a few are on the shelves of supplement outlets. However, a quick Google search indicates that there are many products available. The current Dietary Reference Intake (DRI) for vitamin K is an adequate intake of 90 µg/day, and most of the available supplements contain much more. As an example, the following products and their vitamin K content per pill (manufacturers' names omitted) are readily available by mail: vitamin K-1 (10 µg phytonadione); vitamin K-2 (100 µg of natural MK-7); MK-7 (90 µg as natto extract); vitamin K (500 µg, form not indicated); full spectrum vitamin K (1,000 µg phytadione, 3000 µg vitamin K-2 as menaquinone-4, 50 µg vitamin K-2 as menaquinone-7); vitamin K_2 menatetrenone (5 µg vitamin K_2); vitamin K complex (200 µg phylloquinone, 200 µg menaquinone, MK-7). Although all of these products probably meet

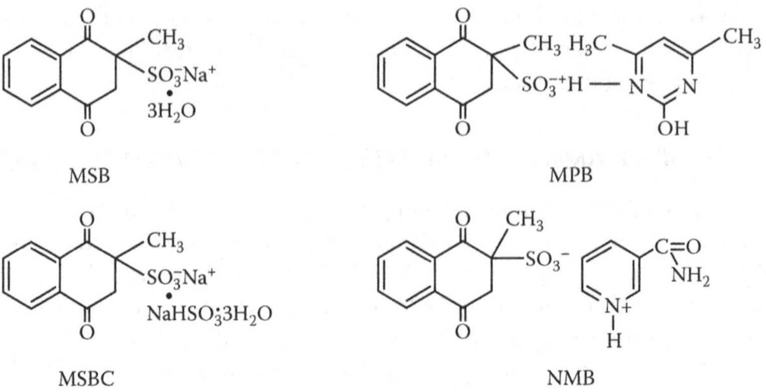

FIGURE 2.12 Menadione adducts used in poultry and swine rations.

the current regulations that cover the sale of dietary supplements, the wide range of intakes and forms of vitamin K would appear to make it very difficult for a consumer to know if their use would result in better health (see Chapter 7).

The major use of vitamin K is in poultry diets. Chicks are very sensitive to vitamin K restriction, and antibiotics that decrease intestinal vitamin synthesis are often added to poultry diets. Supplementation is therefore required to ensure an adequate supply. Phylloquinone would be very expensive for this purpose, and different forms of menadione have been used. Menadione itself possesses high biological activity in a deficient chick, but its effectiveness depends on the presence of lipids in the diet to promote absorption. There are also problems in the stability of menadione in feed products, and because of this, water-soluble forms are used (Figure 2.12). Menadione forms a water-soluble sodium bisulfite addition product, menadione sodium bisulfite (MSB), which has been used commercially, but it can also be somewhat unstable in mixed feeds. In the presence of excess sodium bisulfite, MSB crystallizes as a complex with an additional mole of sodium bisulfite; this complex, known as menadione sodium bisulfite complex (MSBC), has increased stability and is widely used in the poultry industry. Other water-soluble forms of vitamin K are salts formed by the addition of dimethylpyridinol to MSB to form menadione dimethylpyridinol bisulfite (MPB) [62] and menadione nicotinamide bisulfite (MNB) [63]. Comparisons of the relative biopotency of these compounds have often been made on the basis of the weight of the salts rather than on the basis of menadione content, and this has caused some confusion in assessing their value in animal feeds. However, a number of studies [62,64] have indicated that MPB is somewhat more effective in chick rations than is MSBC. This form of the vitamin has also been successfully used in swine rations [65].

2.5 SYNTHESIS OF VITAMIN K

2.5.1 BIOSYNTHESIS

The biosynthesis of vitamin K has been studied most extensively through the elucidation of the metabolic pathway leading to the synthesis of menaquinones in bacteria.

Two prominent cellular isoprenoid quinones, menaquinones and ubiquinones, are components of electron transport pathways leading to oxygen in aerobic organisms and a wide range of fermentation products in anaerobic organisms. Most aerobic gram-negative organisms contain ubiquinones as their sole quinone, and aerobic gram-positive bacteria utilize menaquinones in their electron transport pathways. The majority of all classes of anaerobic bacteria contain only menaquinones. As a facultative anaerobe, *E. coli* contains both and can grow under both aerobic and anaerobic conditions. The majority of the studies leading to the understanding of the pathway of menaquinone biosynthesis were carried out using *E. coli* as a model. The earlier progress in the elucidation of this pathway was reviewed extensively by Bentley and Meganathan in 1988 [66], and the more current understanding of the biosynthesis of both the menaquinones and ubiquinones is available in a 2001 detailed review by Meganathan [67].

The major precursor of the naphthoquinone ring is shikimic acid (Figure 2.13) which forms the cyclohexane ring of the synthesized menaquinone. The carboxyl carbon of shikimate becomes part of the quinone ring, while the other three carbons are derived from 2-ketoglutarate during the conversion of isochorismate to O-succinylbenzoate. Following closure of the ring, the resulting 1,4-dihydroxy-2-naphthoate is decarboxylated and prenylated to a desmethyl menaquinone. The pathway is completed by the insertion of the 2-methyl group by S-adenosylmethionine. Although this pathway has been assumed to apply in general to all organisms synthesizing menaquinones, there is evidence [68] that some organisms are forming menaquinones by an alternate pathway. Synthesis of the polyprenyl side chain of the menaquinones (Figure 2.14) depends on the isomerization of isopentenyl diphosphate to dimethylallyl diphosphate and the subsequent condensation of these two 5-carbon

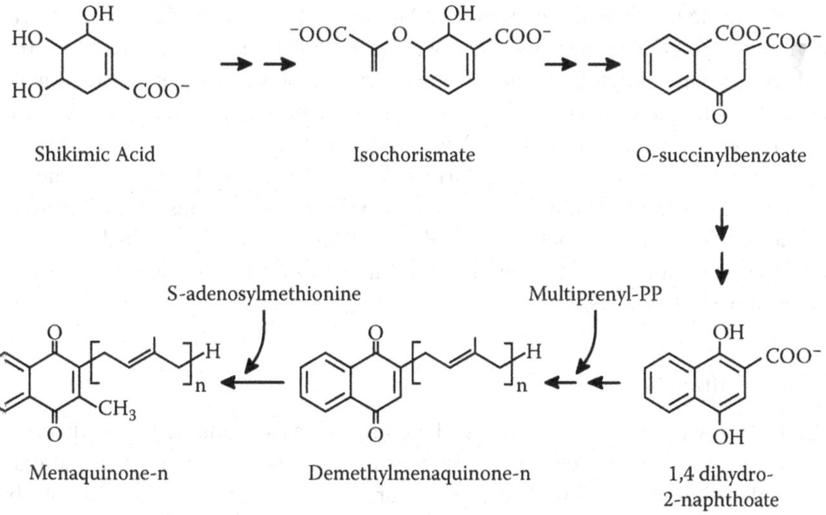

FIGURE 2.13 Pathway of menaquinone synthesis in *E. coli*. A number of intermediates that are known to be present between the structures in the figure are not shown here. For details see Reference [67].

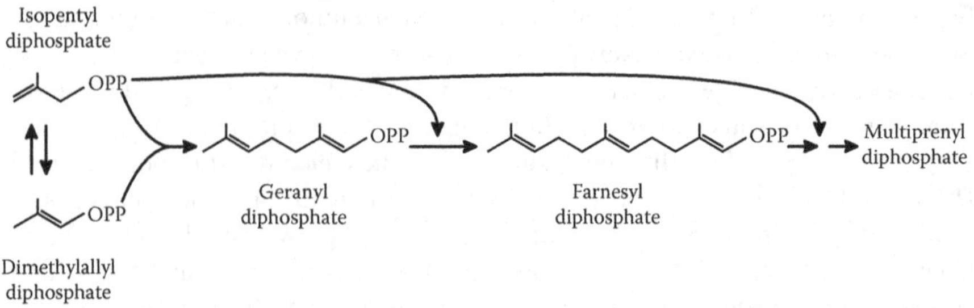

FIGURE 2.14 Metabolic pathway for the biosynthesis of the long-chain multiprenyl side chain of the menaquinones. For details see Meganathan [67].

intermediates to form geranyl diphosphate. Lengthening of the developing side chain results from the repetition of another isopentyl group. The length of the side chain that is attached to the menaquinones is very closely controlled by each organism and is one way of typing this class of organisms. The basis for the selectivity is not completely understood, but appears to be related to very small alterations in the enzyme that catalyze the head to tail condensation beyond the farnesyl diphosphate stage. Phylloquinone, synthesized by green plants, does not participate in electron transfers coupled to substrate oxidation, but is involved in the photosynthetic process as a secondary electron acceptor in photosystem I. Relatively little is known about the pathway of synthesis of phylloquinone in plants, but biochemical and genetic analysis [69] indicate that it is very similar to the pathway of menaquinone production in bacteria. Studies utilizing transgenic plants which have altered the production of some of the early intermediates in the pathway have demonstrated the amount of phylloquinone and can be increased or decreased by this approach [70].

At the time that menadione was found to have antihemorrhagic activity when fed to vitamin K-deficient animals, there was no evidence that it was a natural product and it was assumed that it was not. There are, however, subsequent reports that small amounts of menadione are present in the fern, *Asplenium indicum* [71,72], and in walnut husks [73]; and it is likely that it could be found in other plants if a serious search were made. Whether it is formed by dealkylation of phylloquinone or by an alternate metabolic pathway is not known. The observations that derivatives of menadione formed by demethylation, alternate site methylation, or hydroxylation of the naphthoquinone ring are found in the same species [73] suggests a rather complex pathway of synthesis.

2.5.2 CHEMISTRY

The methods used in the synthesis of vitamin K have remained essentially those originally described in the late 1930s by the investigators involved in the discovery of the vitamin [74–76]. Those procedures involved the condensation of phytol or its bromide with the reduced form of menadione (menadiol) or its salt to form the reduced addition compound, which is then oxidized to the quinone. Substantial amounts of menadione are produced by the chemical industry by the oxidation of 2-methylnaphthalene with CrO_3 and sulfuric acid or some other strong oxidant. The yield of the desired product is in the range of 50% to 80% depending on the oxidant used, and a number of side products that are formed must be separated from the menadione formed. The oxidation of 2-methyl-1-naphthol by a peroxide or molecular oxygen has more recently been used [77] as a pathway for industrial production that would lead to higher yields and fewer side products. Following addition of the side chain at the 3-position, purification of the desired product from unreacted reagents and side products occurs either at the quinol stage or after oxidation. These reactions have been reviewed in considerable detail, as have methods to produce the specific menaquinones rather than phylloquinone [78,79]. The major side reactions in this general scheme are the formation of the *cis* rather than the *trans* isomer at the Δ^2 position and alkylation at the 2- rather than the 3-position to form the 2-methyl-2-phytyl derivative. The use of monoesters of menadiol and newer acid catalysts for the condensation step [80] is the basis for the general method of industrial preparation used at the present time. A new method for the synthesis of compounds of the vitamin K series based on the coupling of polyprenyltrimethyltins to menadione has also been reported [81,82]. This method has been utilized [50] to synthesize a number of potential vitamin K-dependent carboxylase substrates and is also a regio- and stereo-controlled synthesis that gives a high yield of the desired product. It is likely that this method may have particular utility in the synthesis of radiolabeled vitamin K for metabolic studies, as the purification of the desired product appears to be somewhat simpler than with the synthesis currently in use. Although a large number of vitamin K analogs have been synthesized, they have tended to be structural variations related to alkylation of the naphthoquinone ring, or alterations in the number of saturated or unsaturated isoprenoid groups attached to the 3-position of the ring. More recently methods for the synthesis of ω-oxygenated side-chain analogs of menaquinones [15,83]. These ω-oxygenated alcohol and aldehyde derivatives of the vitamin are presumably intermediates in the formation of the only characterized degradative metabolites of vitamin K, the ω-acids (see Chapter 6).

2.6   PHYSICAL AND CHEMICAL PROPERTIES OF VITAMIN K

Compounds with vitamin K activity are substituted 1,4-naphthoquinones and, therefore, have the chemical properties that are common to all quinones. The chemistry of quinoids has been reviewed [84], and a great deal of data related to the spectral and other physical characteristics of phylloquinone and the menaquinones have been summarized [85,86]. The oxidized form of all K vitamers exhibits an ultraviolet (UV) spectrum that is characteristic of the naphthoquinone nucleus, with four distinct peaks between 240 and 280 nm and a less sharp absorption at around 320 to 330 nm. The extinction coefficient ($E_{1cm}^{1\%}$) decreases with chain length and has been used as a means of determining the length of the side chain. The molar extinction value ε for both phylloquinone and the various menaquinones is about 19,000. The absorption spectrum changes drastically upon reduction to the hydroquinone, with an enhancement of the 245 nm peak and disappearance of the 270 nm peak. These compounds also exhibit characteristic infrared and nuclear magnetic resonance (NMR) absorption spectra that are again largely those of the naphthoquinone ring. NMR analysis of phylloquinone has been used to establish firmly that natural phylloquinone is the *trans* isomer and can be used to establish the *cis-trans* ratio in synthetic mixtures of the vitamin. Mass spectroscopy has been useful in determining the length of the

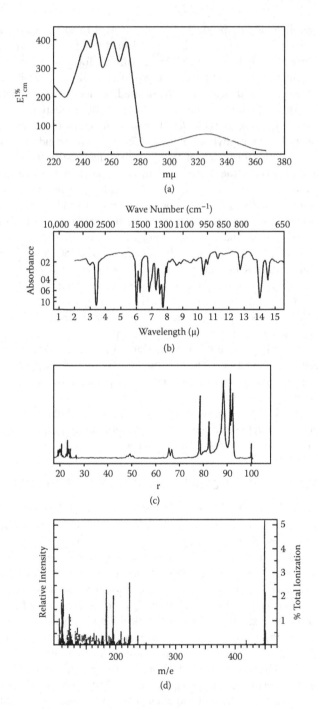

FIGURE 2.15 Physical properties of phylloquinone. (a) Ultraviolet absorption spectra in petroleum ether. (b) Infrared absorption spectra. (c) Nuclear magnetic resonance spectra in CDCl$_3$ at 60 Mc. (d) Mass fragmentation spectrum of the parent molecular ion is seen at m/e = 450.

side chain and the degree of saturation of vitamins of the menaquinone series isolated from natural sources. The UV, infrared, NMR, and mass fragmentation spectra of phylloquinone are presented in Figure 2.15. Phylloquinone is an oil at room temperature, while the various menaquinones can easily be crystallized from organic solvents and have melting points from 35°C to 60°C, depending on the length of the isoprenoid chain.

REFERENCES

1. IUPAC-IUB, Commission on Biochemical Nomenclature. 1975. Nomenclature of quinones with isoprenoid side chains recommendations (1973). *Eur J Biochem* 53:15–18.
2. Fieser, L.F., M. Tishler, and W.L. Sampson. 1941. Vitamin K activity and structure. *J Biol Chem* 137:659–692.
3. Dam, H. 1942. Vitamin K, its chemistry and physiology. *Adv Enzymol* 2:285–324.
4. Weber, F. and O. Wiss. 1971. Vitamin K group: Active compounds and antagonists. In *The Vitamins*, 2nd ed., Vol. 3, ed. W.H. Sebrell and R.S. Harris, 457–466. New York: Academic Press.
5. Brinkhous, K.M. 1940. Plasma prothrombin; vitamin K. *Medicine* 19:329–416.
6. Matschiner, J.T. and R.G. Bell. 1972. Metabolism and vitamin K activity of *cis* phylloquinone in rats. *J Nutr* 102:625–630.
7. Ramotar, K., J.M. Conly, H. Chubb, and T.J. Louie. 1984. Production of menaquinones by intestinal anaerobes. *J Infect Dis* 150:213–218.
8. Conly, J.M. and R.T. Stein. 1992. The production of menaquinones (vitamin K_2) by intestinal bacteria and their role in maintaining coagulation homeostasis. *Prog Food Nutr Sci* 16:307–343.
9. Collins, M.D. and D. Jones. 1981. Distribution of isoprenoid quinone structural types in bacteria and their taxonomic implications. *Microbiol Rev* 45:316–354.
10. Kindberg, C., J.W. Suttie, K. Uchida, K. Hirauchi, and H. Nakao. 1987. Menaquinone production and utilization in germ-free rats following inoculation with specific organisms. *J Nutr* 117:1032–1035.
11. Tindall, B.J., K.O. Stetter, and M.D. Collins. 1989. A novel, fully saturated menaquinone from the thermophilic, sulphate-reducing archaebacterium *Archaeoglobus fulgidus*. *J Gen Microbiol* 135:693–696.
12. Tindall, B.J. 1989. Fully saturated menaquinones in the archaebacterium *Pyrobaculum islandicum*. *FEMS Microbiol Lett* 60:251–254.
13. Collins, M.D., F. Fernandez, and O.W. Howarth. 1985. Isolation and characterization of a novel vitamin-K from *Eubacterium lentum*. *Biochem Biophys Res Commun* 133:322–328.
14. Howarth, O.W., E. Grund, R.M. Kroppenstedt, and M.D. Collins. 1986. Structural determination of a new naturally occurring cyclic vitamin K. *Biochem Biophys Res Commun* 140:916–923.
15. Suhara, Y., Y. Hirota, K. Nakagawa, M. Kamao, N. Tsugawa, and T. Okano. 2008. Design and synthesis of biologically active analogues of vitamin K_2: Evaluation of their biological activities with cultured human cell lines. *Bioorg Med Chem* 16:3108–3117.
16. Kresge, N., R.D. Simoni, and R.L. Hill. 2005. Hemorrhagic sweet clover disease, Dicumarol, and warfarin: The work of Karl Paul Link. *J Biol Chem* 280:e5–e6.
17. Last, J.A. 2002. The missing link: The story of Karl Paul Link. *Toxicol Sci* 66:4–6.
18. Link, K.P. 1959. The discovery of Dicumarol and its sequels. *Circulation* 19:97–107.
19. Campbell, H.A., W.K. Smith, W.L. Roberts, and K.P. Link. 1941. Studies on the hemorrhagic sweet clover disease. II. The bioassay of hemorrhagic concentrates by following the prothrombin level in the plasma of rabbit blood. *J Biol Chem* 138:1–20.

20. Campbell, H.A. and K.P. Link. 1941. Studies on the hemorrhagic sweet clover disease. IV. The isolation and crystallization of the hemorrhagic agent. *J Biol Chem* 138:21–33.

21. Stahmann, M.A., C.F. Huebner, and K.P. Link. 1941. Studies on the hemorrhagic sweet clover disease. V. Identification and synthesis of the hemorrhagic agent. *J Biol Chem* 138:513–527.

22. Overman, R.S., M.A. Stahmann, C.F. Huebner, W.R. Sullivan, L. Spero, D.G. Doherty, M. Ikawa, L. Graf, S. Roseman, and K.P. Link. 1944. Studies on the hemorrhagic sweet clover disease. XIII. Anticoagulant activity and structure in the 4-hydroxycoumarin group. *J Biol Chem*, 153:5–24.

23. Ufer, M. 2005. Comparative pharmacokinetics of vitamin K antagonists. *Clin Pharmacokinet* 44:1227–1246.

24. Almquist, H.J. 1936. Purification of the antihemorrhagic vitamin by distillation. *J Biol Chem* 115:589–591.

25. Boyle, C.M. 1960. Case of apparent resistance of *Rattus norvegicus berkenhout* to anti-coagulant poisons. *Nature* 188:517.

26. Lund, M. 1964. Resistance to warfarin in the common rat. *Nature* 203:778.

27. Jackson, W.B. and D. Kaukeinen. 1972. Resistance of wild Norway rats in North Carolina to warfarin rodenticide. *Science* 176:1343–1344.

28. Hildebrandt, E.F., P.C. Preusch, J.L. Patterson, and J.W. Suttie. 1984. Solubilization and characterization of vitamin K epoxide reductase from normal and warfarin-resistant rat liver microsomes. *Arch Biochem Biophys* 228:480–492.

29. Hermodson, M.A., J.W. Suttie, and K.P. Link. 1969. Warfarin metabolism and vitamin K requirement in the warfarin-resistant rat. *Am J Physiol* 217:1316–1319.

30. O'Reilly, R.A. 1971. Vitamin K in hereditary resistance to oral anticoagulant drugs. *Am J Physiol* 221:1327–1330.

31. Lund, M. 1981. Comparative effect of the three rodenticides warfarin, difenacoum and brodifacoum on eight rodent species in short feeding periods. *J Hyg Camb* 87:101–107.

32. Pelz, H.-J., S. Rost, M. Hunerberg, A. Fregin, A.-C. Heiberg, K. Baert, A.D. MacNicoll, C.V. Prescott, A.-S. Walker, J. Oldenburg, and C.R. Muller. 2005. The genetic basis of resistance to anticoagulants in rodents. *Genetics* 170:1839–1847.

33. Oldenburg, J., M. Watzka, S. Rost, and C.R. Muller. 2007. VKORC1: Molecular target of coumarins. *J Thromb Haemost* 5(Suppl 1):1–6.

34. Lasseur, R., A. Grandemange, C. Longin-Sauvageon, P. Berny, and E. Benoit. 2007. Comparison of the inhibition effect of different anticoagulants on vitamin K epoxide reductase activity from warfarin-susceptible and resistant rat. *Pesticide Biochem Physiol* 88:203–208.

35. Markussen, M.D., A.C. Heiberg, M. Fredholm, and M. Kristensen. 2008. Differential expression of cytochrome P450 genes between bromadiolone-resistant and anticoag-ulant-susceptible Norway rats: A possible role for pharmacokinetics in bromadiolone resistance. *Pest Manag Sci* 64:239–248.

36. Wallin, R., S.M. Hutson, D. Cain, A. Sweatt, and D.C. Sane. 2001. A molecular mecha-nism for genetic warfarin resistance in the rat. *FASEB J* 15:163–186.

37. Markussen, M.D., A.C. Heiberg, M. Fredholm, and M. Kristensen. 2007. Characterization of bromadiolone resistance in a Danish strain of Norway rats, *Rattus norvegicus,* by hepatic gene expression profiling of genes involved in vitamin K-dependent gamma-carboxylation. *J Biochem Mol Toxicol* 21:373–381.

38. Eason, C.T., E.C. Murphy, G.R.G. Wright, and E.B. Spurr. 2002. Assessment of risks of brodifacoum to non-target birds and mammals in New Zealand. *Ecotoxicology* 11:35–48.

39. Stone, W.B., J.C. Okoniewski, and J.R. Stedelin. 2003. Anticoagulant rodenticides and rap-tors: Recent findings from New York, 1998–2001. *Bull Environ Contam Toxicol* 70:34–40.

40. Weitzel, J.N., J.A. Sadowski, B.C. Furie, R. Moroose, H. Kim, M.E. Mount, M.J. Murphy, and B. Furie. 1990. Surreptitious ingestion of a long-acting vitamin K antagonist/rodenticide, brodifacoum: Clinical and metabolic studies of three cases. *Blood* 76:2555–2559.

41. Spahr, J.E., J.S. Maul, and G.M. Rodgers. 2007. Superwarfarin poisoning: A report of two cases and review of the literature. *Am J Hematol* 82:656–660.

42. Chua, J.D. and W.R. Friedenberg. 1998. Superwarfarin poisoning. *Arch Intern Med* 158:1929–1932.

43. Routh, C.R., D.A. Triplett, M.J. Murphy, L.J. Felice, J.A. Sadowski, and E.G.T. Bovill. 1991. Superwarfarin ingestion and detection. *Am J Hematol* 36:50–54.

44. Kabat, H., E.F. Stohlman, and M.I. Smith. 1944. Hypoprothrombinemia induced by administration of indandione derivatives. *J Pharmacol Exp Ther* 80:160–170.

45. O'Reilly, R.A. 1976. Vitamin K and the oral anticoagulant drugs. *Annu Rev Med* 27:245–261.

46. Ren, P., R.E. Laliberte, and R.G. Bell. 1974. Effects of warfarin, phenylindanedione, tetrachloropyridinol, and chloro-vitamin K_1 on prothrombin synthesis and vitamin K metabolism in normal and warfarin-resistant rats. *Mol Pharmacol* 10:373–380.

47. Lowenthal, J., J.A. MacFarlane, and K.M. McDonald. 1960. The inhibition of the anti-dotal activity of vitamin K_1 against coumarin anticoagulant drugs by its chloro analogue. *Experentia* 16:428–429.

48. Lowenthal, J. and R.C.H. Wang. 1971. Formation of plasma clotting factor VII by vitamin K_1 in a cell-free system. *Fed Proc* 30:423.

49. Lowenthal, J. and J.A. MacFarlane. 1965. Vitamin K-like and antivitamin K activity of substituted para-benzoquinones. *J Pharmacol Exp Ther* 147:130–138.

50. Cheung, A. and J.W. Suttie. 1988. Synthesis of menaquinone-2 derivatives as substrates for the liver microsomal vitamin K-dependent carboxylase. *BioFactors* 1:61–65.

51. Thierry, M.J. and J.W. Suttie. 1971. Effect of warfarin and the chloro analog of vitamin K on phylloquinone metabolism. *Arch Biochem Biophys* 147:430–435.

52. Shah, D.V. and J.W. Suttie. 1973. The chloro analog of vitamin K: antagonism of vitamin K action in normal and warfarin-resistant rats. *Proc Soc Exp Biol Med* 143:775–779.

53. Suttie, J.W. 1973. Anticoagulant-resistant rats: Possible control by the use of the chloro analog of vitamin K. *Science* 180:741–743.

54. Marshall, F.N. 1972. 2,3,5,6-Tetrachloro-4-pyridinol: A new chemical structure for anti-coagulant activity. *Proc Soc Exp Biol Med* 139:223–227.

55. Friedman, P.A. and A.E. Griep. 1980. In vitro inhibition of vitamin K-dependent carboxylation by tetrachloropyridinol and the imidazopyridines. *Biochemistry* 19:3381–3386.

56. Grossman, C.P. and J.W. Suttie. 1990. Vitamin K-dependent carboxylase: Inhibitory action of polychlorinated phenols. *Biochem Pharmacol* 40:1351–1355.

57. Bang, N.U., G.O.P. O'Doherty, and R.D. Barton. 1975. Selective suppression of vitamin K-dependent procoagulant synthesis by compounds structurally unrelated to vitamin K. *Clin Res* 23:521A.

58. Grossman, C.P. and J.W. Suttie. 1992. Synthesis of fluoro- and hydroxy-derivatives of vitamin K as substrates or inhibitors of the liver microsomal vitamin K-dependent carboxylase. *BioFactors* 3:205–209.

59. Grossman, C.P., J.W. Suttie, T. Taguchi, Y. Suda, and Y. Kobayashi. 1988. Synthesis of trifluoromethyl analogs of vitamin K as substrates for the liver microsomal vitamin K-dependent carboxylase. *BioFactors* 1:255–259.

60. DeZee, K.J., W.T. Shimeall, K.M. Douglas, N.M. Shumway, and P.G. O'Malley. 2006. Treatment with excessive anticoagulation with phytonadione (vitamin K). *Arch Intern Med* 166:391–397.

61. Helphingstine, C.J. and B.R. Bistrian. 2003. New Food and Drug Administration requirements for inclusion of vitamin K in adult parenteral multivitamins. *J Parenteral Enteral Nutr* 27:220–224.
62. Griminger, P. 1965. Relative vitamin K potency of two water-soluble menadione analogues. *Poultry Sci* 44:211–213.
63. Oduho, G.W., T.K. Chung, and D.H. Baker. 1993. Menadione nicotinamide bisulfite is a bioactive source of vitamin K and niacin activity for chicks. *J Nutr* 123:737–743.
64. Dua, P.N. and E.J. Day. 1966. Vitamin K activity of menadione dimethyl-pyrimidinol bisulfite in chicks. *Poultry Sci* 45:94–96.
65. Seerley, R.W., O.W. Charles, H.C. McCampbell, and S.P. Bertsch. 1976. Efficacy of menadione dimethylpyrimidinol bisulfite as a source of vitamin K in swine diets. *J Animal Sci* 42:599–607.
66. Bentley, R. and R. Meganathan. 1982. Biosynthesis of vitamin K (menaquinone) in bacteria. *Microbiol Rev* 46:241–280.
67. Meganathan, R. 2001. Biosynthesis of menaquinone (vitamin K_2) and ubiquinone (coenzyme Q): A perspective on enzymatic mechanisms. *Vitamins and Hormones* 61:173–218.
68. Seto, H., Y. Jinnai, T. Hiratsuka, M. Fukawa, K. Furihata, N. Itoh, and T. Dairi. 2008. Studies on a new biosynthetic pathway for menaquinone. *J Am Chem Soc* 130:5614–5615.
69. Schultz, G., B.H. Ellerbrock, and J. Soll. 1981. Site of prenylation reaction in synthesis of phylloquinone (vitamin K_1) by spinach chloroplasts. *Eur J Biochem* 117:329–332.
70. Verberne, M.C., K. Sansuk, J.F. Bol, H.J. Linthorst, and R. Verpoorte. 2007. Vitamin K1 accumulation in tobacco plants overexpressing bacterial genes involved in the biosynthesis of salicylic acid. *J Biotechnol* (January 30)128(1):72–79.
71. Rohtagi, B.K., R.B. Gupta, and R.N. Khanna. 1984. Chemical constituents of *Asplenium indicum*. *J Natural Products* 47:901.
72. Gupta, R.B., R.N. Khanna, and N.N. Sharma. 1976. Chemical components of *Asplenium laciniatum*. *Current Sci* 45:44–46.
73. Binder, R.G., M.E. Benson, and R.A. Flath. 1984. Eight 1,4-naphthoquinones from *Juglans*. *Phytochemistry* 28:2799–2802.
74. Almquist, H.J. 1979. Vitamin K: Discovery, identification, synthesis, functions. *Fed Proc* 38:2687–2689.
75. Binkley, S.B., L.C. Cheney, W.F. Holcomb, R.W. McKee, S.A. Thayer, D.W. MacCorquodale, and E.A. Doisy. 1939. The constitution and synthesis of vitamin K_1. *J Am Chem Soc* 61:2558–2559.
76. Fieser, L.F. 1939. Synthesis of 2-methyl-3-phytyl-1,4-naphthoquinone. *J Am Chem Soc* 61:2559–2561.
77. Kholdeeva, O.A., O.V. Zalomaeva, A.B. Sorokin, I.D. Ivanchikova, C.D. Pina, and M. Rossi. 2007. New routes to vitamin K_3. *Catalysis Today* 121:58–64.
78. Mayer, H. and O. Isler. 1971. Vitamin K group: Chemistry. In *The Vitamins,* 2nd ed., Vol. 3, ed. W.H. Sebrell and R.S. Harris, 418–443. New York: Academic Press.
79. Mayer, H. and O. Isler. 1971. Synthesis of vitamins K. *Meth Enzymol* 18C:491–547.
80. Mayer, H. and O. Isler. 1971. Vitamin K group: Industrial. In *The Vitamins,* 2nd ed., Vol. 3, ed. W.H. Sebrell and R.S. Harris, 444–445. New York: Academic Press.
81. Naruta, Y. 1980. Allylation of quinones with allyltin reagents. *J Am Chem Soc* 102:3774–3783.
82. Naruta, Y. and K. Maruyama. 1979. Regio- and stereocontrolled polyprenylation of quinones. A new synthetic method of vitamin K series. *Chem Lett*:881–884.

83. Suhara, Y., A. Murakami, M. Kamao, S. Mimatsu, K. Nakagawa, N. Tsugawa, and T. Okano. 2007. Efficient synthesis and biological evaluation of omega-oxygenated analogues of vitamin K_2: Study of modification and structure-activity relationship of vitamin K_2 metabolites. *Bioorg Med Chem Lett* 17:1622–1625.
84. Patai, S. 1974. *The Chemistry of the Quinonoid Compounds,* Parts 1 & 2. New York: John Wiley & Sons.
85. Sommer, P. and M. Kofler. 1966. Physicochemical properties and methods of analysis of phylloquinones, menaquinones, ubiquinones, phostoquinones, menadione, and related compounds. *Vitamins and Hormones* 24:349–399.
86. Dunphy, P.J. and A.F. Brodie. 1971. The structure and function of quinones in respiratory metabolism. *Meth Enzymol* 18C:407–461.
87. Matschiner, J.T. and W.V. Taggart. 1968. Bioassay of vitamin K by intracardial injection in deficient adult male rats. *J Nutr* 94:57–59.

3 Dietary Intake of Vitamin K and the Vitamin K Content of Foods and Plasma

3.1 METHODOLOGY

The lack of good analytical methodology and the relatively infrequent observation of insufficient intake of vitamin K within the population hampered the development of accurate databases relevant to the amount of vitamin K in foods or biological tissues until the mid-1980s. Pure or nearly pure samples of vitamin K can be analyzed by the classical chemical techniques of ultraviolet spectroscopy or polarography, and these techniques, as well as the relatively nonspecific color reactions that were available during early attempts to isolate and characterize the vitamin, have been reviewed [1]. The number of interfering substances present in crude extracts of foods and tissues is such that a significant amount of preliminary separation is required before these methods can be applied to the measurement of vitamin K, and they have been of little practical value. Determinations of the vitamin K content of foods were, therefore, historically dependent on a biological assay. The chick is the species most susceptible to development of a vitamin K deficiency and is the species that has most often been used for vitamin K bioassays. It has a relatively high vitamin K requirement, and vitamin K intake via coprophagy is not the problem that it is with most small mammals. Vitamin K-deficient chicks were utilized, and the material to be assayed was either inserted into the crop or fed over a short period. Improvements in clotting times of vitamin K-deficient chicks were then compared to a standard curve prepared from administration of known amounts of the vitamin. Either whole blood clotting times [2] in early studies, or various types of one-stage prothrombin times in more recent studies [3,4] were used to follow the response. All oral bioassay procedures are complicated by the effects that variations in the composition of the administered substance may have on the rate and extent of absorption of the desired nutrient, and these and other factors influencing the sensitivity of these assays have been discussed by Griminger [5] and Almquist [6]. Many reviews of the nutritional aspects of vitamin K published before the early 1980s contain food composition data that have apparently been recalculated in an unspecified way from early bioassay results [7,8] and should be considered no more than a rough estimate of the vitamin K content of foods.

Separation of phylloquinone and menaquinone isoprenalogs was initially accomplished by various thin-layer and paper chromatographic systems, and reviews of this methodology are available [1,9–12]. At the present time, high-performance liquid chromatography (HPLC) is the standard analytical tool used to determine vitamin K concentration in various sources. This method was first demonstrated to be applicable to the separation of vitamin K by Williams, Schmit, and Henry [13], and early progress in this analytical field has been comprehensively reviewed by Shearer [14]. Both adsorptive HPLC and reversed-phase partition chromatography have been utilized in various methods developed to separate vitamin K from interfering lipids and to separate the various homologs of the vitamin, but only the latter is in widespread use at this time. Early reports [15,16] of the utilization of HPLC to determine the vitamin K content of biological samples utilized spectrophotometric detectors or electrochemical detection [17]. Although the sensitivity of spectrophotometric detection is marginal for the determination of vitamin K in animal tissues and plasma, some early reports utilized this approach [18], and others [19,20] utilized electrochemical detection.

Electrochemical reduction detection has been improved by the use of a dual-electrode coulometric detector [21], and at the present time, this method [22] or assays that depend on the fluorimetric detection of the reduced hydronaphthoquinone form of the vitamin are widely used. The postcolumn reduction of the naturally stable quinone form of the vitamin can be accomplished by electrochemical [23] or dry chemical [24] reduction. The latter method is widely utilized at the present time [25]. Photochemical reduction under aerobic conditions has also been reported as a means to utilize fluorescence detection [26] but has not been widely used. A recent report [27] has demonstrated the ability to determine the concentrations of vitamin K homologs in plasma by the utilization of HPLC and chemiluminescence (PO-CL) detection following online ultraviolet (UV) irradiation. The value of this procedure for large studies also remains to be determined.

Plant material contains vitamin K in the form of phylloquinone, but animal products and bacterial sources often contain an extensive mixture of various isoprenalogs of the menaquinone series. Vitamin K analyses are always complicated by the small amount of vitamin in the initial extracts. Initial extractions are usually made with the use of some type of dehydrating conditions, such as chloroform-methanol, or by first grinding the wet tissue with anhydrous sodium sulfate and then extracting it with acetone followed by hexane or ether. Sample preparations for various types of foods differ in some respects [28], and the various protocols have been summarized [29]. Determination of vitamin K from difficult to assay food matrices by lipase and α-amylase digestion followed by C_{18} solid-phase extraction (SPE) has also been reported [30] as a method of increasing the reproducibility of the assay. Vitamin K is sensitive to ultraviolet radiation, and all separations involving concentrated extracts of vitamin K should be carried out in subdued light to minimize decomposition of the vitamin. Compounds with vitamin K activity are also sensitive to alkali but are relatively stable to an oxidizing atmosphere and to heat.

Gas chromatography has also been explored as a method for vitamin K assay [31], and a protocol for the determination of the vitamin K content of green vegetables by this method has been published [32]. This method has seldom been used, but further improvements [33] may lead to useful assay techniques. A method for the determination of vitamin K in plasma utilizing stable isotope dilution gas chromatography/mass spectrometry (GC/MS) has been described [34] employing 2-methyl-deuterated phylloquinone as the internal standard. This method has been used in one study [35] of vitamin K status of infants and GC/MS has also been used to specifically follow the absorption of deuterium-labeled broccoli in the presence of endogenous phylloquinone in human serum [34]. In an attempt to more accurately measure the various forms of vitamin K in human plasma, a method employing ^{18}O-labeled vitamers as internal standards, and HPLC-tandem mass-mass spectrometry with atmospheric pressure chemical ionization (LC-APCI-MS/MS) has been developed [36], and a similar approach utilizing methyl-^{13}C- or ring-D_4-labeled phylloquinone has been described [37]. These methods have the potential for more accurate measurement of the less common forms of vitamin K but have not yet gained wide acceptance. There have also been attempts to develop an enzyme-linked immunosorbent assay (ELISA) that would allow the assay of vitamin K in foods or plasma with less laborious sample preparation [38], but no workable protocol has been developed.

3.2   VITAMIN K IN FOODS

3.2.1   PHYLLOQUINONE CONTENT OF FOODS

Following the development of standardized assays for vitamin K in foods, numerous reports of the phylloquinone content of various foods became available. The first attempt to bring these together in a more useful format was a provisional table [39] published in 1993. It was based largely on assays available in the 1980s or early 1990s [15,40–45] and analyses carried out in the authors' laboratories. The data shown in Table 3.1 are taken from the 2001 Institute of Medicine (IOM) Food and Nutrition Report which contains the dietary reference intakes for a number of micronutrients, including vitamin K [46]. The values in the table are the mean of the medians of the values in the older provisional table [39], and four more recent analytical reports [47-50]. A very extensive list of the phylloquinone content of foods is also available as a component of the U.S. Department of Agriculture's National Nutrient Database for Standard Reference, Release 18 (http://www.nal.usda.gov/fnic/foodcomp). The phylloquinone content values in the USDA database are those obtained by analyses of the U.S. Food and Drug Administration's total diet study representing for the most part North American dietary components, and are updated as new values become available [51]. Much of the currently available data has been obtained by Sadowski and Booth at the USDA/ARS Nutrition Center in Boston, but substantial amounts are also available from the United Kingdom [50,52], The Netherlands [53,54], Finland [49,55], and Japan [56,57]. There are also data from various geographic locations which are related to specific types of foods (Table 3.2).

The reliability of the vitamin K content of a food based on assays of a limited number of samples is questionable. As indicated in Table 3.3, there are substantial differences in the reported phylloquinone content of commonly consumed foods analyzed in different laboratories. For the few foods used as an example in Table 3.3, the highest value shown varies from 150% to 285% of the lowest, and the median

TABLE 3.1

Phylloquinone Content of Common Foods[a]

Food Item	µg/100 g	Food Item	µg/100 g
Vegetables		**Fats and Oils**	
Collards	440	Soybean oil	193
Spinach	380	Canola oil	127
Salad greens	315	Cottonseed oil	60
Broccoli	180	Olive oil	55
Brussels sprouts	177	Margarine	42
Cabbage	145	Butter	7
Bib lettuce	122	Corn oil	3
Asparagus	60	**Prepared Foods**	
Okra	40	Salad dressings	100
Iceberg lettuce	35	Coleslaw	80
Green beans	33	Mayonnaise	41
Green peas	24	Beef chow mein	31
Cucumbers	20	Muffins	25
Cauliflower	20	Doughnuts	10
Carrots	10	Potato chips	15
Tomatoes	6	Apple pie	11
Potatoes	1	French fries	5
Protein Sources		Macaroni/cheese	5
Dry soybeans	47	Lasagna	5
Dry lentils	22	Pizza	4
Liver	5	Hamburger/bun	4
Eggs	2	Hot dog/bun	3
Fresh meats	<1	Baked beans	3
Fresh fish	<1	Bread	3
Whole milk	<1		

[a] Modified from Reference [46]. Values are the median of values reported in other primary sources [39, 47–50] and both raw and cooked values are included. The vitamin K content of prepared foods is greatly influenced by the source of fat or oil in the product.

value is 30% to 50% different than the extremes. Analytical methodology has become more standardized, and most recent reports are of replicate analyses where the coefficient of variation (CV). is 15% or less. The basis for the wide discrepancy in reported values is therefore not obvious. A study [41] of green vegetables grown from the same seeds in Montreal or in Boston indicated significant differences in most cases with leaf lettuce grown in Montreal containing twice as much phyllo-quinone as that grown in Boston. Whether climate, soil, or growing conditions were

TABLE 3.2
Vitamin K Content of Specialized Foods

Food Source	References
Animal products, fresh and processed	54, 93, 112, 113
Baby food products	114
Cereal products	115
Fast foods and snack foods	116
Fats and oils	117
Fruits and berries	49, 118
Margarine and dairy products	48, 113, 119
Mixed dishes, soups, and cheeses	112
Nuts	118
Tea and coffee	120
Vegetables	51

TABLE 3.3
Variation in Phylloquinone Content of Foods from Different Published Sources[a]

Literature	µg Phylloquinone/100 g Food			
Ref.	Broccoli	Spinach	Olive Oil	Peas
52	179	381	55	–
39	205	400	49	36
50	179	380	80	34
47	113	360	28	24
48, 49	110	270	44	28
54	156	387	53	36
121	101	483	60	23
Median	156	381	53	31
Range	101–205	270–483	28–80	23–36
Mean ± SD	149 ± 41	382 ± 63	53 ± 16	30 ± 6

[a] Values for both raw and cooked foods are included, and the USDA data [121] have been recalculated from portion data.

responsible for these differences was not determined. The study also demonstrated that phylloquinone tended to increase with plant maturity, but these differences were minor compared to the geographic differences. The content of both phylloquinone and chlorophyll have been measured [56] in 28 green vegetables. In about 75% of these there was a molar ratio of phylloquinone to chlorophyll of about 1:100, but in a few cases there was 10% as much phylloquinone as chlorophyll. The effect of heat processing (canning) or sterilization by ionizing radiation on the vitamin K content of asparagus, broccoli, cabbage, cauliflower, green beans, and spinach has been assessed by utilizing a chick bioassay [58,59], and vitamin K activity did not differ consistently from that of the fresh frozen food. Storage of any of the products for 15 months also failed to have a significant effect. These data would suggest that the general assumption that vitamin K in food is relatively stable is warranted, and a recent limited study of the influence of boiling or microwaving carrots or spinach [51] indicates that the vitamin is not destroyed by these processes. However, substantial losses in phylloquinone have been reported during industrial juice production from berries [60]. The vitamin is not stable when exposed to ultraviolet light, and exposure of edible oils to daylight or fluorescent light in clear glass containers has been demonstrated [42] to rapidly destroy phylloquinone.

A substantial amount of dietary vitamin K is contributed by only a limited number of foods. Data obtained from the U.S. FDA total diet study [61] indicate that 56% of adult male and 60% of adult female phylloquinone consumption was obtained from the top 10 contributors. For men (in the order of contribution) these were: spinach, iceberg lettuce, collards, broccoli, coleslaw with dressing, cabbage, French salad dressing, green peas, beef chow mein, and stick margarine; and for women they were spinach, collards, broccoli, iceberg lettuce, coleslaw with dressing, French salad dressing, green beans, brussels sprouts, and green peas. In a study limited to Caucasian postmenopausal women in the Boston, Massachusetts area [62], the top 10 contributors to the total diet (in order of contribution) were: broccoli, iceberg lettuce, spinach, other lettuces, greens, salad dressings, asparagus, brussels sprouts, and cabbage. These 10 foods represented 78% of the total intake.

Differences in the dietary sources of vitamin K between different national or geographic groups are for the most part determined by the relative intakes of various green leafy vegetables and cooking oils with a high content of phylloquinone. A study conducted in Shenyang, China, and in Cambridge, England [63] indicated that the food groups "green leafy vegetables," "other vegetables," and "cooking fats" comprised respectively 69%, 12%, and 13% of total phylloquinone intake in China, but 50%, 15%, and 3% in the United Kingdom. These values are consistent with a report of a study of vitamin K intake by older adult women in Ireland [64] where broccoli, cabbage, and lettuce contributed 44% of the total phylloquinone consumed. It is apparent that substantial amounts of vitamin K are not widely distributed in foods commonly consumed in many countries, but are limited to green vegetables and selected vegetable oils. It is, however, rather difficult to consume what most authorities would label as a "healthy diet" without obtaining an amount of vitamin K that would be considered adequate by most nutritionists. It has also been found (see Chapter 7) that it is difficult for researchers to produce a clinically significant deficiency of vitamin K by offering subjects a low vitamin K diet that in other respects would be nutritionally adequate.

3.2.2 Dietary Intake of Phylloquinone

The rather limited distribution of vitamin K with only a few foods containing substantial amounts results in calculations of intakes in both populations and individuals that are probably less accurate than they appear to be from a casual survey of the literature. Data from the "Framingham Offspring" study [65], which were based on usual dietary intakes for the last 12 months as reported on a semiquantitative food frequency questionnaire by 2900 male and female subjects with a mean age of 54, has indicated a mean daily phylloquinone intake of 162 ± 114 µg (mean ± S.D.). The distribution within the population was large, and median intakes for quintiles ranged from 63 to 282 µg/day (Figure 3.1). Daily vitamin K intakes based on dietary records and existing databases are extremely variable, and a study of 362 postmenopausal women [62] reported individual daily intakes ranging from 3 to 276 µg, and the mean three consecutive day intake was 156 ± 147 µg (mean ± S.D.). The authors of this study have recommended a minimum of five days of dietary recording to obtain a good estimate of individual subject intakes. A reasonably constant intake of vitamin K has been found to be beneficial in maintaining a stable prothrombin time in patients receiving oral anticoagulant therapy, and a self-assessment instrument has been developed [66] to aid patients in monitoring their vitamin K intake.

The accuracy of the calculated total phylloquinone content of diets based on two commonly used food composition databases has been assessed by direct laboratory analysis of a number of metabolic diets [67]. A daily diet formulated to contain 400 µg/day of phylloquinone was shown to contain 377 µg by direct analysis and 352 µg or 713 µg by the two food databases, a difference of –25% or +89% from the determined value. Four diets formulated to contain 100 µg/day of phylloquinone furnished 93 to 106 µg by direct analysis, and the calculations of phylloquinone content ranged from –21% to +22% when one of the databases was used and from –5% to +62% for the other. Five diets formulated to contain 10 µg/day of phylloquinone contained 10 to 22 µg by direct analysis and database estimates substantially differed from the determined amount. These data suggest that attempts to calculate vitamin K intake of individuals from food frequency questionnaires or dietary histories and existing food nutrient composition databases will yield values that are questionable at best. Estimates of phylloquinone intake in various populations are probably more accurate and there is a substantial difference in the reported intakes from a number of countries (Table 3.4) which seems to be related to food consumption practices in different areas. These estimates of mean population intake range from about

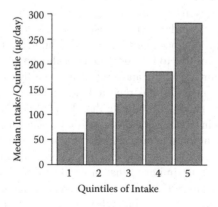

FIGURE 3.1 Distribution of phylloquinone intake in a large population based on a food frequency questionnaire. See Reference [65] for details.

TABLE 3.4
Estimates of Mean Phylloquinone Intake of Adults from Different Countries

Location	Ref.	Age (years)	n	Phylloquinone/day (Mean µg) Male	Phylloquinone/day (Mean µg) Female
United States (NHANES III)	46	51–70	3,999	120	97
Great Britain	122	65–74	325	72[a]	66[a]
Ireland	123	51–64	335	86	81
Japan	124	20–23	125		155
The Netherlands	53	65–69	1,135		254[b]
Shengyang, China	63	67 (mean)	176		247[b]
Cambridge, United Kingdom	63	69 (mean)	134		117[b]

[a] Geometric mean.
[b] Combined male and female subjects.

70 to 250 µg/day with a large variation in individual intakes. Although the current message of the nutrition community to the public encourages the consumption of green leafy vegetables, alterations in cultural eating habits are difficult to achieve. A recent extensive study of the changes in phylloquinone intake of 16- to 64-year-old adults in Great Britain [68,69] indicates a slight decrease over a 15-year period.

3.2.3 VITAMIN K IN MILK

Hemorrhagic disease of the newborn (see Chapter 7) is a vitamin K deficiency that has been largely eliminated by vitamin K administration at birth and phylloquinone supplementation of infant formulas [70]. It is, however, related to the relatively low content of vitamin K in human milk [71], and it has historically been regarded as a disease of breastfed infants. Milk is not an important dietary source of vitamin K; and, as the vitamin is located in the fat portion of whole milk [72], reduced-fat products or skim milk have even less. Milk from other species has been reported to have a vitamin K content [73] similar to that measured in humans.

Most reports of phylloquinone concentrations in human milk [74–77] are in the range of 1.0 to 1.5 ng/ml (0.1 to 0.15 µg/100 ml) although values about double this amount have been reported [40,78], and a recent analysis by liquid chromatography-tandem mass spectrometry [79] has reported values in the range of 3 to 4 ng/ml. More recent databases [52,54,80] indicate that the phylloquinone content of whole (3.5% fat) cow milk is in the range of 4 to 6 ng/100 ml. The phylloquinone content of maternal milk has been found to be somewhat, but not greatly, higher in colostrum than in mature milk [72,75]. Two studies have reported that the content of MK-4 in human and cow milk is similar to that of phylloquinone [54,78], but additional studies are needed to confirm these observations. Although normal variations in the dietary intake of vitamin K within a population do not substantially alter maternal milk phylloquinone [74], supplementation of 2.5 mg/day of phylloquinone has been shown to increase milk phylloquinone content 25- to 30-fold [76,81].

3.2.4   Dihydrophylloquinone in Foods

Dihydrophylloquinone (2′,3′-dihydrophylloquinone, dK) was first detected in foods as an interfering peak when it was used as an internal analytical standard [28]. This form of vitamin K is not a natural product but the saturated side-chain form of the vitamin is formed during the industrial process involved in the conversion of liquid oils containing a high proportion of unsaturated fatty acids to semisolid fats by hydrogenation. This process increases the oxidative stability of the oil and converts a substantial amount of the remaining polyunsaturated fatty acids from the *cis* to the *trans* form. The amount of dihydrophylloquinone in the product is related to the extent of hydrogenation, and in more heavily treated products the majority of endogenous phylloquinone is either converted to the dihydro form or destroyed [82]. The quantities of dihydrophylloquinone in the diet are therefore rather variable and are a function of the amount of various lipid sources used in food preparation or incorporated into processed foods (see Table 3.5).

Dihydrophylloquinone can be a substantial contributor to the total vitamin K content of a diet. Data from the U.S. FDA total diet study have been used [83] to calculate that dihydrophylloquinone comprises about 28% of the total vitamin K intake of 14- to 16-year-old boys and girls, and about 18% of the total vitamin K intake of 60- to 65-year-old men and women. Another study [84] based on the 14-day food

TABLE 3.5

Content of Phylloquinone and Dihydrophylloquinone in Oils, Fats, Processed Foods, and "Fast Foods"

Foods	µg/100 g Food[a]	
	Phylloquinone	**Dihydrophylloquinone**
Commercial soybean oil[b]	314	<1
Lightly hydrogenated soybean oil[b]	71	85
Heavily hydrogenated soybean oil[b]	1	52
Butter	10	<1
"Tub" margarine	161	83
"Stick" margarine	90	165
Cheese crackers with cheese	21	64
French fries	11	42
Chicken nuggets	11	22
Taco salad	11	10
Fish sticks	7	8
Cheese pizza	7	5
Hamburger with cheese	6	<1
Beef hot dog	4	1

[a] Values from various sources [82,83,112,116,117,119]. Analyses of processed foods from different sources may be substantially different.

[b] All products from the same source of soybean oil.

diaries of nearly 5000 men, women, and children found a mean intake of 77 μg/day of phylloquinone and 17 μg/day of dihydrophylloquinone, about 18% of the total. These data suggest that, at least in the United States, adults are consuming an additional 20% to 25% of this form of the vitamin above the intakes of phylloquinone that would be calculated from existing databases. The teenaged population, because of a higher consumption of foods containing or cooked in hydrogenated fats, may be consuming an additional 30% or 40% of this form of vitamin K.

The nutritional significance of the ingestion of this form of vitamin K has not yet been established. There is no evidence that this compound has inhibitory properties, but its activity relative to phylloquinone has not yet been firmly established in experimental animals or in humans. An early report based on a chick bioassay [85] has indicated that dihydrophylloquinone was about 10% as active as phylloquinone. A more recent study comparing dihydrophylloquinone and phylloquinone for their ability to counteract a warfarin-induced deficiency in rats [86] demonstrates that dihydrophylloquinone is well absorbed and has some biological activity as measured by its ability to increase vitamin K-dependent clotting factor activity in the model. However, the experimental design of this study, with a single high dose of both forms of the vitamin, makes it impossible to accurately determine the relative effectiveness of the two forms. A more detailed study of the absorption and tissue distribution of phylloquinone and dihydrophylloquinone in different aged rats [87] has shown that the two forms of vitamin K are present in differing amounts in the tissues assayed and that the distribution is to some extent age dependent (Table 3.6). Although prothrombin times were not measured in this study, there were no apparent coagulation disorders as characterized by bleeding episodes, suggesting that dihydrophylloquinone was

---

TABLE 3.6

Serum and Tissue Concentrations of Phylloquinone and Dihydrophylloquinone When They Were Fed Similar Amounts of Each Form of Vitamin K

	12-Month-Old Rats		24-Month-Old Rats	
Tissue	Phylloquinone	Dihydrophylloquinone	Phylloquinone	Dihydrophylloquinone
Serum (nmol/L)	<1	<1	2 ± 3	2 ± 1
Liver (nmol/kg)	20 ± 7	54 ± 26	52 ± 17	106 ± 39
Kidney (nmol/kg)	8 ± 2	1 ± 1	12 ± 5	2 ± 1
Heart (nmol/kg)	11 ± 3	1 ± 1	11 ± 3	2 ± 1
Spleen (nmol/kg)	18 ± 4	11 ± 1	15 ± 4	11 ± 9

Note: Each form of vitamin K was added to a vitamin K-deficient diet (~190 μg/kg diet) and fed to the 12- or 24-month-old rats (10/group) for 28 days. For details, see Reference [87].

functioning to some extent during the month-long comparison of the two forms of vitamin K. Only a limited amount of data is available to assess the activity of dihydrophylloquinone in human studies. Ingestion of dihydrophylloquinone by young adult subjects has shown that it is absorbed, although circulating plasma concentrations of dihydrophylloquinone are lower than those observed following the ingestion of a similar amount of phylloquinone [88]. The same study found that circulating under-γ-carboxy osteocalcin was decreased, and urinary excretion of Gla was increased following phylloquinone administration to vitamin K-restricted subjects, but that this response was not observed when dihydrophylloquinone was administered. As this study did not utilize a range of intakes, it was not possible to determine if the hydrogenated form had partial activity. Additional studies will be needed to establish whether or not dihydrophylloquinone has sufficient biological activity to be a significant factor in calculating vitamin K intake. It is likely that consumption of diets containing substantial amounts of dihydrophylloquinone will tend to decrease with time. The recognition that diets with a high content of transfatty acids, which are also produced during hydrogenation of food oils, are a risk factor for coronary heart disease [89,90] has resulted in a decrease in the use of partially hydrogenated fats in many food products [91,92], and this will result in a lowering of consumption of this form of vitamin K.

3.2.5 MENAQUINONES IN FOODS

Although the majority of biologically active dietary vitamin K is in the form of phylloquinone, menaquinones can in some cases substantially contribute to the total intake. Only a few foods contain significant amounts of menaquinones, with cheese being the most commonly consumed source (Table 3.7). When menadione is utilized as a source of vitamin K activity in poultry rations, a large amount of MK-4 is formed, and chicken meat [93] and egg yolk [54] can contain relatively high amounts of MK-4. The amount undoubtedly varies a great deal as chicken meat has been reported to contain 60 μg/100 g in Finland [93], and 9 μg/100 g in the Netherlands [54]. The bacterially produced long-chain menaquinones are found mainly in cheeses and, again, the amounts reported are quite variable when obtained from different sources [54,93]. In the Netherlands, a country where the intake of eggs and cheese is relatively high, the mean intake of an elderly population has been reported to be 7 μg/day of MK-4 and 22 μg/day of long-chain menaquinones [53]. A rather unique source of vitamin K is the traditional Japanese food, natto. It contains very high concentrations of MK-7 and is produced by growing *Bacillus natto* on cooked soybeans. It is a food consumed mainly in eastern Japan where it may constitute the major source of vitamin K for many individuals [94]. The data in Table 3.8 demonstrate the large variance in MK-7 intake in the Japanese population. Natto was consumed by only 42% of the subjects in this study, and this is responsible for the large variation seen not only in the MK-7 intake, but also in the total vitamin K intake. Much of the MK-7 in natto is apparently bound to a water-soluble protein [95], while the majority of phylloquinone in plant material is associated with internal cellular membranes.

TABLE 3.7

Phylloquinone and Menaquinone Content of Selected Foods

	μg/100 g of Food[a]			
Food	Phylloquinone	MK-4	MK-7	Other MK[b]
Butter[c]	15	15	<1	<1
Hard cheese[c]	10	5	1	70
Soft cheese[c]	3	4	1	52
Chicken meat[d]	<1	30	<1	<1
Beef roast[e]	1	3	<1	<1
Egg yolk[f]	2	37	<1	1
Beef liver[d]	6	1	3	5
Natto[c]	35	<1	998	105

[a] Values are means of three to seven samples.
[b] Sum of MK-5, MK-6, MK-8, MK-9, and MK-10.
[c] Values from Reference [54].
[d] Value from MK-4 is a mean of values from References [54,113,115, and 124].
[e] Values from Reference [93].
[f] Value for MK-4 is a mean of values from References [54,113, and 124].

TABLE 3.8

Vitamin K Intake in a Young Female Adult Japanese Population

			Range (μg/day)	
Form of Vitamin	Mean ± SD (μg/day)	Median (μg/day)	Min	Max
Total vitamin K	230 ± 143	205	24	726
Phylloquinone	156 ± 91	141	11	461
MK-4	17 ± 10	15	1	67
MK-7	57 ± 84	<1	0	340

Note: Data are based on 3 days of dietary records obtained from 125 young women aged
20–23 years. See Reference [124] for details.

3.3   VITAMIN K CONTENT OF HUMAN PLASMA

3.3.1   PLASMA PHYLLOQUINONE

The earliest attempts to quantitate the small amounts of phylloquinone in human plasma (or serum) utilized separation by HPLC and quantitation by ultraviolet (UV) absorption. Values reported ranged from 5 to 30 ng/ml, which may have been post-absorptive values [16], to a reported mean of 2.6 ng/ml [96] or 0.26 ng/ml [18] for fasting values. An early study utilizing reductive electrochemical detection [20] reported a mean of 1.11 ng/ml in 24 fasting adults.

These early reports were obtained from small populations and most utilized UV detectors, which lacked the sensitivity needed to accurately quantitate the small amount of phylloquinone present in the plasma of some individuals. Electrochemical reduction or fluorescence detection of the reduced form of the vitamin following chemical or electrochemical reduction has replaced this methodology. Comprehensive reviews of the procedures utilized to determine plasma phylloquinone concentrations by both detection methodologies are available [22,25]. The most commonly used methodology at the present time involves fluorescence detection following postcolumn reduction with zinc. Continued modification of this technique [97] has greatly increased its sensitivity and reproducibility. Although earlier reports of plasma phylloquinone concentrations were somewhat higher, it now appears that normal fasting values are around or below 0.5 ng/ml (1.1 nmol/L). There is a strong positive correlation between plasma triglycerides and plasma phylloquinone [98], and the variation between samples measured at different days from the same subject is much higher than for the other fat-soluble vitamins [99]. Because of this, extreme caution should be used in attempts to determine vitamin K status of an individual from a single day's sample of plasma. Circulating phylloquinone concentrations respond to daily changes in intake and fall rather rapidly when intake is restricted and demonstrate increases when dietary intake is increased [100–102].

When data from some of the larger populations studied are considered, it appears that, as would be expected, mean plasma phylloquinone concentrations are positively related to mean intake. The data in Table 3.9 indicate that, in general, higher plasma phylloquinone concentrations are observed in studies where the estimated vitamin K intake was also higher. However, the within population variability of both estimated intake and circulating phylloquinone is large, and it is not possible to obtain

TABLE 3.9

Fasting Plasma Phylloquinone Concentrations and Estimated Phylloquinone Intake of Selected Populations

Location	n	Phylloquinone	
		µg/day	nmol/L plasma
New England[a]	402	156[b]	1.12[b]
Great Britain[c]	834	65[d]	0.36[d]
Shengyang, China[e]	178	244[d]	2.17[d]
Cambridge, United Kingdom[f]	134	103[d]	0.69[d]
Framingham Offspring Study[g]	369	115[d]	0.99[d]

[a] Postmenopausal Caucasian women [62].
[b] Mean.
[c] "Free-living British people over 65 years" [122,125].
[d] Geometric mean.
[e] 65 years (mean) men and women [63].
[f] 68 years (mean); men and women [63].
[g] Adult males [103].

a meaningful estimate of an individual's circulating phylloquinone concentration
from an estimate of daily intake. In studies utilizing large numbers of subjects [103],
the statistical relationship between vitamin K intake and circulating phylloquinone
may appear rather strong, but the individual responses vary substantially. When the
relationship of plasma phylloquinone intake to daily phylloquinone intake is plotted as a relationship of the intakes of population deciles to plasma phylloquinone
(Figure 3.2), the response appears to be reasonably good across the range of intakes
that represents most of the population. However, when plotted as plasma concentrations and intakes of individuals (Figure 3.3), it is apparent that this relationship does

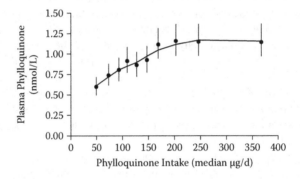

FIGURE 3.2   Relationship between plasma phylloquinone concentrations and phylloquinone
intake expressed as deciles of intake. (From McKeown, N.M., et al. 2002. *J Nutr* 1329–1334.
With permission.)

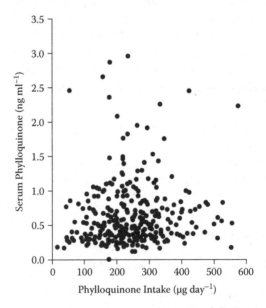

FIGURE 3.3   Serum phylloquinone concentration as a function of dietary phylloquinone intake
for 310 adult men and women [52]. Intake was obtained from a food frequency questionnaire and
interviews. (From Schurgers, L. J., et al. 1999. *J Nutr Env Med* 115 –122. With permission.)

not extend to individuals in a population, as both intake and plasma concentrations of phylloquinone vary substantially from day to day. These presumed markers of vitamin K status have little value unless relatively large populations are considered.

3.3.2 PLASMA CONCENTRATIONS OF OTHER K VITAMERS

Although the emphasis has been on plasma phylloquinone, reports of the circulating concentrations of various menaquinones are also available. The available data are from relatively small populations and for the most part have concentrated on MK-4 which appears to be a normal tissue-specific metabolite of phylloquinone (see Chapter 6) and MK-7, which is present in high concentrations in natto, a fermented soybean product. The plasma concentration of MK-4 has been reported in one study [104] to be very low and not statistically increased by administration of sufficient phylloquinone to nearly double the fasting concentration of plasma phylloquinone in three hours. Similar low concentrations of MK-4 (<0.1 ng/ml) have been reported by some other investigators [105,106], but substantially higher concentrations have been reported by others [107,108], who have found MK-4 plasma concentrations to exceed 0.3 ng/ml. Substantial amounts (0.3 to 0.5 ng/ml) of both MK-7 and MK-8 have been reported in young adults in a population not likely to be consuming natto [109], and decreases in these two vitamers have been related to increased age [109] and osteoporotic fractures [110]. Menaquinones MK-5 and MK-6 have also been reported to be present in human plasma in concentrations that are well within the analytical capability of the methods employed. The impact of increased intakes of these menaquinones has been assessed in one study [107] with a limited number of subjects (Table 3.10). The coefficient of variation within the small group was about 20% to 30%, and the ingestion of the fermented soybean product, natto, resulted in an increase of plasma MK-7 of about 100% in four hours. There was a wide range of plasma MK-7 in the individuals, and the mean increase in MK-7 of each individual was about 170%. Alterations in the concentrations of MK-4 and MK-5 were minor, while phylloquinone and MK-6 were increased 45% and 70%. The basis for these changes is not apparent. New technology utilizing HPLC-tandem mass-mass spectrometry and atmospheric pressure chemical ionization [36] has verified some of the other published data, and values reported for phylloquinone, MK-4, and MK-7 are similar to those presented in Table 3.7.

TABLE 3.10
Effect of Natto Ingestion on Circulating Vitamin K in Human Volunteers

Time	Plasma Concentration (ng/ml)				
	Phylloquinone	MK-4	MK-5	MK-6	MK-7
Fasting	1.04 ± 0.22	0.41 ± 0.18	0.31 ± 0.09	0.42 ± 0.16	1.18 ± 0.22
4 h after feeding	1.52 ± 0.12	0.53 ± 0.53	0.42 ± 0.14	0.72 ± 0.20	2.41 ± 0.43

Note: Six fasting subjects were fed 50 g of natto (~500 µg of MK-7) resulting in alterations in the plasma concentration of various forms of vitamin K. For details see Reference [107].

With the exception of MK-4 and MK-7, the dietary contribution to the other long-chain menaquinones is limited to aged cheeses. Major contributors to the vitamin K stores in human liver and the menaquinone pool within the human gut are MK-8, MK-10, and MK-11 (see Chapter 6). There are insufficient data to establish circulating concentrations of these longer menaquinones, although a rat study has established that when fed at equimolar amounts, MK-9 was present in plasma at about 50% the concentration of phylloquinone [111]. The presence of substantial amounts of the longer-chain menaquinones would suggest that the absorption of bacterially produced menaquinones from the lower bowel might be more extensive than currently thought. As the amount of data available is minimal, there is a clear need for a careful assessment of the distribution of the complete spectrum of K vitamers in a large population.

3.4   CURRENT STATUS OF RESEARCH EFFORTS

The current status of research efforts to accurately establish the daily intake of vitamin K within the population and to accurately measure the plasma concentration of vitamin K as one measure of vitamin K adequacy represents reasonable progress. The methodology currently used for determining the vitamin K content of various foods appears to be reproducible within a given laboratory, although there is considerable variation between different reports of the phylloquinone content of individual foods. This lack of confidence in calculated intake data can probably be resolved by additional data directed at those few foods that furnish a significant amount of our daily dietary intake. More recently a substantial amount of data directed toward the vitamin K content of prepared foods with multiple ingredients provides some assistance to research in the area. Although there are claims that some long-chain menaquinones might provide benefits not provided by phylloquinone, their intake within a population is heavily skewed toward individuals consuming higher amounts of aged cheeses, and the vast majority of the population does not consume a sufficient amount of these forms of the vitamin to have any nutritional impact. Although some data are available, additional studies that compare the amount of vitamin K in daily meals, measured by direct analysis, to the estimates based on the values in food composition databases would be valuable.

Although there are problems with current calculations of a daily dietary intake of vitamin K, they are probably reasonable estimates to use in most nutritional studies. The major problem in the currently available studies is the large differences in vitamin K intakes from day to day and the lack of sufficient daily dietary records or completed food frequency questionnaires to calculate an average daily value that is representative of an extended period of time. The other factor that brings a lack of validity to currently available data consumption is the very limited available data on the bioavailability of vitamin K in various foods (see Chapter 6). At the present time there has been no attempt to make adjustments based on this critical factor. As long as diets contain substantial amounts of hydrogenated oils, dihydrophylloquinone will be consumed in amounts that are easily detected, and depending on the diets of individuals, may be equivalent to as much as a third of the calculated content of phylloquinone. Although the limited data available indicate that this form of vitamin K has low biological activity and is not an inhibitor of vitamin K action, additional studies are needed to more accurately assess its biological activity in humans, and to determine if its contribution to the total amount of vitamin K in the diet is sufficient to require its inclusion in calculations of intake.

The assay of circulating vitamin K by HPLC with fluorescence detection of the reduced form of the vitamin following postcolumn reduction of vitamin K quinone has been the standard method of quantification for the last decade with only small changes in this technique. This method, or HPLC followed by electrochemical detection, appears to be capable of reproducible measurements, and the various laboratories involved have tended to get reasonably similar values for human fasting phylloquinone concentrations. These values show some relationship to mean dietary intake, but there is a great deal of individual variation in this relationship which depends on a number of factors. The most important is probably related to the rapid turnover of the vitamin and the large variation in vitamin K intake from day to day. These factors have made it impossible to use plasma phylloquinone concentrations, now a rather routine assay, as a measure of vitamin K status in attempts to set dietary reference intakes for the vitamin.

There are few available reports of the circulating concentrations of various menaquinones, and although some earlier reports indicated the presence of long-chain menaquinones, they did not appear to be conclusive. Newer methodology appears to be capable of measuring circulating menaquinones at concentrations substantially below the level usually seen for phylloquinone. Unfortunately the majority of the available data deals with MK-4, which is produced in tissues from phylloquinone, and with MK-7, which is found in very high quantities in a single food, natto, consumed only in Japan. With the techniques now available, it would be possible to determine if any significant amount of the long-chain menaquinones that are present in the human lower bowel are present in the circulation of individuals who consume a diet free of these forms of vitamin K. These data would be very relevant to the continuing discussion of the importance, if any, of this potential source of vitamin K in meeting the total requirement of this vitamin.

REFERENCES

1. Sommer, P. and M. Kofler. 1966. Physicochemical properties and methods of analysis of phylloquinones, menaquinones, ubiquinones, phostoquinones, menadione, and related compounds. *Vitamins and Hormones* 24:349–399.
2. Dam, H. and E. Sondergaard. 1967. The determination of vitamin K. In *The Vitamins*, 2nd ed., Vol. 6, ed. P. Gyorgy and W.N. Pearson, 245–260. New York: Academic Press.
3. Griminger, P. and O. Donis. 1960. Potency of vitamin K_1 and two analogs in counteracting the effects of dicumarol and sulfaquinoxaline in the chick. *J Nutr* 70:361–368.
4. Matschiner, J.T. and E.A. Doisy, Jr. 1966. Bioassay of vitamin K in chicks. *J Nutr* 90: 87–100.
5. Griminger, P. 1971. Nutritional requirements for vitamin K-animal studies. In *Symposium Proceedings on the Biochemistry, Assay, and Nutritional Value of Vitamin K and Related Compounds*, 39–59. Chicago: Association of Vitamin Chemists.
6. Almquist, H.J. 1966. Vitamin K group: IV. Estimation in foods and food supplements. In *The Vitamins, 2nd ed.*, ed. W.H. Sebrell and R.S. Harris, 445–447. New York: Academic Press.
7. Dam, H. and F. Schonheyder. 1936. The occurrence and chemical nature of vitamin K. *Biochem J* 30:897–901.
8. Dam, H. and J. Glavind. 1938. Vitamin K in the plant. *Biochem J* 32:485–487.
9. Mayer, H. and O. Isler. 1971. Isolation of vitamin K. *Meth Enzymol* 18C:469–491.

10. Mayer, H. and O. Isler. 1971. Vitamin K group: Chemistry In *The Vitamins,* 2nd ed., ed. W.H. Sebrell and R.S. Harris, 418–443. New York: Academic Press.

11. Dunphy, P.J. and A.F. Brodie. 1971. The structure and function of quinones in respiratory metabolism. *Meth Enzymol* 18C:407–461.

12. Matschiner, J.T. and J.M. Amelotti. 1968. Characterization of vitamin K from bovine liver. *J Lipid Res* 9:176–179.

13. Williams, R.C., J.A. Schmit, and R.A. Henry. 1972. Quantitative analysis of fat-soluble vitamins by high-speed liquid chromatography. *J Chromatog Sci* 10:494–501.

14. Shearer, M.J. 1983. High-performance liquid chromatography of K vitamins and their antagonists. *Adv Chromatog* 21:243–301.

15. Shearer, M.J., V. Allan, Y. Haroon, and P. Barkhan. 1980. Nutritional aspects of vitamin K in the human. In *Vitamin K Metabolism and Vitamin K-Dependent Proteins*, ed. J.W. Suttie, 317–327. Baltimore: University Park Press.

16. LeFevere, M.F., A.P.D. Leenheer, and A.E. Claeys. 1979. High-performance liquid chromatographic assay of vitamin K in human serum. *J Chromatog* 186:749–762.

17. Ikenoya, S., K. Abe, T. Tsuda, Y. Yamano, O. Hiroshima, M. Ohmae, and K. Kawabe. 1979. Electrochemical detector for high-performance liquid chromatography. II. Determination of tocopherols, ubiquinones, and phylloquinone in blood. *Chem Pharm Bull* 27:1237–1244.

18. Shearer, M.J., S. Rahim, P. Barkhan, and L. Stimmler. 1982. Plasma vitamin K_1 in mothers and their newborn babies. *Lancet* ii:460–463.

19. Hart, J.P., M.J. Shearer, P.T. McCarthy, and S. Rahim. 1984. Voltammetric behaviour of phylloquinone (vitamin K_1) at a glassy-carbon electrode and determination of the vitamin in plasma using high-performance liquid chromatography with electrochemical detection. *Analyst* 109:477–481.

20. Ueno, T. and J.W. Suttie. 1983. High-pressure liquid chromatographic-electrochemical detection analysis of serum trans-phylloquinone. *Anal Biochem* 133:62–67.

21. Haroon, Y., C.A.W. Schubert, and P.V. Hauschka. 1984. Liquid chromatographic dual electrode detection system for vitamin K compounds. *J Chromatog Sci* 22:89–93.

22. McCarthy, P.T., D.J. Harrington, and M.J. Shearer. 1997. Assay of phylloquinone in plasma by high-performance liquid chromatography with electrochemical detection. *Meth Enzymol* 282:421–433.

23. Langenberg, J.P. and U.R. Tjaden. 1984. Determination of (endogenous) vitamin K_1 in human plasma by reversed-phase HPLC using fluorometric detection after post-column electrochemical reduction. Comparison with ultraviolet, single and dual electrochemical detection. *J Chromatog* 305:61–72.

24. Haroon, Y., D.S. Bacon, and J.A. Sadowski. 1986. Liquid-chromatographic determination of vitamin K_1 in plasma, with fluorometric detection. *Clin Chem* 32:1925–1929.

25. Davidson, K.W. and J.A. Sadowski. 1997. Determination of vitamin K compounds in plasma or serum by high-performance liquid chromatography using postcolumn chemical reduction and fluorimetric detection. *Meth Enzymol* 282:408–421.

26. Perez-Ruiz, T., C. Martinez-Lozano, M.D. Garcia, and J. Martin. 2007. High-performance liquid chromatography: Photochemical reduction in aerobic conditions for determination of K vitamins using fluorescence detection. *J Chromatogr A* 1141:67–72.

27. Ahmed, S., N. Kishikawa, K. Nakashima, and N. Kuroda. 2007. Determination of vitamin K homologues by high-performance liquid chromatography with on-line photoreactor and peroxyoxalate chemiluminescence detection. *Anal Chim Acta* 591:148–154.

28. Booth, S.L., K.W. Davidson, and J.A. Sadowski. 1994. Evaluation of an HPLC method for the determination of phylloquinone (vitamin K_1) in various food matrices. *J Agric Food Chem* 42:295–300.

29. Booth, S.L. and J.A. Sadowski. 1997. Determination of phylloquinone in foods by high-performance liquid chromatography. *Meth Enzymol* 282:446–456.

30. Ware, G.M. and G.W. Chase. 2000. Determination of vitamin K_1 in medical foods by liquid chromatography with postcolumn reduction and fluorometric detection. *J AOAC Int* 83:957–962.

31. Sheppard, A.J., A.R. Prosser, and W.D. Hubbard. 1972. Gas chromatography of the fat-soluble vitamins: A review. *J Am Oil Chem Soc* 49:619–633.

32. Seifert, R.M. 1979. Analysis of vitamin K_1 in some green leafy vegetables by gas chromatography. *J Agric Food Chem* 27:1301–1304.

33. Reto, M., M.E. Figueira, H.M. Filipe, and C.M.M. Almeida. 2007. Analysis of vitamin K in green tea leafs and infusion by SPME-GC-FID. *Food Chem* 100:405–411.

34. Dolnikowski, G.G., Z. Sun, M.A. Grusak, J.W. Peterson, and S.L. Booth. 2002. HPLC and GC/MS determination of deuterated vitamin K (phylloquinone) in human serum after ingestion of deuterium-labeled broccoli. *J Nutr Biochem* 13:168–174.

35. Raith, W., G. Fauler, G. Pichler, and W. Muntean. 2000. Plasma concentrations after intravenous administration of phylloquinone (vitamin K_1) in preterm and sick neonates. *Thrombosis Res* 99:467–472.

36. Suhara, Y., M. Kamao, N. Tsugawa, and T. Okano. 2005. Method for the determination of vitamin K homologues in human plasma using high-performance liquid chromatography-tandem mass spectrometry. *Anal Chem* 77:757–763.

37. Jones, K.S., L.J.C. Bluck, and W.A. Coward. 2006. Analysis of isotope ratios in vitamin K_1 (phylloquinone) from human plasma by gas chromatography/mass spectrometry. *Rapid Commun Mass Spectrom* 20:1894–1898.

38. Payne, R.J., A.M. Daine, B.M. Clark, and A.D. Abell. 2004. Synthesis and protein conjugation studies of vitamin K analogues. *Bioorg Med Chem* 12:5785–5791.

39. Booth, S.L., J.A. Sadowski, J.L. Weihrauch, and G. Ferland. 1993. Vitamin K_1 (phylloquinone) content of foods: A provisional table. *J Food Comp Anal* 6:109–120.

40. Canfield, L.M., J.M. Hopkinson, A.F. Lima, G.S. Martin, K. Sugimoto, J. Burri, L. Clark, and D.L. McGee. 1990. Quantitation of vitamin K in human milk. *Lipids* 25:406–411.

41. Ferland, G. and J.A. Sadowski. 1992. Vitamin K_1 (phylloquinone) content of green vegetables: Effects of plant maturation and geographical growth location. *J Agric Food Chem* 40:1874–1877.

42. Ferland, G. and J.A. Sadowski. 1992. Vitamin K_1 (phylloquinone) content of edible oils: Effects of heating and light exposure. *J Agric Food Chem* 40:1869–1873.

43. Ferland, G., D.L. MacDonald, and J.A. Sadowski. 1992. Development of a diet low in vitamin K-1 (phylloquinone). *J Am Dietet Assoc* 92:593–597.

44. Langenberg, J.P., U.R. Tjaden, E.M. De Vogel, and D.I.S. Langerak. 1986. Determination of phylloquinone (vitamin K_1) in raw and processed vegetables using reversed phase HPLC with electrofluorometric detection. *Acta Alimentaria* 15:187–198.

45. Sakano, T., S. Notsumoto, T. Nagaoka, A. Morimoto, K. Fujimoto, S. Masuda, Y. Suzuki, and K. Hirauchi. 1988. Measurement of K vitamins in food by high-performance liquid chromatography with fluorometric detection. *Vitamins (Japan)* 62:393–398.

46. Food and Nutrition Board, Institute of Medicine. 2001. *Dietary Reference Intakes: Vitamin A, Vitamin K, Arsenic, Boron, Chromium, Copper, Iodine, Iron, Manganese, Molybdenum, Nickel, Silicon, Vanadium, and Zinc*, Washington, D.C.: National Academy Press.

47. Booth, S.L., J.A. Sadowski, and A.T. Pennington. 1995. Phylloquinone (vitamin K1) content of foods in the U.S. Food and Drug Administration's total diet study. *J Agric Food Chem* 43:1574–1579.

48. Piironen, V., T. Koivu, O. Tammisalo, and P. Mattila. 1997. Determination of phylloquinone in oils, margarines and butter by high-performance liquid chromatography with electrochemical detection. *Food Chem* 59:473–480.

49. Koivu, T.J., V.I. Piironen, S.K. Henttonen, and P.H. Mattila. 1997. Determination of phylloquinone in vegetables, fruits, and berries by high-performance liquid chromatography with electrochemical detection. *J Agric Food Chem* 45:4644–4649.

50. Shearer, M.J., A.U. Bach, and M. Kohlmeier. 1996. Chemistry, nutritional sources, tissue distribution and metabolism of vitamin K with special reference to bone health. *J Nutr* 126:1181S–1186S.
51. Damon, M., N.Z. Zhang, D.B. Haytowitz, and S.L. Booth. 2005. Phylloquinone (vitamin K₁) content of vegetables. *J Food Comp Anal* 18:751–758.
52. Bolton-Smith, C., R.J.G. Price, S.T. Fenton, D.J. Harrington, and M.J. Shearer. 2000. Compilation of a provisional UK database for the phylloquinone (vitamin K₁) content of foods. *Brit J Nutr* 83:389–399.
53. Schurgers, L.J., J.M. Geleijnse, D.E. Grobbee, H.A.P. Pols, A. Hofman, J.C.M. Witteman, and C. Vermeer. 1999. Nutritional intake of vitamins K₁ (phylloquinone) and K₂ (menaquinone) in The Netherlands. *J Nutr Env Med* 9:115–122.
54. Schurgers, L.J. and C. Vermeer. 2000. Determination of phylloquinone and menaquinones in food. *Haemostasis* 30:298–307.
55. Piironen, V. and T. Koivu. 2000. Quality of vitamin K analysis and food composition data in Finland. *Food Chem* 68:223–226.
56. Kodaka, K., T. Ujiie, T. Ueno, and M. Saito. 1986. Contents of vitamin K₁ and chlorophyll in green vegetables. *J Jap Soc Nutr Food Sci* 39:124–126.
57. Sumi, H., K. Osada, C. Yatagi, S. Naito, and Y. Yanagisawa. 2003. High concentration of vitamin K₁ proved in the seaweeds and sweet potato leaves. *Nippon Shokuhin Kagaku Kogaku Kaishi* 50:63–66.
58. Richardson, L.R., P. Woodworth, and S. Coleman. 1956. Effect of ionizing radiations on vitamin K. *Fed Proc* 15:924–926.
59. Richardson, L.R., S. Wilkes, and S.J. Ritchey. 1961. Comparative vitamin K activity of frozen, irradiated and heat-processed foods. *J Nutr* 73:369–373.
60. Gutzeit, D., G. Baleanu, P. Winterhalter, and G. Jerz. 2007. Determination of processing effects and of storage stability on vitamin K₁ (phylloquinone) in sea buckthorn berries (*Hippophae rhamnoides* L ssp *rhamnoides*) and related products. *J Food Sci* 72:C491–C497.
61. Booth, S.L., A.T. Pennington, and J.A. Sadowski. 1996. Food sources and dietary intakes of vitamin K-1 (phylloquinone) in the American Diet: Data from the FDA Total Diet Study. *J Am Dietet Assoc* 96:149–154.
62. Booth, S.L., L.J. Sokoll, M.E. O'Brien, K.L. Tucker, B. Dawson-Hughes, and J.A. Sadowski. 1995. Assessment of dietary phylloquinone intake and vitamin K status in postmenopausal women. *Eur J Clin Nutr* 49:832–841.
63. Yan, L., B. Zhou, D. Greenberg, L. Wang, S. Nigidikar, C. Prynne, and A. Prentice. 2004. Vitamin K status of older individuals in Northern China is superior to that of older individuals in the UK. *Brit J Nutr* 92:939–945.
64. Collins, A., K.D. Cashman, and M. Kiely. 2006. Phylloquinone (vitamin K₁) intakes and serum undercarboxylated osteocalcin levels in Irish postmenopausal women. *Brit J Nutr* 95:982–988.
65. Braam, L., N. McKeown, P. Jacques, A. Lichtenstein, C. Vermeer, P. Wilson, and S. Booth. 2004. Dietary phylloquinone intake as a potential marker for a heart-healthy dietary pattern in the Framingham offspring cohort. *J Am Diet Assoc* 104:1410–1414.
66. Couris, R.R., G.R. Tataronis, S.L. Booth, G.E. Dallal, J.B. Blumberg, and J.T. Dwyer. 2000. Development of a self-assessment instrument to determine daily intake and variability of dietary vitamin K. *J Am Coll Nutr* 19:801–806.
67. McKeown, N.M., H.M. Rasmussen, J.M. Charnley, R.J. Wood, and S.L. Booth. 2000. Accuracy of phylloquinone (vitamin K-1) data in 2 nutrient databases as determined by direct laboratory analysis of diets. *J Am Dietet Assoc* 100:1201–1204.
68. Thane, C.W., C. Bolton-Smith, and W.A. Coward. 2006. Comparative dietary intake and sources of phylloquinone (vitamin K₁) among British adults in 1986–7 and 2000–1. *Brit J Nutr* 96:1105–1115.

69. Thane, C.W., L.Y. Wang, and W.A. Coward. 2006. Plasma phylloquinone (vitamin K_1) concentration and its relationship to intake in British adults aged 19–64 years. *Brit J Nutr* 96:1116–1124.

70. Greer, F.R. 1995. The importance of vitamin K as a nutrient during the first year of life. *Nutr Res* 15:289–310.

71. Canfield, L.M. and J.M. Hopkinson. 1989. State of the art vitamin K in human milk. *J Pediatr Gastroenterol Nutr* 8:430–441.

72. Canfield, L.M., J.M. Hopkinson, A.F. Lima, B. Silva, and C. Garza. 1991. Vitamin K in colostrum and mature human milk over the lactation period: A cross-sectional study. *Am J Clin Nutr* 53:730–735.

73. Indyk, H.E. and D.C. Woollard. 1997. Vitamin K in milk and infant formulas: Determination and distribution of phylloquinone and menaquinone-4. *Analyst* 122:465–469.

74. Pietschnig, B., F. Haschke, H. Vanura, M. Shearer, V. Veitl, S. Kellner, and E. Schuster. 1993. Vitamin K in breast milk: No influence of maternal dietary intake. *Eur J Clin Nutr* 47:209–215.

75. von Kries, R., M. Shearer, P.T. McCarthy, M. Haug, G. Harzer, and U. Gobel. 1987. Vitamin K_1 content of maternal milk: Influence of the stage of lactation, lipid composition, and vitamin K1 supplements given to the mother. *Pediatr Res* 22:513–517.

76. Greer, F.R., S. Marshall, A. Foley, and J.W. Suttie. 1997. Improving the vitamin K status of breast-feeding infants with maternal vitamin K_1 supplements. *Pediatrics* 99:88–92.

77. Greer, F.R., S. Marshall, J. Cherry, and J.W. Suttie. 1991. Vitamin K status of lactating mothers, human milk, and breastfeeding infants. *Pediatrics* 88:751–756.

78. Kojima, T., M. Asoh, N. Yamawaki, T. Kanno, H. Hasegawa, and A. Yonekubo. 2004. Vitamin K concentrations in the maternal milk of Japanese women. *Acta Paediatr* 93:457–463.

79. Kamao, M., N. Tsugawa, Y. Suhara, A. Wada, T. Mori, K. Murata, R. Nishino, T. Ukita, K. Uenishi, K. Tanaka, and T. Okano. 2007. Quantification of fat-soluble vitamins in human breast milk by liquid chromatography-tandem mass spectrometry. *J Chromatogr B Anal Technol Biomed Life Sci* 859:192–200.

80. Jakob, E. and I. Elmadfa. 2000. Rapid and simple HPLC analysis of vitamin K in food, tissues and blood. *Food Chem* 68:219–221.

81. Bolisetty, S., J.M. Gupta, G.G. Graham, C. Salonikas, and D. Naidoo. 1998. Vitamin K in preterm breastmilk with maternal supplementation. *Acta Paediatr* 87:960–962.

82. Davidson, K.W., S.L. Booth, G.D. Dolnikowski, and J.A. Sadowski. 1996. Conversion of vitamin K_1 to 2′,3′-dihydrovitamin K_1 during the hydrogenation of vegetable oils. *J Agric Food Chem* 44:980–983.

83. Booth, S.L., J.A.T. Pennington, and J.A. Sadowski. 1996. Dihydro-vitamin K_1: Primary food sources and estimated dietary intakes in the American diet. *Lipids* 31:715–720.

84. Booth, S.L., D.R. Webb, and J.C. Peters. 1999. *Assessment of phylloquinone and dihydrophylloquinone dietary intakes among a nationally representative sample of U.S. consumers using 14-day food diaries.* J Am Dietet Assoc 99:1072–1076.

85. Fieser, L.F., M. Tishler, and W.L. Sampson. 1941. Vitamin K activity and structure. *J Biol Chem* 137:659–692.

86. Sato, T., R. Ozaki, S. Kamo, Y. Hara, S. Konishi, Y. Isobe, S. Saitoh, and H. Harada. 2003. The biological activity and tissue distribution of 2′,3′-dihydrophylloquinone in rats. *Biochim Biophys Acta* 1622:145–150.

87. Booth, S.L., J.W. Peterson, D. Smith, M.K. Shea, J. Chamberland, and N. Crivello. 2008. Age and dietary form of vitamin K affect menaquinone-4 concentrations in male Fischer 344 rats. *J Nutr* 138:492–496.

88. Booth, S.L., A.H. Lichtenstein, M.E. O'Brien-Morse, N.M. McKeown, R.J. Wood, E.J. Saltzman, and C.M. Gundberg. 2001. Effects of a hydrogenated form of vitamin K on bone formation and resorption. *Am J Clin Nutr* 74:783–790.

89. Woodside, J.V. and D. Kromhout. 2005. *Fatty acids and CHD*. Proc Nutr Soc 64: 554–564.

90. Lichtenstein, A.H., A.T. Erkkila, B. Lamarche, U.S. Schwab, S.M. Jalbert, and L.M Ausman. 2003. *Influence of hydrogenated fat and butter on CVD risk factors: Remnant-like particles, glucose and insulin, blood pressure and C-reactive protein.* Atherosclerosis, 171:97–107.

91. Tarrago-Trani, M.T., K.M. Phillips, L.E. Lemar, and J.M. Holden. 2006. New and existing oils and fats used in products with reduced trans-fatty acid content. *J Am Dietet Assoc* 106:867–880.

92. Upritchard, J.E., M.J. Zeelenberg, H. Huizinga, P.M. Verschuren, and E.A. Trautwein. 2005. Modern fat technology: What is the potential for heart health? *Proc Nutr Soc* 64:379–386.

93. Koivu-Tikkanen, T.J., V. Ollilainen, and V.I. Piironen. 2000. Determination of phylloquinone and menaquinones in animal products with fluorescence detection after postcolumn reduction with metallic zinc. *J Agric Food Chem* 48:6325–6331.

94. Kaneki, M., S.J. Hedges, T. Hosoi, S. Fujiwara, A. Lyons, S.J. Crean, N. Ishida, M. Nakagawa, M. Takechi, Y. Sano, Y. Mizuno, S. Hoshino, M. Miyao, S. Inoue, K. Horiki, M. Shiraki, Y. Ouchi, and H. Orimo. 2001. Japanese fermented soybean food as the major determinant of the large geographic difference in circulating levels of vitamin K_2: Possible implications for hip-fracture risk. *Nutrition* 17:315–321.

95. Yanagisawa, Y. and H. Sumi. 2005. *Natto bacillus* contains a large amount of water-soluble vitamin K (menaquinone-7). *J Food Biochem* 29:267–277.

96. LeFevere, M.F., A.P.D. Leenheer, A.E. Claeys, I.V. Claeys, and H. Steyaert. 1982. Multidimensional liquid chromatography: A breakthrough in the assessment of physiological vitamin K levels. *J Lipid Res* 23:1068–1072.

97. Wang, L.Y., C.J. Bates, L. Yan, D.J. Harrington, M.J. Shearer, and A. Prentice. 2004. Determination of phylloquinone (vitamin K_1) in plasma and serum by HPLC with fluorescence detection. *Clin Chim Acta* 347:199–207.

98. Sadowski, J.A., S.J. Hood, G.E. Dallal, and P.J. Garry. 1989. Phylloquinone in plasma from elderly and young adults: Factors influencing its concentration. *Am J Clin Nutr* 50:100–108.

99. Booth, S.L., K.L. Tucker, N.M. McKeown, K.W. Davidson, G.E. Dallal, and J.A. Sadowski. 1997. Relationships between dietary intakes and fasting plasma concentrations of fat-soluble vitamins in humans. *J Nutr* 127:587–592.

100. Usui, Y., H. Tanimura, N. Nishimura, N. Kobayashi, T. Okanoue, and K. Ozawa. 1990. Vitamin K concentrations in the plasma and liver of surgical patients. *Am J Clin Nutr* 51:846–852.

101. Ferland, G., J.A. Sadowski, and M.E. O'Brien. 1993. Dietary induced subclinical vitamin K deficiency in normal human subjects. *J Clin Invest* 91:1761–1768.

102. Booth, S.L., M.E. O'Brien-Morse, G.E. Dallal, K.W. Davidson, and C.M. Gundberg. 1999. Response of vitamin K status to different intakes and sources of phylloquinone-rich foods: Comparison of younger and older adults. *Am J Clin Nutr* 70:368–377.

103. McKeown, N.M., P.F. Jacques, C.M. Gundberg, J.W. Peterson, K.L. Tucker, D.P. Kiel, P.W.F. Wilson, and S.L. Booth. 2002. Dietary and nondietary determinants of vitamin K biochemical measures in men and women. *J Nutr* 132:1329–1334.

104. Hirauchi, K., T. Sakano, T. Nagaoka, and A. Morimoto. 1988. Simultaneous determination of vitamin K_1, vitamin K_1 2,3-epoxide and menaquinone-4 in human plasma by high-performance liquid chromatography with fluorimetric detection. *J Chromatogr* 430:21–29.

105. Hiraike, H., M. Kimura, and Y. Itokawa. 1988. Distribution of K vitamins (phylloquinone and menaquinones) in human placenta and maternal and umbilical cord plasma. *Am J Obstet Gynecol* 158:564–569.

106. Tsugawa, N., M. Shiraki, Y. Suhara, M. Kamao, K. Tanaka, and T. Okano. 2006. Vitamin K status of healthy Japanese women: Age-related vitamin K requirement for gamma-carboxylation of osteocalcin. *Am J Clin Nutr* 83:380–386.

107. Wakabayashi, H., K. Onodera, S. Yamato, and K. Shimada. 2003. Simultaneous determination of vitamin K analogs in human serum by sensitive and selective high-performance liquid chromatography with electrochemical detection. *Nutrition* 19:661–665.

108. Kamao, M., Y. Suhara, N. Tsugawa, and T. Okano. 2005. Determination of plasma vitamin K by high-performance liquid chromatography with fluorescence detection using vitamin K analogs as internal standards. *J Chromatogr B* 816:41–48.

109. Hodges, S.J., M.J. Pilkington, M.J. Shearer, L. Bitensky, and J. Chayen. 1990. Age-related changes in the circulating levels of congeners of vitamin K_2, menaquinone-7 and menaquinone-8. *Clin Sci* 78:63–66.

110. Hodges, S.J., M.J. Pilkington, T.C.B. Stamp, A. Catterall, M.J. Shearer, L. Bitensky, and J. Chayen. 1991. Depressed levels of circulating menaquinones in patients with osteoporotic fractures of the spine and femoral neck. *Bone* 12:387–389.

111. Will, B.H. and J.W. Suttie. 1992. Comparative metabolism of phylloquinone and menaquinone-9 in rat liver. *J Nutr* 122:953–958.

112. Dumont, J.F., J. Peterson, D. Haytowitz, and S.L. Booth. 2003. Phylloquinone and dihydrophylloquinone contents of mixed dishes, processed meats, soups and cheeses. *J Food Comp Anal* 16:595–603.

113. Elder, S.J., D.B. Haytowitz, J. Howe, J.W. Peterson, and S.L. Booth. 2006. Vitamin K contents of meat, dairy, and fast food in the U.S. Diet. *J Agric Food Chem* 54:463–467.

114. Majchrzak, D. and I. Elmadfa. 2001. Phylloquinone (vitamin K_1) content of commercially-available baby food products. *Food Chem* 74:275–280.

115. Koivu, T., V. Piironen, and P. Matilla. 1998. Phylloquinone (vitamin K_1) in cereal products. *Cereal Chem* 75:113–116.

116. Weizmann, N., J.W. Peterson, D. Haytowitz, P.R. Pehrsson, V.P. de Jesus, and S.L. Booth. 2004. Vitamin K content of fast foods and snack foods in the U.S. diet. *J Food Comp Anal* 17:379–384.

117. Peterson, J.W., K.L. Muzzey, D. Haytowicz, J. Exler, L. Lemar, and S.L. Booth. 2002. Phylloquinone (vitamin K_1) and dihydrophylloquinone content of fats and oils. *J Am Oil Chem Soc* 79:641–646.

118. Dismore, M.L., D.B. Haytowitz, S.E. Gebhardt, J.W. Peterson, and S.L. Booth. 2003. Vitamin K content of nuts and fruits in the U.S. diet. *J Am Dietet Assoc* 103:1650–1652.

119. Cook, K.K., G.V. Mitchell, E. Grundel, and J.I. Rader. 1999. HPLC analysis for trans-vitamin K_1 and dihydro-vitamin K in margarines and margarine-like products using the C_{30} stationary phase. *Food Chem* 67:79–88.

120. Booth, S.L., H.T. Madabushi, K.W. Davidson, and J.A. Sadowski. 1995. Tea and coffee brews are not dietary sources of vitamin K-1 (phylloquinone). *J Am Dietet Assoc* 95:82–83.

121. USDA and ARS. 2005. USDA National Nutrient Database for Standard Reference, Release 18. Nutrient Data Laboratory Home Page, http://www.nal.usda.gov/fnic/foodcomp.

122. Thane, C.W., A.A. Paul, C.J. Bates, C. Bolton-Smith, A. Prentice, and M.J. Shearer. 2002. Intake and sources of phylloquinone (vitamin K_1): Variation with socio-demographic and lifestyle factors in a national sample of British elderly people. *Brit J Nutr* 87:605–613.

123. Duggan, P., K.D. Cashman, A. Flynn, C. Bolton-Smith, and M. Kiely. 2004. Phylloquinone (vitamin K1) intakes and food sources in 18–64-year-old Irish adults. *Brit J Nutrition* 92:151–158.

124. Kamao, M., Y. Suhara, N. Tsugawa, M. Uwano, N. Yamaguchi, K. Uenishi, H. Ishida, S. Sasaki, and T. Okano. 2008. Vitamin K content of foods and dietary vitamin K intake in Japanese young women. *J Nutr Sci Vitaminol (Tokyo)* 53:464–470.

125. Thane, C.W., C.J. Bates, M.J. Shearer, N. Unadkat, D.J. Harrington, A.A. Paul, A. Prentice, and C. Bolton-Smith. 2002. Plasma phylloquinone (vitamin K_1) concentration and its relationship to intake in a national sample of British elderly people. *Brit J Nutr* 87:615–622.

4 Vitamin K-Dependent Carboxylase and Vitamin K Epoxide Reductase

4.1 VITAMIN K-DEPENDENT CARBOXYLASE

4.1.1 DISCOVERY OF γ-CARBOXYGLUTAMIC ACID (GLA)

It is understandable that a period of approximately 40 years separated the discovery of vitamin K and the demonstration of its biochemical role. As the metabolic pathway leading to the synthesis of proteins was unknown when the vitamin was discovered, it was difficult to elucidate the mechanism by which a low-molecular-weight lipophilic compound such as vitamin K could influence either the activity or the amount of a specific plasma protein such as prothrombin. Various roles for the involvement of vitamin K in prothrombin production were, however, postulated. In the 1930s, Dam, Schonheyder, and Tage-Hansen postulated [1] that vitamin K, or a portion of it, might be part of the prothrombin molecule, and in the 1950s Martius and Nitz-Litzow proposed [2] that vitamin K might be involved in mammalian electron transport and that a vitamin K deficiency could lead to a low cellular ATP level and an inability to maintain normal physiological concentrations of proteins with a rapid turnover rate. In the mid 1960s, as an understanding of protein synthesis and its control was being developed, Olson [3] postulated that the rate of prothrombin synthesis is regulated by an effect of vitamin K on DNA transcription. In the late 1960s, Johnson [4] proposed that vitamin K was a precursor of a protein cofactor that was involved in the removal of prothrombin from polysomes and guiding it to its biologically active tertiary structure. Little evidence to support these early hypotheses was ever developed.

For a period of time beginning in the late 1960s, substantial research efforts were directed toward determining if vitamin K regulated the rate of *de novo* synthesis of specific proteins or if it functioned posttranslationally to convert inactive protein precursors to biologically active proteins. The time course of plasma prothrombin appearance when vitamin K was administered to vitamin K-deficient hypoprothrombinemic rats, a rapid burst followed by a slow increase, was suggestive of the activation of an existing precursor pool of this protein [5], and this initial burst of prothrombin was only slightly decreased by the prior administration of the protein

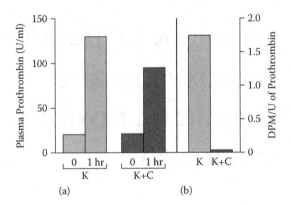

FIGURE 4.1   Effect of the protein synthesis inhibitor cycloheximide on prothrombin synthesis in vitamin K-deficient rats. Vitamin K-deficient rats were given radioactive amino acids and vitamin K (K) or vitamin K + cycloheximide (K+C) at 0 time, and blood was drawn after 1 h. Prothrombin was adsorbed from plasma with $BaSO_4$, eluted with citrate, purified by polyacrylamide gel electrophoresis, and radioactivity determined. (a) Prothrombin production in the presence or absence of cycloheximide. (b) Specific radioactivity of purified prothrombin. See References [5,6] for details.

synthesis inhibitor cycloheximide to the rats. More evidence of the presence of a liver precursor protein was obtained when it was demonstrated [6] that the prothrombin produced when hypoprothrombinemic rats were given vitamin K and cycloheximide was not radiolabeled if radioactive amino acids were administered at the same time as the vitamin (Figure 4.1). These data were consistent with the hypothesis that vitamin K was required for the conversion of an inactive form of prothrombin within the liver to the biologically active plasma form. The postulated liver precursor was subsequently isolated [7] and characterized [8]. A number of reviews published in the 1970s describe these efforts in more detail [9–14].

The observation [15,16] that there was a biologically inactive form of prothrombin in the plasma of patients treated with the vitamin K antagonist warfarin (see Chapter 5), strongly suggested that a vitamin K-dependent modification of a liver prothrombin precursor was needed to form active prothrombin and that at least some of the inactive forms reached the circulation. The subsequent demonstration [17] that large quantities of this protein could be obtained from the plasma of warfarin-treated cattle provided a pathway to identify the alteration needed. Studies of this inactive bovine "abnormal" prothrombin (see Reference [12]) demonstrated that it contained normal thrombin, had the same molecular weight and amino acid composition, but did not adsorb to insoluble barium salts as did normal prothrombin [18–20]. This difference, and the altered calcium-dependent electrophoretic and immunochemical properties, suggested a difference in calcium binding properties of these two proteins. This potential modification in one of the two proteins was subsequently demonstrated by direct calcium-binding measurements [21,22]. The late 1960s and early 1970s were also periods when much effort was being made to determine the structure of prothrombin and to elucidate the pathway by which the active protease, thrombin, was generated from the prothrombin [13]. These efforts

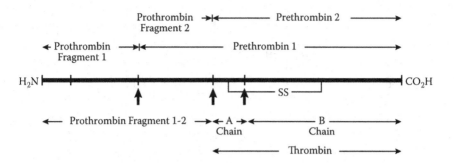

FIGURE 4.2 Schematic structure of prothrombin. Proteolytic cleavage at the points of the three arrows generates two fragments without biological activity and the 2-chain protease, thrombin. The vitamin K-dependent modification of specific Glu residues during prothrombin synthesis occurs within prothrombin fragment-1 (see Chapter 5).

led to a schematic structure (Figure 4.2) that aided researchers in this area to incorporate the vitamin K-dependent modification of prothrombin during its formation into the overall function of this protease. The critical vitamin K-dependent difference in the properties of the active and "abnormal" form of prothrombin was eventually shown to be the inability of the abnormal protein to participate in the calcium-dependent phospholipid-stimulated activation of prothrombin by factor X [23]. Acidic, Ca^{2+}-binding peptides were isolated from tryptic digests of the amino terminal (prothrombin fragment 1) domain of normal bovine prothrombin [24,25], but they could not be obtained when similar isolation procedures were applied to preparations of abnormal prothrombin.

Based on these studies, researchers in this field were directing their efforts toward the identification of some type of calcium-binding prosthetic group which needed vitamin K for its attachment to prothrombin. The general hypothesis was correct, but the modification of prothrombin was much simpler than what investigators working on this problem were probably looking for. Stenflo et al. [26] succeeded in isolating an acidic tetrapeptide (residues 6–9 of prothrombin) and demonstrated through the use of NMR spectra that the glutamic acid residues of this peptide were modified so that they were present as γ-carboxyglutamic acid (3-amino-1,1,3-propanetricarboxylic acid) residues (Figure 4.3). Nelsestuen, Zytkovicz, and Howard [27] independently characterized γ-carboxyglutamic acid (Gla) from a dipeptide (residues 33 and 34 of prothrombin) by mass spectral analysis. These characterizations of the modified glutamic acid residues in prothrombin were confirmed by Magnusson et al. [28], who later demonstrated that all of the 10 Glu residues in the first 33 residues of prothrombin were modified in this fashion.

4.1.2 DEMONSTRATION OF THE VITAMIN K-DEPENDENT γ-GLUTAMYL CARBOXYLASE

Although the publications identifying the posttranslational formation of Gla as the vitamin K-dependent step in prothrombin formation were published in late 1974, Stenflo had presented the structure to a relatively small group of investigators at

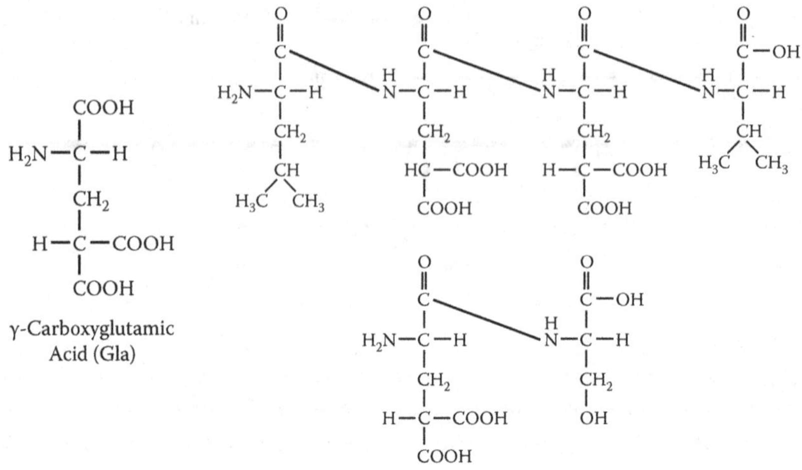

FIGURE 4.3 Structure of γ-carboxyglutamic acid and the two peptides obtained from pro-thrombin which were initially shown to contain this posttranslational modification: residues 6–9 and 33, 34.

a Boorhava Conference in Liden some months before the publications [29]. Not all of the audience was convinced. At this point in the efforts to determine the molecular role of vitamin K, it had also been demonstrated [30] that prothrombin activity could be generated in vitro by the addition of vitamin K to a crude liver microsomal preparation obtained from warfarin-treated or vitamin K-deficient rats. These preparations contained the postulated precursor of prothrombin, and the final step in the discovery of the metabolic role of vitamin K was the addition of $H^{14}CO_3^-$ to these microsomal incubations and the demonstration that the $^{14}CO_2$ had been fixed into microsomal proteins [31]. The $^{14}CO_2$ which was fixed into these proteins in a vitamin K-dependent manner was shown to be present in a deter-gent-solubilized extract of the incubated microsomes (Table 4.1) and was found to be related to the amount of prothrombin activity generated during the incu-bation. The vitamin K-dependent clotting factors were known to be adsorbed to $BaSO_4$, and adsorption and subsequent elution of these proteins from the detergent extract demonstrated that the fixed CO_2 had similar properties. It was known that acid hydrolysis of Gla would release one of the two acidic groups attached to the γ-carbon of Gla and convert it to glutamic acid. The fixed $^{14}CO_2$ in the detergent extract was shown to lose 50% of its activity when subjected to acid hydrolysis, and the remainder of the radioactivity was shown to be associated with glutamic acid. These data clearly established the role of vitamin K as an essential factor in a previously unknown carboxylase reaction.

Initial studies [32] of this crude carboxylase preparation demonstrated that Gla for-mation required O_2, vitamin K, HCO_3^-, and some component of the post-microsomal supernatant. This cytosolic component appeared to be reduced pyridine nucleotides or a reduced pyridine nucleotide generating system, and it was found that the enzymati-cally active form of the vitamin was the hydronaphthoquinone reduced form (vitamin KH_2). Although the initial demonstration of the vitamin K-dependent carboxylase

TABLE 4.1

Demonstration of the Vitamin K-Dependent Incorporation of $^{14}CO_2$ and the Generation of Active Prothrombin in Liver Microsomal Proteins of Vitamin K-Deficient and Warfarin-Treated Rats

Rats Used to Obtain Microsomes	Vitamin K in Incubation	Microsomal Extract		BaSO$_4$ Eluate	
		^{14}C (dpm)	Prothrombin (U)	^{14}C (dpm)	Prothrombin (U)
Vit K def	−	1,500	4	300	<1
Vit K def	+	16,200	78	9,600	30
Warf treated	−	2,400	2	30	<1
Warf treated	+	16,800	48	2,600	12

Note: Following incubation, a postmitochondrial supernatant was centrifuged to obtain a microsomal pellet which was extracted in buffered detergent. This extract was treated with BaSO$_4$ and the adsorbed proteins eluted. Fixed $^{14}CO_2$ and prothrombin present in the initial extract and in the BaSO$_4$ eluate were determined. For details, see Reference [31].

utilized a dispersed microsomal pellet, it was soon shown that carboxylase activity was retained in detergent-solubilized microsomal preparations [33]. As the substrate for the carboxylase in the early studies was the uncarboxylated precursor proteins of vitamin K-dependent proteins, it was not possible to study the kinetics of the reaction because the substrate concentration could not be altered. It was soon demonstrated that a synthetic peptide which represented residues 5–9 of bovine prothrombin (Phe-Leu-Glu-Glu-Val) was an effective substrate for the solubilized enzyme [34]. A number of similar low-molecular-weight peptides were subsequently synthesized [35], and it was found that peptides with only a single Glu or two Glu residues separated by different amino acids were poor substrates and that a hydrophobic amino acid prior to the Glu-Glu sequence improved the substrate activity of a peptide. These were not high affinity substrates, and the peptide Phe-Leu-Glu-Glu-Leu (FLEEL) which came to be used for most early studies of the properties of the carboxylase had a K_m of only about 4 mM. The rough microsomal fraction of liver was found to be highly enriched in carboxylase activity, and lower but significant activity was found in smooth microsomes. These initial studies were consistent with the hypothesis that the carboxylation event occurs on the lumenal side of the rough endoplasmic reticulum [36]. The same microsomal preparations and incubation conditions that would support the posttranslational formation of Gla also converted vitamin K to its 2,3-epoxide [37] supporting Willingham and Matschiner's [38] earlier suggestion that formation of this metabolite of vitamin K might be related to prothrombin production.

4.1.3 GENERAL PROPERTIES OF THE CARBOXYLASE SYSTEM

A general understanding of the properties of the vitamin K-dependent carboxylase was gained from studies utilizing the crude detergent-solubilized microsomal

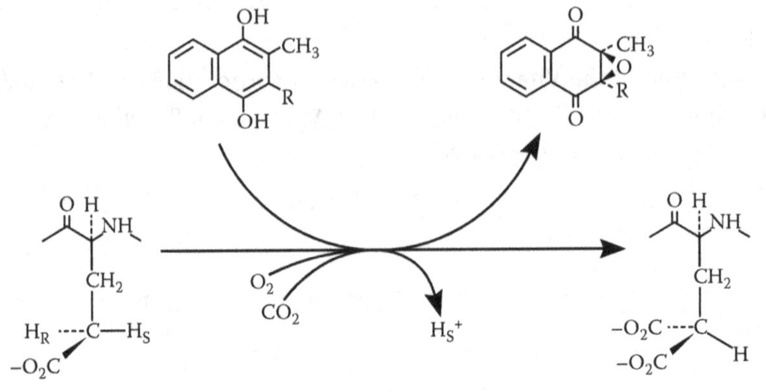

FIGURE 4.4 The vitamin K-dependent carboxylase reaction. In the presence of reduced vitamin K, O_2, and CO_2, the enzyme stereospecifically converts a protein-bound Glu residue to a γ-carboxyglutamyl residue and generates vitamin K 2,3-epoxide.

preparation as a source of enzyme activity, and small Glu-containing peptides as substrates. These data have been adequately reviewed [14,39–44]. The vitamin K-dependent carboxylation reaction was found to not require ATP, and the energy to drive this carboxylation reaction was shown to be derived from the oxidation of vitamin KH_2 by O_2 to form vitamin K-2,3-epoxide (Figure 4.4). The lack of a requirement for biotin, studies of the CO_2/HCO_3^- requirement, and the inhibition of the reaction by cyanide [45] indicated that carbon dioxide rather than HCO_3^- was the active species in the carboxylation reaction. Studies of the substrate specificity at the vitamin K binding site of the enzyme have shown that those vitamers with biological activity are 2-methyl-1,4-naphthoquinones substituted at the 3-position with a rather hydrophobic group. Although some differences in carboxylase activity can be measured, phylloquinone, MK-4, and the predominant intestinal forms of the vitamin, MK-6 through MK-9, were all found to be effective substrates. The 2-ethyl and des-methyl analogs of the vitamin have little activity, and methyl substitution of the benzenoid ring was shown to have little effect, or to decrease substrate binding (see Chapter 2). The vitamin K antagonist, 2-chloro-3-phytyl-1,4-naphthoquinone, is an antagonist of the enzyme, and its reduced form has been shown to be a competitive inhibitor. Synthesis and assay of a large number of rather high K_m low-molecular-weight peptides that are substrates of the enzyme have failed to reveal any unique sequences surrounding the Glu residue that are needed as a signal for carboxylation.

Only a small fraction of the total hepatic secretory protein pool is dependent on the action of vitamin K to γ-carboxylate specific Glu residues to form Gla residues within the vitamin K-dependent clotting factors. The basis for this selectivity lies not with the ability of the enzyme to recognize the specific Glu residues of the precursor protein which should be carboxylated, but in a domain of the primary gene product of these proteins that is lost prior to secretion. Cloning of the vitamin K-dependent proteins revealed that their primary gene products contained a very homologous, approximately 18 amino acid, "propeptide" between the amino terminus Gla domain of the mature protein and the signal peptide [46]. Deletion of this propeptide abolished γ-carboxylation of, but not secretion of, these proteins [47]. Early in vitro and in vivo lines of evidence from the Furie laboratory [48,49] suggested that this propeptide performed a "recognition," or "docking," site function, often called a "carboxylase recognition site" (CRS) to bring these proteins to the carboxylase. Small Glu-containing substrates were found to have high K_m values and to be poor substrates for the carboxylase when compared to Glu substrates attached to a propeptide (Figure 4.5). Further studies demonstrated that three hydrophobic residues of the propeptide (–16Phe, –10Ala, and –6Leu) were critical to the function of the hepatic propeptide in its carboxylase recognition role [50]. It was also found [51] that Glu-containing peptides, domains of other non-vitamin K-dependent proteins, or the thrombin domain of prothrombin were carboxylase substrates if attached to a propeptide.

Although the propeptides of all the vitamin K-dependent plasma proteins are very similar, studies from the Stafford laboratory [52] utilized the ability of chemically synthesized propeptide from various vitamin K-dependent proteins to inhibit the rate of carboxylation of a carboxylase substrate composed of the propeptide from factor IX and the Gla domain of prothrombin to assess the relative affinity of each propeptide for the enzyme (Table 4.2). These studies demonstrated that there was a wide variation in the strength of binding of each of the propeptides to the carboxylase. Factor X was the most tightly bound, most were from 2 to 10 times less tightly bound, and protein C and prothrombin were about 100 times less tightly bound than factor X. The propeptide of the bone protein osteocalcin was shown to have a very low affinity for the carboxylase. These differences in the affinity of the propeptide of clotting factor precursors would suggest that there may be situations where competition for the enzyme would impact the balance of the various factors synthesized, and it has been shown that in warfarin-treated cultured cells of cattle, the uncarboxylated form of factor X accumulates to a much greater extent than expected from its normal concentration in plasma [53,54]. Mutations in the propeptide of human factor IX which result in a lower affinity for the carboxylase have also been shown to greatly increase the sensitivity to warfarin. Although the vitamin K-dependent bone protein osteocalcin is synthesized with a propeptide that is very similar in sequence to the plasma clotting factors, the very low affinity of this propeptide for the enzyme suggests that it does not bind to the carboxylase through this region. However, the uncarboxylated form of osteocalcin does bind tightly to the carboxylase [55] and is a good substrate for the enzyme. This high affinity binding site within osteocalcin itself is not the active site for the conversion of Glu to Gla residues carried out by the carboxylase, but rather it provides for the tethering of the Glu substrate in the absence of an effective propeptide [56].

In addition to its function of binding the protein substrates of the carboxylase to the enzyme, it has also been shown that the propeptide can modulate the activity of the enzyme. During attempts to purify the rat liver microsomal carboxylase through the use of a factor X propeptide-based affinity column, it was found that attempts to elute the carboxylase with a high concentration of factor X propeptide resulted in an apparent increase in the amount of carboxylase activity. It was then found that the addition of the factor X propeptide to the detergent-solubilized microsomal preparation prior to any attempt to purify the carboxylase from it would increase the carboxylase activity about 10-fold at microsomal concentrations of propeptide [57].

Substrate		Km
A	FLEEL	Phe Leu Glu Glu Leu	2200.0
B	PT10	Ala Asn Thr Phe Leu Glu Glu Val Arg Lys	1000.0
C	proPT28	His Val Phe Leu Ala Pro Gln Gln Ala Arg Ser Leu Leu Gln Arg Val Arg Ala Asn Thr Phe Leu Glu Glu Val Arg Lys	3.6
D	proPT28/FA-16	His Val Ala Leu Ala Pro Gln Gln Ala Arg Ser Leu Gln Arg Val Arg Arg Ala Asn Thr Phe Leu Glu Glu Val Arg Lys	20.0
E	proPT20	Ala Arg Ser Leu Leu Gln Arg Val Arg Arg Ala Asn Thr Phe Leu Glu Glu Val Arg Lys	850.0

FIGURE 4.5 Importance of the propeptide of the vitamin K-dependent proteins in their interaction with the carboxylase. (A) The commonly used substrate FLEEL; (B) the decopeptide which is the first 10 residues of prothrombin; (C) the decopeptide attached to the prothrombin propeptide; (D) the same substrate as C with a switch of Ala for Phe at position –16; and (E) a truncated form of C which removes a portion of the propeptide, including –16 Phe. For details, see Reference [49].

TABLE 4.2

Amino Acid Sequences and Inhibition Constants of the Propeptides of Vitamin K-Dependent Proteins

	−16				−10	−6			−1		K_i (nM)
Prothrombin	H V F L A P Q Q A R S L L Q R V R R										277 ± 122
Factor VII	R V F V T Q E E A H G V L H R R R R										11.1 ± 0.8
Factor IX	T V F L D H E N A N K I L N R P K R										33.6 ± 4.5
Factor X	S L F I R R E Q A N N I L A R V T R										$2.6 \pm .12$
Protein C	S V F S S S E R A H Q V L R I R K R										230 ± 18
Protein S	A N F L S K Q Q A S Q V L V R K R R										12.2 ± 2.3
Matrix Gla Protein	N P F I N R R N A N T F I S P Q Q R										5.8 ± 1.4
Osteocalcin	K A F V S K Q E G S E V V K R P R R										$>500 \times 10^3$

Note: Propeptides of the various proteins were chemically synthesized and their ability to inhibit the activity of the carboxylasle was determined. The substrate used consisted of the factor IX propeptide and the Gla domain of prothrombin. The inhibitive constants determined from these assays is directly related to the affinity of the propeptide for the carboxylase. For details see Reference [50].

Subsequent studies [58] demonstrated that the same structural features of the propeptide domain that are important in stimulating the activity of the enzyme, (-16 Phe, -10 Ala, and −6 Leu), were those that had been shown to be involved in targeting these proteins for carboxylation. The basis for the increase in activity of the carboxylase is a decrease in the apparent K_m of the carboxylase substrate. In these early studies, less than micromolar concentrations of the factor X propeptide decreased the K_m of the Glu substrate used, Boc-Glu-Glu-Leu-OMe, by about 10-fold. Further studies [59] of the basis for the propeptide-related increase in carboxylase activity have demonstrated an acceleration of the formation of the carbanion which is generated on the γ-carbon of the Glu substrate during the carboxylation reaction. The interaction between the carboxylase and its propeptide containing protein substrates is complex, and it has been shown that binding of the Glu or vitamin K co-substrates to the enzyme has an influence on the affinity of the propeptide for the carboxylase [60].

The typical amino-terminal propeptide (CRS) that is cleaved from the mature carboxylated protein before it is released from the endoplasmic reticulum is not present on all vitamin K-dependent proteins. Two proteins originating in bone have been found to differ from this pathway. The CRS on matrix Gla protein is located within the mature protein [61,62], and periostin, a previously known protein secreted from the bone marrow, which has now been claimed [63] to be a vitamin K-dependent protein, may have a similar structure. Based on reaction with an anti-Gla antibody, four domains of this protein contain Gla residues, and, based on homology to other proteins, CRSs within with the mature protein have been identified. Another deviation from the typical propeptide domain of vitamin K-dependent proteins is the identification of a carboxy-terminal recognition site within the precursor of a novel Gla containing conatoxin [64].

The overall reaction catalyzed by the vitamin K-dependent carboxylase (Figure 4.5) is the abstraction of a hydrogen to form an anion on the γ-carbon of the glutamyl substrate to allow attack of CO_2 at this position; and, in the presence of the substrate [65,66], this action is coupled to conversion of the vitamin to its 2,3-epoxide. The stereochemistry of the reaction at the glutamyl residue has been determined by the incorporation of *threo-* or *erythro-*γ-fluoroglutamate into a peptide substrate, which demonstrated a stereospecific hydrogen abstraction corresponding to the elimination of the 4-pro-*S*-hydrogen of the glutamyl residues [67–70]. The mechanism by which epoxide formation is coupled to γ-hydrogen abstraction is key to a complete understanding of the role of vitamin K. The utilization of substrates tritiated at the γ-carbon of each Glu residue [71–73] has demonstrated that the carboxylase catalyzes a vitamin KH_2- and O_2-dependent, but CO_2-independent release of tritium from the substrate, and at saturating concentrations of CO_2 there is an apparent equivalent stoichiometry between vitamin K-2,3-epoxide formation and Gla formation. The enzyme has been shown to catalyze a vitamin KH_2- and O_2-dependent exchange of ^3H from ^3H_2O into the γ-position of a Glu residue, and this exchange reaction is decreased as the concentration of HCO_3^- in the media is increased. The reaction efficiency defined as the ratio of Gla residues formed to γ-C-H bonds cleaved has been shown to be independent of Glu substrate concentrations, and to approach unity at high CO_2 concentrations [74]. Studies with tritium-labeled substrates have also established that the hydrogen exchange catalyzed by the enzyme in the absence of CO_2 proceeds with a stereospecific abstraction of the same 4-pro-*S*-hydrogen of the glutamyl residue that is eliminated in the carboxylation reaction, and that the carboxylation proceeds with the inversion of configuration [75]. The majority of the studies that utilized modified or tritium-labeled substrates to follow the course of stoichiometry of the reaction were conducted with very crude preparations of the carboxylase, but more recent studies [59] employing recombinant carboxylase have yielded very similar results.

4.1.4 PURIFICATION, CLONING, AND DISTRIBUTION OF THE CARBOXYLASE

Following the discovery of this vitamin K-dependent reaction, progress in purifying the carboxylase that was associated with the endoplasmic reticulum and was present in relatively small amounts was slow. Early efforts based on utilization of a propeptide affinity column [76] or attraction of the carboxylase/precursor complex to a prothrombin antibody and elution with a propeptide [77] resulted in increases of specific activity of only 500- to 1,000-fold. The enzyme was eventually purified to near homogeneity from bovine liver microsomes by Stafford [78], and the human carboxylase was soon cloned and expressed by the same group [79]. The carboxylase was found to be a unique 758 amino acid residue protein with a sequence suggestive of an integral membrane protein with a number of membrane spanning domains in the N-terminus and a C-terminal domain located in the lumen of the endoplasmic reticulum. The human carboxylase gene is 13 kb long, contains 15 exons [80] and genetic mapping places it at p12 of chromosome 2 [81]. As might be expected, heterozygous mice carrying a null mutation for the carboxylase do exhibit normal development, but an intercross of these mice results in the null/null offspring failing to survive to term or dying from hemorrhage soon after birth [82].

Expression of the carboxylase has been demonstrated in essentially all human tissues, and the gene is distributed widely across animal phyla [83–85]. The gene is developmentally regulated [86] and carboxylase mRNA is expressed early in rat embryogenes in the central nervous system, mesenchymal, and skeletal tissue, and later in hepatocytes. In studies where the properties of the carboxylase present in various species have been studied [87], the enzyme has been shown to carboxylate low-molecular-weight Glu-containing peptides as does the mammalian enzyme, and attachment of mammalian propeptides to these peptides increases the affinity of the substrate for the enzyme. The carboxylase from the poisonous marine snail *Conus* functions in the synthesis of a large number of toxic peptides. This enzyme has been studied extensively [88], and although it has many common properties, its propeptide does not stimulate the activity of the enzyme to the same extent as the mammalian enzyme. The carboxylase has been identified in *Drosophila* [89,90], and when this gene is expressed in insect cell lines, carboxylation of synthetic Glu-containing substrates can be demonstrated. However, no Gla-containing proteins or any endogenous precursors to a vitamin K-dependent protein have been identified in these flies [91].

At the present time the vitamin K-dependent carboxylase has not been identified in any single-celled organism, but an ortholog of the carboxylase has been identified in the bacterial pathogen *Leptospira* [92]. This carboxylase ortholog has been isolated, expressed in baculovirus, and studied by Berkner [93]. This protein, which appears to have been acquired by horizontal transfer, does have vitamin K epoxidase activity, but no demonstrable carboxylase activity, suggesting that the strong base generated during epoxide formation might be used for an alternate purpose.

4.1.5 ENZYMATIC ACTION AND PROCESSIVITY

Details of the pathway by which the energy obtained from the oxidation of the reduced form of vitamin K to its 2,3-epoxide could be coupled to the carboxylation of glutamyl residues are not yet finalized, but the general nature of the scheme appears to be established. Although some attention was at one time given to the possibility of a free radical-driven reaction, a preponderance of early data supported an attack of CO_2 on a carbanion generated at the γ-position of the glutamyl residue. The problem then became one of identifying an intermediate chemical form of vitamin K that was sufficiently basic (pk of ~25) to abstract the γ-hydrogen of the Glu substrate. The first clearly defined mechanism to be considered was proposed by Dowd [94] in 1991. They hypothesized a "base amplification" model that would utilize a weak catalytic base of a carboxylase amino acid residue to deprotonate the reduced vitamin (KH_2) and allow O_2 to interact with the vitamin and generate the strong base needed. It was suggested [95] that an initial attack of O_2 at the naphthoquinone carbonyl carbon adjacent to the methyl group would result in the formation of a dioxetane ring that could generate an alkoxide intermediate. This intermediate is hypothesized to be the strong base that abstracts the γ-methylene hydrogen and leaves a carbanion that can interact with CO_2. This pathway leads to the possibility that a second atom of molecular oxygen can be incorporated into the carbonyl group of the epoxide product as well as the epoxide oxygen, and this partial dioxygenase activity has been verified by Dowd and other investigators [96,97], which provides very strong support for the proposed pathway. Although the general scheme [98] (Figure 4.6) is consistent with all of the available data, there is no direct chemical proof of the postulated intermediates, and the mechanism remains a hypothesis at this time. Additional support is, however, given by recent quantum chemical studies of the carboxylase [99–101] that indicate that the most energetic step in the pathway is the initial deprotonation of the hydroquinone after which the reaction proceeds downhill in free energy to form the critical alkoxide species. The authors suggest that the enzyme is probably involved in reducing the energy required for the initial hydroquinone deprotonation.

The vitamin K-dependent proteins contain multiple Gla residues, and mature proteins from vitamin K-replete animals are carboxylated at all of the potential Gla sites. Two scenarios could accomplish this. Both the initial gene product and partially carboxylated species could be released from the enzyme and then reinteract with the enzyme multiple times until the carboxylase is complete, or the primary gene product could be tethered to the carboxylase until complete carboxylation

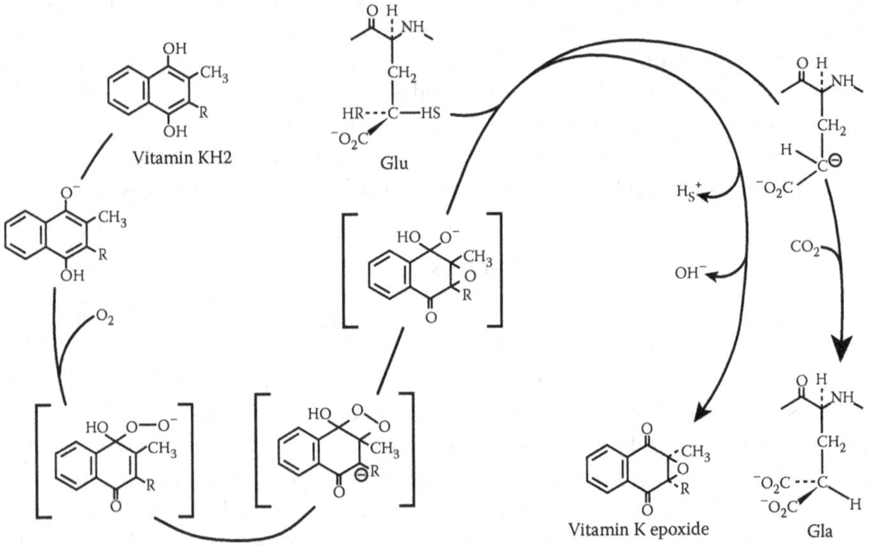

FIGURE 4.6 The postulated mechanism of action of the vitamin K-dependent γ-glutamyl carboxylase. An interaction of O_2 with vitamin KH_2, the reduced (hydronaphthoquinone) form of vitamin K, generates intermediates eventually leading to an oxygenated metabolite that is sufficiently basic to abstract the γ-hydrogen of the glutamyl residue. The products of this reaction are vitamin K 2,3-epoxide and a glutamyl carbanion. Attack of CO_2 on the carbanion leads to the formation of a γ-carboxyglutamyl residue (Gla). The bracketed peroxy, dioxetane, and alkoxide intermediates have not been identified in the enzyme-catalyzed reaction but are postulated based on model organic reactions. The available data are consistent with their presence.

is achieved. The later possibility has been demonstrated to be the pathway utilized. In in vitro studies utilizing a substrate composed of a propeptide attached to the uncarboxylated Gla domain of factor IX and recombinant carboxylase as an enzyme source, Stafford [102] has found that the carboxylated products identified were fully or only slightly undercarboxylated. These data suggested that once a substrate is carboxylated, it does not equilibrate with the uncarboxylated substrate pool. The suggested processivity of the process was further established by Berkner [103], who demonstrated that the rate of, and completeness of, the carboxylation of an undercarboxylated factor IX/carboxylase complex was not altered by the presence of uncarboxylated factor IX in the incubation. The tethered processivity carboxylation model requires that the rate of dissociation of the protein substrate from the carboxylase is much slower than the rate of Glu carboxylation, which was consistent with the data obtained in this study. It appears that the relatively high affinity of the substrate propeptide for the carboxylase, a second binding site on the carboxylase which recognizes the Glu binding site [104], and an allosteric response of the enzyme to this binding site [105] are all involved in the tethering event. The combined affinity of these three interactions could be responsible for the 3000-fold difference in the off-rate of factor IX propeptide from the carboxylase and the rate of the carboxylation event [60]. If sufficient amounts of reduced vitamin K are not available because of insufficient amounts of the vitamin or inhibition of the recycling of the vitamin K epoxide to the reduced form, partially γ-carboxylated forms of the protein substrates are released to the circulation (see Chapter 5). The overall process of producing biologically active vitamin K-dependent proteins is, therefore, one that involves the carboxylase, the vitamin K-epoxide reductase, an electron donor, and the complex series of chaperones and cargo receptors that are involved in transferring endoplasmic reticulum-synthesized proteins through the golgi and into the circulation (Figure 4.7).

4.1.6 Topology and Physiological Control of the Carboxylase

The vitamin K-dependent carboxylase is a resident protein of the endoplasmic reticulum whose topology within the membrane has not yet been firmly established. Analysis of the amino acid sequence of the carboxylase indicates seven hydrophobic regions in the protein, and it has been proposed that the enzyme has five transmembrane regions spanning the endoplasmic reticulum [106]. Alternative models of the topology are, however, possible [107], and additional data are needed to establish the relationship of the various hydrophobic regions (Figure 4.8) of the enzyme to the membrane. The two-dimensional crystallization of the human vitamin K-dependent carboxylase has been reported [108], but little information regarding the structure is currently available. Progress in more clearly defining the structure continues, and studies of a two-chain carboxylase joined by a disulfide bond [109] have been used to locate specific residues that are involved in the stabilization of the tertiary structure of the enzyme. Although a three-dimensional structure of the carboxylase is not yet available to confirm them, a number of studies have been directed toward the location of both the propeptide and the substrate binding sites of the enzyme (see [107,110,111]). To generate the strong vitamin K base needed to generate a carbanion

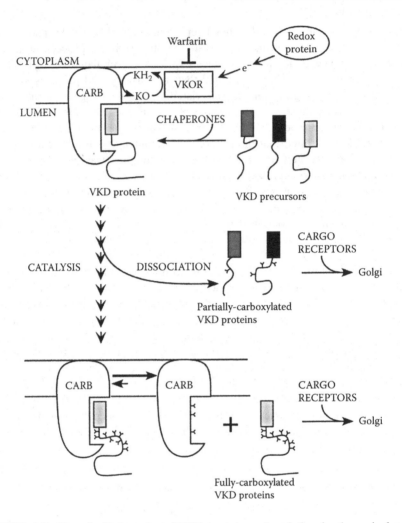

FIGURE 4.7 Vitamin K-dependent (VKD) protein carboxylation in the endoplasmic reticulum. VKD proteins contain propeptides with different affinities (indicated by altered shading) for the carboxylase (CARB). This binding results in the conversion of multiple Glu residues to Gla residues (the grey "Y"s). A VKD protein undergoing nine modifications is shown as an example. The carboxylase is also carboxylated (see Chapter 5), subsequent to the carboxylation of the VKD substrate. Each Glu to Gla conversion requires one reduced vitamin K (KH_2) which is recycled from the vitamin K epoxide (KO) product of carboxylation by the vitamin K epoxide reductase (VKOR) and a redox protein which may be the endoplasmic reticulum protein disulfide isomerase. KH_2 availability supports a high rate of catalysis and low rate of dissociation that result in processive carboxylation, and warfarin disrupts normal carboxylation by blocking the supply of KH_2. Quality control components that affect carboxylation are chaperones, which mediate VKD protein-carboxylase assembly, and cargo receptors, which transport fully and partially carboxylated VKD proteins out of the endoplasmic reticulum. The quality control components specific to carboxylation have not yet been identified. (From Berkner, K.L. 2005. *Annu Rev Nutr* 25:127. With permission.)

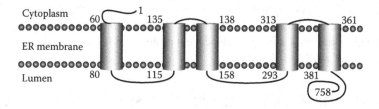

FIGURE 4.8 Proposed topology of the vitamin K-dependent carboxylase. The carboxylation of precursor proteins occurs on the lumenal side of the endoplasmic reticulum membrane, and the amino acid sequence of the enzyme is consistent with a topology containing five transmembrane domains.

on the γ-carbon of the Glu residue would require deprotonation of the reduced form of the vitamin so that it could react with O_2, and early evidence suggested that a Cys residue was used to deprotonate vitamin KH_2. There are 10 Cys residues in the protein, two of which are present as a disulfide bond, and a number of attempts to identify the Cys residue involved in the carboxylation event have been made. However, more recent data have proposed an activated amine as the catalytic base [112] and it has been identified by Berkner as Lys 218 [113]. Progress in definitively locating other active site amino acid residues is slow, but more information is becoming available. It has recently been shown [114] that a mutation of His160 to an Ala residue results in an enzyme that has nearly normal vitamin K-epoxide formation, but much lower Gla formation. When a peptide substrate with Glu residues tritiated at the γ-carbon position was used, the ratio of tritium release to epoxidation was 10-fold lower when the mutant enzyme was used rather than the wild type. The data have clearly established that His160 is involved in the formation of the transition state needed for carbanion formation.

The use of recombinant vitamin K-dependent clotting factors produced in cultured mammalian cells as drugs has led to efforts to improve yields, and it has been found that low-level expression of these proteins results in full carboxylation of the product, but increased expression leads to poorly carboxylated proteins with low biological activity. Early attempts to increase the yield of biologically active products by overexpression of the carboxylase itself in the same cell lines did not substantially increase the production of fully carboxylated product. Co-expression of the vitamin K epoxide reductase in cell lines expressing recombinant factor X [115] or factor IX [116] has been shown to increase the yield of functional products and has led to the conclusion that the production of vitamin KH_2 by this enzyme is the rate-limiting factor in the production of fully carboxylated proteins. More recent data [117] suggest that although the flux of vitamin KH_2 is a factor, overexpression of the epoxide reductase is limited in vivo, and that some other factor may be the rate-limiting step [117]. The endoplasmic reticulum chaperone protein calumenin has been reported to be associated with the carboxylase and to inhibit its activity [118], and siRNA silencing of calumenin in cells engineered to overexpress both the epoxide reductase and hfIX has been demonstrated to increase the production of functional r-hIX [119]. At the present time, the mechanism by which calumenin inhibits carboxylase activity or the physiological responses that might control its concentration are not known, nor is it known if it plays any role in the synthesis of vitamin K-dependent proteins in intact animals. It is, however, apparent that a complete understanding of the control of full carboxylation of vitamin K-dependent proteins and of their secretion from the cell is still not available.

4.2 THE VITAMIN K-EPOXIDE REDUCTASE

4.2.1 DEMONSTRATION OF THE EPOXIDE REDUCTASE

Gla residues which are one of the end products of the intracellular degradation of vitamin K-dependent proteins are not further metabolized, but are excreted in the urine [120]. In the adult human the extent of Gla excretion is in the range of 50 μmol/day, indicating that a similar amount must be formed each day to maintain a steady-state cellular concentration of vitamin K-dependent proteins. At least a mole of vitamin K is oxidized for each mole of Gla formed by the carboxylase, and the average daily dietary intake of the vitamin is in the range of 0.1 to 0.3 μmole/day. These observations suggest that to maintain functional concentrations of the reduced vitamin K substrate for the carboxylase, the vitamin K 2,3-epoxide generated by the carboxylase must be actively recycled. The epoxide had been shown by Matschiner and coworkers [121] to be a major liver metabolite of vitamin K before it was demonstrated that it was a co-product of Gla formation, and the hepatic ratio of the epoxide relative to that of the vitamin had been found to be increased in animals administered the 4-hydroxycoumarin anticoagulant warfarin [122]. Some early observations suggested that the anticoagulant activity of warfarin and other 4-hyroxycoumarins (see Chapter 2) was based on a competitive inhibition of vitamin K action by its epoxide, but later studies [123,124] supported the hypothesis that warfarin interfered with the activity of an enzyme which came to be called the vitamin K-epoxide reductase and now is commonly referred to as VKOR. Inhibition of this reductase would prevent the reduction of the epoxide to the quinone form of the vitamin and eventually to the carboxylase substrate, vitamin KH_2.

About 10 years before the epoxide was identified as a vitamin K metabolite, widespread use of warfarin as an anticoagulant rodenticide led to the appearance of strains of warfarin-resistant rats [125,126], and the study of the activity of the epoxide reductase in livers of these animals was key to an understanding [127–129] of the details of what is now referred to as the "vitamin K cycle" (Figure 4.9). Three forms of vitamin K [the quinone (K), the hydronaphthoquinone (KH_2), and the 2,3-epoxide (KO)] can feed into this liver vitamin K cycle. In normal liver, the ratio of vitamin K-2,3-epoxide to the less oxidized forms of the vitamin is about 1:10 but can increase to a majority of epoxide in an anticoagulated animal. The quinone and hydronaphthoquinone forms of the vitamin can be interconverted by NAD(P)H-linked reductases [130], including one that appears to be a microsomal-bound form of the extensively studied liver DT-diaphorase activity [131]. There are a number of these flavin containing, NAD(P)H linked quinone oxidoreductases in tissues that will reduce vitamin K quinone to vitamin KH_2 by a two-electron transfer and cytochrome p450-linked reductases which transfer single electrons to generate vitamin K semiquinone, which could lead to the formation of reactive oxygen species. None of these reductases are

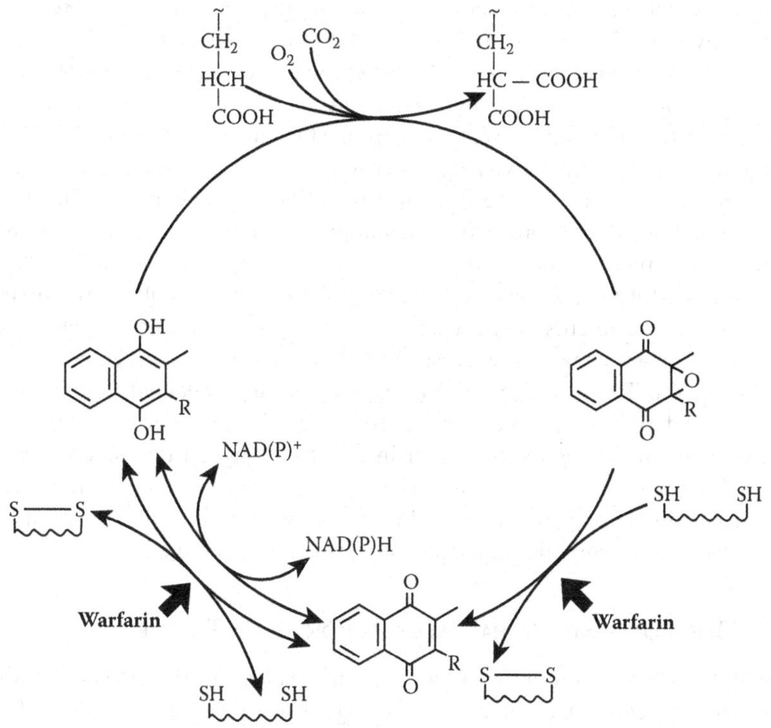

FIGURE 4.9 Tissue recycling of vitamin K. Vitamin K epoxide formed in the carboxylation reaction is reduced to the quinone form of the vitamin by a warfarin-sensitive enzyme, the vitamin K epoxide reductase. This reaction is driven by a reduced dithiol. The naphthoquinone form of the vitamin can be reduced to the hydronaphthoquinone form either by the same warfarin-sensitive dithiol-driven reductase or by one or more of the hepatic NADH- or NADPH-linked quinone reductases that are less sensitive to warfarin.

capable of reducing vitamin K-epoxide to vitamin KH_2. Various forms of vitamin K have been used in pharmacological amounts in anticancer drugs, and their activity is likely dependent on the activity of these reductases. The distribution and mechanism of action of these enzymes have been recently reviewed [132,133].

4.2.2 PURIFICATION AND PROPERTIES OF THE ENZYME

Efforts to purify and characterize the protein or proteins responsible for the reductase activity soon after it was identified were not successful. Although present in most tissues studied, the activity was found to be much higher in liver [134] than in other tissues. The activity of the hepatic enzyme and its kinetic parameters [135] has been compared to and was found to be rather similar in eight species that have been studied. Early studies of the properties of the enzyme, which have been reviewed [136], were successful in establishing that thiols are involved in the catalytic activity, and that warfarin binding appeared to interfere with the oxidized thiol redox center and therefore prevented reduction of this center by an unknown electron donor. Early attempts to determine if a single protein or a multiprotein complex was responsible for the activity of the enzyme and for the ability of warfarin to block the activity of the enzyme were not successful. As the epoxide reductase was demonstrated to be a component of the endoplasmic reticulum, it was necessary to solubilize this membrane before it could be separated from other membrane proteins. Attempts to solubilize the enzyme activity by either ionic or nonionic detergents led to loss of activity, and this was assumed by most investigators to be an indicator that the epoxidase activity was the property of a multiprotein complex that had been dissociated by the detergent. Efforts in a number of laboratories over a period of 20 years were unsuccessful in substantially increasing the specific activity of the reductase from a crude liver microsomal preparation, and these efforts have been reviewed [133]. Recombinant epoxidase expressed in insect cells has, however, been purified over 90% [137]. The identification by the Stafford and Oldenburg laboratories of the human and rat genes for the epoxide reductase [138,139] and the presence of the identified gene in *Drosophila* and other insects [140] suggest that this activity may be as widespread as the carboxylase. The demonstration that the rate-limiting step in the production of recombinant proteins in mammalian cell culture systems is the epoxide reductase clearly defines an essential role for its presence.

4.2.3 TOPOLOGY AND MECHANISM OF ACTION OF THE ENZYME

Recent efforts have led to attempts to map the topology of the enzyme within the endoplasmic reticulum membrane [141], resulting in a model (Figure 4.10) that has a short amino-terminal domain in the lumen of the endoplasmic reticulum, three transmembrane domains, and the majority of the protein in the cytoplasm. The data currently available would indicate that both the active site of the enzyme and the warfarin-binding site are located within one of these transmembrane domains, presumably near the luminal surface. Although early efforts to purify the vitamin K-epoxide reductase were carried out with the expectation that the enzyme activity was a function of two distinct proteins, it is now clear that this is not the case. The small 18-kDa protein expressed by this gene has now been shown to be sufficient for the reduction of the epoxide to the quinone form of vitamin K and also the quinone to the hydronaphthoquinone [137], confirming early data [142–144] that the reductase could carry out both of these essential functions. The epoxide reductase has been shown to harbor a thioredoxin-like Cys-X-X-Cys center utilizing Cys132 and Cys135 of the 163 amino acid residue protein [137,145] which is involved in the reduction of the epoxide. Subsequently, the same two cysteines of the enzyme that had been demonstrated to be involved in epoxide to quinone reduction were shown to carry out the quinone to hydronaphthoquinone reduction [146]. The initial source of the electrons needed to reduce this center has been difficult to identify. Assays of the reductase have typically utilized dithiothreitol (DTT) as the reductant for the overall reaction, and this serves to reduce the critical disulfide. Identification of the physiologically important reductant needed to allow the continued recycling of the epoxide generated by the carboxylase has been an important question. A number of early studies [143,147,148] proposed that thioredoxin, which will drive the reaction, was the physiologically important component, although there are reasons to

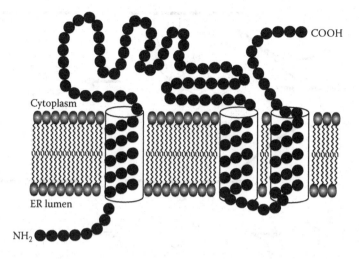

FIGURE 4.10 Proposed topology of VKOR within the endoplasmic reticulum (ER) membrane. Based on the known amino acid sequence of the protein and computer program-based comparisons to the structures of known membrane proteins, it has been proposed that the topology of VKOR includes three transmembrane domains (residues 10–29, 101–123, and 127–149) with a small amino-terminal segment of the protein in the ER lumen and the majority of the protein within the cytoplasm. The proposed redox center, C-X-X-C, is located within the most carboxy-terminal transmembrane domain and near the lumenal surface. For details see Reference [133].

question this role [149]. Protein disulfide isomerase (PDI) has been shown [150] to substantially enhance the activity of the thioredoxin-driven reaction, and in a recent report Wallin [151] has presented evidence that would support the theory that PDI, the enzyme involved in the dithiol-dependent oxidative folding of proteins in the endoplasmic reticulum, is the source of electrons needed for the reduction. Much of the more recent data dealing with the properties of the reductase are available in more detailed reviews [133,136,152,153].

The mechanisms initially proposed for the action of the epoxide reductase [154,155] have more recently been found [156] to be energetically feasible by quantum chemical calculations. Additional quantum chemical studies [157] have, however, indicated that the first step in the reduction of the epoxide would involve an initial protonation of the epoxide oxygen by a free mercapto group rather than a water molecule. Although further study may provide additional detail, the pathway for the reduction of the epoxide shown in Figure 4.11 is consistent with the available data. The interaction of anticoagualnt drugs such as warfarin with the epoxide reductase has been of great interest. Although early studies suggested that warfarin bound irreversibly to a site on the reductase not related to the active site, more recent data [158] are consistent with the view that warfarin acts by blocking the binding of vitamin K epoxide to the active site of the enzyme. The newer data show that the 4-hydroxy group is critical to the activity of the 4-hydroxycoumarins, and deprotonation of this group appears to allow warfarin to attack the active site of the enzyme. The constituent on the 3-position is also involved. This would be consistent with

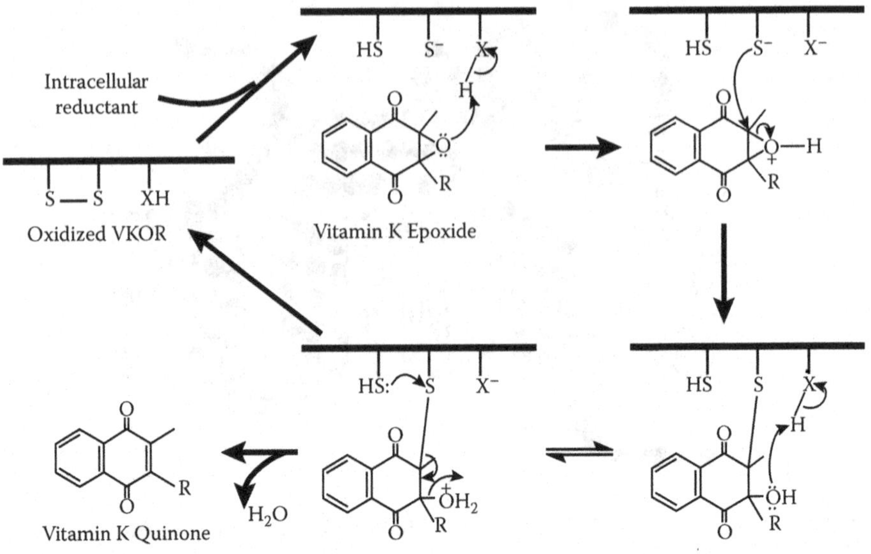

FIGURE 4.11 Proposed mechanism of action of the vitamin K epoxide reductase. The substrate epoxide binds to the reduced form of the enzyme, and protonation of the ring oxygen allows formation of the thiol bound 3-hydroxy intermediate. Reformation of the oxidized active site dithiol and elimination of the ring oxygen as H_2O results in the formation of the vitamin K quinone product. The same enzyme can also reduce the quinone to the reduced form of the vitamin, vitamin KH_2.

the demonstration that Ferulenol, a 4-hydroxycoumarin natural product that has a 15-carbon isoprenyl side chain, is one of the more potent of this class of anticoagulants to be tested [158].

Both an adequate amount of vitamin K from the diet and a functional vitamin K epoxide reductase are needed for the synthesis of normal amounts of biologically active vitamin K-dependent proteins. A hypothetical model based on current information linking the activities of the vitamin K-dependent carboxylase and the epoxide reductase has been proposed [159].

4.3 CURRENT STATUS OF RESEARCH EFFORTS

Although the mechanism of action of the vitamin K-dependent carboxylase appears to be that originally proposed by Dowd, details remain, and there will undoubtedly be continued efforts to more clearly define the interactions of the enzyme with its substrate and to develop a more complete understanding of the enzyme's tertiary structure. Similar efforts are needed to more fully understand the mechanism and structure of the vitamin K-epoxide reductase. Because of the current interest in the public health aspects of vitamin K-dependent proteins (see Chapter 7), it is likely that interest in genetic variants of these two enzymes will continue.

The relationship between these two enzymes has suggested that the rate-limiting factor in substrate carboxylation is based not only on the cellular concentration of vitamin K, but also on the rate of production of the reduced form of vitamin K from the epoxide. The reports that the endoplasmic reticulum chaperone calumenin and a currently unidentified protein are involved in regulating the rate of carboxylation are of great interest and an understanding of the basis of these observations is important to a full characterization of the control mechanisms involved in important posttranslational modification.

REFERENCES

1. Dam, H., F. Schonheyder, and E. Tage-Hansen. 1936. Studies on the mode of action of vitamin K. *Biochem J* 30:1075–1079.
2. Martius, C. and D. Nitz-Litzow. 1954. Oxydative phosphorylierung und vitamin K mangel. *Biochim Biophys Acta* 13:152–153.
3. Olson, R.E. 1964. Vitamin K induced prothrombin formation: Antagonism by actinomycin D. *Science* 145:926–928.
4. Hill, R.B., S. Gaetani, A.M. Paolucci, P.B. RamaRao, R. Alden, G.S. Ranhotra, V.K. Shah, and B.C. Johnson. 1968. Vitamin K and biosynthesis of protein and prothrombin. *J Biol Chem* 243:3930–3939.
5. Suttie, J.W. 1970. The effect of cycloheximide administration on vitamin K-stimulated prothrombin formation. *Arch Biochem Biophys* 141:571–578.
6. Shah, D.V. and J.W. Suttie. 1971. Mechanism of action of vitamin K: Evidence for the conversion of a precursor protein to prothrombin in the rat. *Proc Natl Acad Sci USA* 68:1653–1657.
7. Suttie, J.W. 1973. Mechanism of action of vitamin K: Demonstration of a liver precursor of prothrombin. *Science* 179:192–194.
8. Esmon, C.T., G.A. Grant, and J.W. Suttie. 1975. Purification of an apparent rat liver prothrombin precursor: Characterization and comparison to normal rat prothrombin. *Biochemistry* 14:1595–1600.
9. Suttie, J.W. 1974. Metabolism and properties of a liver precursor to prothrombin. *Vitamins and Hormones* 32:463–481.
10. Olson, R.E. 1974. New concepts relating to the mode of action of vitamin K. *Vitamins and Hormones* 32:483–511.
11. Olson, R.E., G. Philipps, and N. Wang. 1968. The regulatory action of vitamin K. *Adv Enz Reg* 6:213–225.
12. Stenflo, J. and J.W. Suttie. 1977. Vitamin K-dependent formation of gamma-carboxyglutamic acid. *Annu Rev Biochem* 46:157–172.
13. Suttie, J.W. and C.M. Jackson. 1977. Prothrombin structure, activation, and biosynthesis. *Physiol Rev* 57:1–70.
14. Suttie, J.W. 1978. Vitamin K. In *Handbook of Lipid Research: The Fat-Soluble Vitamins*, ed. H.F. DeLuca, 211–277. New York: Plenum Press.
15. Ganrot, P.O. and J.E. Nilehn. 1968. Plasma prothrombin during treatment with dicumarol. II. Demonstration of an abnormal prothrombin fraction. *Scand J Clin Lab Invest* 22:23–28.
16. Josso, F., J.M. Lavergne, M. Gouault, O. Prou-Wartelle, and J.P. Soulier. 1968. Differents etsts moleculaires du facteur II (prothrombine). Leur etude a l'aide de la staphylocoagulase et d'anticorps anti-facteur II. *Thrombos Diathes Haemorrh* 20:88–98.
17. Stenflo, J. and P.O. Ganrot. 1972. Vitamin K and the biosynthesis of prothrombin. I. Identification and purification of a dicoumarol-induced abnormal prothrombin from bovine plasma. *J Biol Chem* 247:8160–8166.
18. Nelsestuen, G.L. and J.W. Suttie. 1972. The purification and properties of an abnormal prothrombin protein produced by dicoumarol-treated cows. A comparison to normal prothrombin. *J Biol Chem* 247:8176–8182.

19. Stenflo, J. 1972. Vitamin K and the biosynthesis of prothrombin. II. Structural comparison of normal and dicoumarol-induced bovine prothrombin. *J Biol Chem* 247:8167–8175.

20. Stenflo, J. 1973. Vitamin K and the biosynthesis of prothrombin. III. Structural comparison of an NH_2 terminal fragment from normal and from dicoumarol-induced bovine prothrombin. *J Biol Chem* 248:6325–6332.

21. Nelsestuen, G.L. and J.W. Suttie. 1972. Mode of action of vitamin K. Calcium binding properties of bovine prothrombin. *Biochemistry* 11:4961–4964.

22. Owen, W.G. and C.T. Esmon. 1981. Functional properties of an endothelial cell cofactor for thrombin-catalyzed activation of protein C. *J Biol Chem* 256:5532–5535.

23. Esmon, C.T., J.W. Suttie, and C.M. Jackson. 1975. The functional significance of vitamin K action. Difference in phospholipid binding between normal and abnormal prothrombin. *J Biol Chem* 250:4095–4099.

24. Stenflo, J. 1974. Vitamin K and the biosynthesis of prothrombin. IV. Isolation of peptides containing prosthetic groups from normal prothrombin and the corresponding peptides from dicoumarol-induced prothrombin. *J Biol Chem* 249:5527–5535.

25. Nelsestuen, G.L. and J.W. Suttie. 1973. The mode of action of vitamin K. Isolation of a peptide containing the vitamin K-dependent portion of prothrombin. *Proc Natl Acad Sci USA* 70:3366–3370.

26. Stenflo, J., P. Fernlund, W. Egan, and P. Roepstorff. 1974. Vitamin K dependent modifications of glutamic acid residues in prothrombin. *Proc Natl Acad Sci USA* 71:2730–2733.

27. Nelsestuen, G.L., T.H. Zytkovicz, and J.B. Howard. 1974. The mode of action of vitamin K. Identification of gamma-carboxyglutamic acid as a component of prothrombin. *J Biol Chem* 249:6347–6350.

28. Magnusson, S., L. Sottrup-Jensen, T.E. Petersen, H.R. Morris, and A. Dell. 1974. Primary structure of the vitamin K-dependent part of prothrombin. *FEBS Lett* 44:189–193.

29. Stenflo, J. 2006. From gamma-carboxy-glutamate to protein C. *J Thromb Haemost* 4:2521–2526.

30. Shah, D.V. and J.W. Suttie. 1974. The vitamin K dependent, in vitro production of prothrombin. *Biochem Biophys Res Commun* 606:1397–1402.

31. Esmon, C.T., J.A. Sadowski, and J.W. Suttie. 1975. A new carboxylation reaction. The vitamin K-dependent incorporation of $H^{14}CO_3^-$ into prothrombin. *J Biol Chem* 250:4744–4748.

32. Sadowski, J.A., C.T. Esmon, and J.W. Suttie. 1976. Vitamin K-dependent carboxylase. Requirements of the rat liver microsomal enzyme system. *J Biol Chem* 251:2770–2775.

33. Esmon, C.T. and J.W. Suttie. 1976. Vitamin K-dependent carboxylase: Solubilization and properties. *J Biol Chem* 251:6238–6243.

34. Suttie, J.W., J.M. Hageman, S.R. Lehrman, and D.H. Rich. 1976. Vitamin K-dependent carboxylase: Development of a peptide substrate. *J Biol Chem* 251:5827–5830.

35. Suttie, J.W., S.R. Lehrman, L.O. Geweke, J.M. Hageman, and D.H. Rich. 1979. Vitamin K-dependent carboxylase: Requirements for carboxylation of soluble peptide substrates and substrate specificity. *Biochem Biophys Res Commun* 86:500–507.

36. Carlisle, T.L. and J.W. Suttie. 1980. Vitamin K dependent carboxylase: Subcellular location of the carboxylase and enzymes involved in vitamin K metabolism in rat liver. *Biochemistry* 19:1161–1167.

37. Sadowski, J.A., H.K. Schnoes, and J.W. Suttie. 1977. Vitamin K epoxidase: Properties and relationship to prothrombin synthesis. *Biochemistry* 16:3856–3863.

38. Willingham, A.K. and J.T. Matschiner. 1974. Changes in phylloquinone epoxidase activity related to prothrombin synthesis and microsomal clotting activity in the rat. *Biochem J* 140:435–441.

39. Johnson, B.C. 1981. Post-translational carboxylation of preprothrombin. *Mol Cell Biochem* 38:77–121.
40. Olson, R.E. and J.W. Suttie. 1978. Vitamin K and gamma-carboxyglutamate biosynthesis. *Vitamins and Hormones* 35:59–108.
41. Olson, R.E. 1984. The function and metabolism of vitamin K. *Annu Rev Nutr* 4:281–337.
42. Suttie, J.W. 1985. Vitamin K-dependent carboxylase. *Annu Rev Biochem* 54:459–477.
43. Vermeer, C. and M.A.G. de Boer-van den Berg. 1985. Vitamin K-dependent carboxylase. *Haematologia* 18:71–97.
44. Vermeer, C. 1990. Gamma-carboxyglutamate-containing proteins and the vitamin K-dependent carboxylase. *Biochem J* 266:625–636.
45. Dowd, P. and S.W. Ham. 1991. Mechanism of cyanide inhibition of the blood-clotting, vitamin K-dependent carboxylase. *Proc Natl Acad Sci USA* 88:10583–10585.
46. Ichinose, A. and E.W. Davie. 1994. The blood coagulation factors: Their cDNAs, genes, and expression. In *Hemostasis and Thrombosis: Basic Principles and Clinical Practice*, 3rd ed., ed. R.W. Colman, J. Hirsh, V.J. Marder, and E.W. Salzman, 19–54. Philadelphia: Lippincott.
47. Jorgensen, M.J., A.B. Cantor, B.C. Furie, C.L. Brown, C.B. Shoemaker, and B. Furie. 1987. Recognition site directing vitamin K-dependent gamma-carboxylation residues on the propeptide of factor IX. *Cell* 48:185–191.
48. Furie, B. and B.C. Furie. 1992. Molecular and cellular biology of blood coagulation. *New Engl. J. Med.* 326:800–806.
49. Furie, B. and B.C. Furie. 1990. Molecular basis of vitamin K-dependent gamma-carboxylation. *Blood* 75:1753–1762.
50. Huber, P., T. Schmitz, J. Griffin, M. Jacobs, C. Walsh, B. Furie, and B.C. Furie. 1990. Identification of amino acids in the gamma-carboxylation recognition site on the propeptide of prothrombin. *J Biol Chem* 265:12467–12473.
51. Furie, B.C., J.V. Ratcliffe, J. Tward, M.J. Jorgensen, L.S. Blaszkowsky, D. DiMichele, and B. Furie. 1997. The gamma-carboxylation recognition site is sufficient to direct vitamin K-dependent carboxylation on an adjacent glutamate-rich region of thrombin in a propeptide-thrombin chimera. *J Biol Chem* 272:28258–28262.
52. Cham, B.E., J.L. Smith, and D.M. Colquhoun. 1999. What happens to vitamin K_1 in serum after bone fracture? *Clin Chem* 45:2261–2263.
53. Metz, M.D., C. Vermeer, B.A.M. Soute, G.J.M.V. Scharrenburg, A.J. Slotboom, and H.C. Hemker. 1981. Partial purification of bovine liver vitamin K-dependent carboxylase by immunospecific adsorption onto antifactor X. *FEBS Lett* 123:215–218.
54. Stanton, C., P.J. Ross, S. Hutson, and R. Wallin. 1995. Evidence for competition between vitamin K-dependent clotting factors for intracellular processing by the vitamin K-dependent gamma-carboxylase. *Thrombosis Res* 80:63–73.
55. Houben, R.J.T.J., D. Jin, D.W. Stafford, P. Proost, H.M. Ebberink, C. Vermeer, and B.A.M. Soute. 1999. Osteocalcin binds tightly to the gamma-glutamylcarboxylase at a site distinct from that of the other known vitamin K-dependent proteins. *Biochem J* 341:265–269.
56. Houben, R.J.T.J., D.T.S. Rijkers, T.B. Stanley, F. Acher, R. Azerad, S.-M. Kakonen, C. Vermeer, and B.A.M. Soute. 2002. Characteristics and composition of the vitamin K-dependent gamma-glutamyl carboxylase-binding domain on osteocalcin. *Biochem J* 364:323–328.
57. Knobloch, J.E. and J.W. Suttie. 1987. Vitamin K-dependent carboxylase. Control of enzyme activity by the "propeptide" region of factor X. *J Biol Chem* 262:15334–15337.
58. Cheung, A., J.W. Suttie, and M. Bernatowicz. 1990. Vitamin K-dependent carboxylase: Structural requirements for propeptide activation. *Biochim Biophys Acta* 1039:90–93.

59. Li, S., B.C. Furie, B. Furie, and C.T. Walsh. 1997. The propeptide of the vitamin K-dependent carboxylase substrate accelerates formation of the gamma-glutamyl carbanion intermediate. *Biochemistry* 36:6384–6390.

60. Presnell, S.R., A. Tripathy, B.R. Lentz, D.-Y. Jin, and D.W. Stafford. 2001. A novel fluorescence assay to study propeptide interaction with gamma-glutamyl carboxylase. *Biochemistry* 40:11723–11733.

61. Price, P.A. and M.K. Williamson. 1985. Primary structure of bovine matrix Gla protein, a new vitamin K-dependent bone protein. *J Biol Chem* 260:14971–14975.

62. Price, P.A., J.D. Fraser, and G. Metz-Virca. 1987. Molecular cloning of matrix gla protein: Implications for substrate recognition by the vitamin K-dependent gamma-carboxylase. *Proc Natl Acad Sci USA* 84:8335–8339.

63. Coutu, D.L., J.H. Wu, A. Monette, G.-E. Rivard, M.D. Blostein, and J. Galipeau. 2008. Periostin: A member of a novel family of vitamin K-dependent proteins is expressed by mesenchymal stromal cells. *J Biol Chem* 238:17991–18001.

64. Brown, M.A., G.S. Begley, E. Czerwiec, L.M. Stenberg, M. Jacobs, D.E. Kalume, P. Roepstorff, J. Stenflo, B.C. Furie, and B. Furie. 2005. Precursors of novel gla-containing conotoxins contain a carboxy-terminal recognition site that directs gamma-carboxylation. *Biochemistry* 44:9150–9159.

65. Suttie, J.W., L.O. Geweke, S.L. Martin, and A.K. Willingham. 1980. Vitamin K epoxidase: Dependence of epoxidase activity on substrates of the vitamin K-dependent carboxylation reaction. *FEBS Lett* 109:267–270.

66. Sugiura, I., B. Furie, C.T. Walsh, and B.C. Furie. 1997. Propeptide and glutamate-containing substrates bound to the vitamin K-dependent carboxylase convert its vitamin K epoxidase function from an inactive to an active state. *Proc Natl Acad Sci USA* 94:9069–9074.

67. Azerad, R., P. Decottignies-LeMarechal, C. Ducrocq, A. Righini-Tapie, A. Vidal-Cros, S. Bory, M. Gaudry, and A. Marquet. 1988. The vitamin K-dependent carboxylation of peptidic substrates: Stereochemical features and mechanistic studies with substrate analogues. In *Current Advances in Vitamin K Research*, ed. J.W. Suttie, 17–23. New York: Elsevier Science Publishing.

68. Decottignies-LeMarechal, P., H. Rikong-Adie, and R. Azerad. 1979. Vitamin K-dependent carboxylation of synthetic substrates. Nature of the products. *Biochem Biophys Res Commun* 90:700–707.

69. Decottignies-LeMarechal, P., P. LeMarechal, and R. Azerad. 1984. Nature of products formed in the vitamin K-dependent carboxylation of synthetic peptides. *Biochem Biophys Res Commun* 119:836–840.

70. Vidal-Cros, A., M. Gaudry, and A. Marquet. 1990. Vitamin K-dependent carboxylation. Mechanistic studies with 3-fluoroglutamate-containing substrates. *Biochem J* 266:749–755.

71. Friedman, P.A., M.A. Shia, P.M. Gallop, and A.E. Griep. 1979. Vitamin K-dependent gamma-carbon-hydrogen bond cleavage and the non-mandatory concurrent carboxylation of peptide bound glutamic acid residues. *Proc Natl Acad Sci USA* 76:3126–3129.

72. Larson, A.E., P.A. Friedman, and J.W. Suttie. 1981. Vitamin K-dependent carboxylase: Stoichiometry of carboxylation and vitamin K 2,3-epoxide formation. *J Biol Chem* 256:11032–11035.

73. McTigue, J.J. and J.W. Suttie. 1983. Vitamin K-dependent carboxylase: Demonstration of a vitamin K- and O_2-dependent exchange of ^3H from ^3H_2O into glutamic acid residues. *J Biol Chem* 258:12129–12131.

74. Wood, G.M. and J.W. Suttie. 1988. Vitamin K-dependent carboxylase. Stoichiometry of vitamin K epoxide formation, gamma-carboxyglutamyl formation, and gamma-glutamyl-^3H cleavage. *J Biol Chem* 263:3234–3239.

75. Dubois, J., C. Dugave, C. Foures, M. Kaminsky, J.C. Tabet, S. Bory, M. Gaudry, and A. Marquet. 1991. Vitamin K dependent carboxylation: Determination of the stereochemical course using 4-fluoroglutamyl-containing substrate. *Biochemistry* 30:10506–10512.

76. Hubbard, B.R., M.M.W. Ulrich, M. Jacobs, C. Vermeer, C. Walsh, B. Furie, and B.C. Furie. 1989. Vitamin K-dependent carboxylase: Affinity purification from bovine liver by using a synthetic propeptide containing the gamma-carboxylation recognition site. *Proc Natl Acad Sci USA* 86:6893–6897.

77. Harbeck, M.C., A.Y. Cheung, and J.W. Suttie. 1989. Vitamin K-dependent carboxylase: Partial purification of the enzyme by antibody affinity techniques. *Thrombosis Res* 56:317–323.

78. Wu, S.M., D.P. Morris, and D.W. Stafford. 1991. Identification and purification to near homogeneity of the vitamin K-dependent carboxylase. *Proc Natl Acad Sci USA* 88:2236–2240.

79. Wu, S.M., W.F. Cheung, D. Frazier, and D. Stafford. 1991. Cloning and expression of the cDNA for human gamma-glutamyl carboxylase. *Science* 254:1634–1636.

80. Wu, S.-M., D.W. Stafford, L.D. Frazier, Y.-Y. Fu, K.A. High, K. Chu, B. Sanchez-Vega, and J. Solera. 1997. Genomic sequence and transcription start site for the human gamma-glutamyl carboxylase. *Blood* 89:4058–4062.

81. Kuo, W.-I., D.W. Stafford, J. Cruces, J. Gray, and J. Solera. 1995. Chromosomal localization of the gamma-glutamyl carboxylase gene at 2p12. *Genomics* 25:746–748.

82. Zhu, A., H. Sun, R.M. Raymond, Jr, B.C. Furie, B. Furie, M. Bronstein, R.J. Kaufman, R. Westrick, and D. Ginsburg. 2007. Fatal hemorrhage in mice lacking gamma-glutamyl carboxylase. *Blood* 109:5270–5275.

83. Bandhyopadhyay, P.K., J.E. Garrett, R.P. Shetty, T. Keate, C.S. Walker, and B.M. Olivera. 2002. Gamma-glutamyl carboxylation: An extracellular posttranslational modification that antedates the divergence of molluscs, arthropods, and chordates. *Proc Natl Acad Sci USA* 99:1264–1269.

84. Wang, C.-P., K. Yagi, P.J. Lin, D.Y. Jin, K.W. Makabe, and D.W. Stafford. 2002. Identification of a gene encoding a typical gamma-carboxyglutamic acid domain in the tunicate *Halocynthia roretzi*. *J Thromb Haemostas* 1:118–123.

85. Begley, G.S., B.C. Furie, B. Czerwiec, K.L. Taylor, G.L. Furie, L. Bronstein, J. Stenflo, and B. Furie. 2000. A conserved motif within the vitamin K-dependent carboxylase gene is widely distributed across animal phyla. *J Biol Chem* 275:36245–36249.

86. Oldenburg, J. and R. Schwaab. 2001. Molecular biology of blood coagulation. *Sem Thromb Hemostas* 27:313–324.

87. Bandyopadhyay, P.K. 2008. Vitamin K-dependent gamma-glutamylcarboxylation: An ancient posttranslational modification. In *Vitamin K*, ed. G. Litwack, 157–185. New York: Academic Press.

88. Czerwiec, E., G.S. Begley, M. Bronstein, J. Stenflo, K.L. Taylor, B.C. Furie, and B. Furie. 2002. Expression and characterization of recombinant vitamin K-dependent gamma-glutamyl carboxylase from an invertebrate, *Conus textile*. *Eur J Biochem* 269:6162–6172.

89. Li, T., C.-T. Yang, D. Jin, and D.W. Stafford. 2000. Identification of a *Drosophila* vitamin K-dependent gamma-glutamyl carboxylase. *J Biol Chem* 275:18291–18296.

90. Walker, C.S., R.P. Shetty, K. Clark, S.G. Kazuko, A. Letsou, B.M. Olivera, and P.K. Bandyopadhyay. 2001. On a potential global role for vitamin K-dependent gamma-carboxylation in animal systems. *J Biol Chem* 276:7769–7774.

91. Bandyopadhyay, P.K., K. Clark, B.J. Stevenson, J.E. Rivier, B.M. Olivera, K.G. Golic, and Y.S. Rong. 2006. Biochemical characterization of *Drosophila* gamma-glutamyl carboxylase and its role in fly development. *Insect Mol Biol* 15:147–156.

92. Schultz, J. 2004. HTTM, a horizontally transferred transmembrane domain. *Trends Biochem Sci* 29:4–7.

93. Rishavy, M.A., K.W. Hallgren, A.V. Yakubenko, R.L. Zuerner, K.W. Runge, and K.L. Berkner. 2005. The vitamin K-dependent carboxylase has been acquired by *Leptospira* pathogens and shows altered activity that suggests a role other than protein carboxylation. *J Biol Chem* 280:34870–34877.

94. Dowd, P., R. Hershline, S.W. Ham, and S. Naganathan. 1995. Vitamin K and energy transduction: A base strength amplification mechanism. *Science* 269:1684–1691.

95. Dowd, P., S.W. Ham, and S.J. Geib. 1991. Mechanism of action of vitamin K. *J Am Chem Soc* 113:7734–7743.

96. Dowd, P., S.W. Ham, and R. Hershline. 1992. Role of oxygen in the vitamin K-dependent carboxylation reaction: Incorporation of a second atom of ^{18}O from molecular oxygen $^{18}O_2$ into vitamin K oxide during carboxylase activity. *J Am Chem Soc* 114:7613–7617.

97. Kuliopulos, A., B.R. Hubbard, Z. Lam, I.J. Koski, B. Furie, B.C. Furie, and C.T. Walsh. 1992. Dioxygen transfer during vitamin K dependent carboxylase catalysis. *Biochemistry* 31:7722–7729.

98. Dowd, P., S.W. Ham, S. Naganathan, and R. Hershline. 1995. The mechanism of action of vitamin K. *Annu Rev Nutr* 15:419–440.

99. Davis, C.H., D. Deerfield II, T. Wymore, D.W. Stafford, and L.G. Pedersen. 2007. A quantum chemical study of the mechanism of action of vitamin K carboxylase (VKC). III. Intermediates and transition states. *J Mol Graph Model* 26:409–414.

100. Silva, P.J. and M.J. Ramos. 2007. Reaction mechanism of the vitamin K-dependent glutamate carboxylase: A computational study. *J Phys Chem B* 111:12883–12887.

101. Davis, C.H., D.D. Ti, D.W. Stafford, and L.G. Pedersen. 2007. Quantum chemical study of the mechanism of action of vitamin K carboxylase (VKC). IV. Intermediates and transition states. *J Phys Chem A* 111:7257–7261.

102. Morris, D.P., P.D. Stevens, D.J. Wright, and D.W. Stafford. 1995. Processive post-translational modification. Vitamin K-dependent carboxylation of a peptide substrate. *J Biol Chem* 270:30491–30498.

103. Stenina, O., B.N. Pudota, B.A. McNally, E.L. Hommema, and K.L. Berkner. 2001. Tethered processivity of the vitamin K-dependent carboxylase: Factor IX is efficiently modified in a mechanism which distinguishes Gla's from Glu's and which accounts for comprehensive carboxylation in vivo. *Biochemistry* 40:10301–10309.

104. Pudota, B.N., E.L. Hommema, K.W. Hallgren, B.A. McNally, S. Lee, and K.L. Berkner. 2001. Identification of sequences within the gamma-carboxylase that represent a novel contact site with vitamin K-dependent proteins and that are required for activity. *J Biol Chem* 276:46878–46886.

105. Lin, P.-J., D.L. Straight, and D.W. Stafford. 2004. Binding of the factor IX gamma-carboxyglutamic acid domain to the vitamin K-dependent gamma-glutamyl carboxylase active site induces an allosteric effect that may ensure processive carboxylation and regulate the release of carboxylated product. *J Biol Chem* 279:6560–6566.

106. Tie, J.-K., S.M. Wu, D. Jin, C.V. Nicchitta, and D.W. Stafford. 2000. A topological study of the human gamma-glutamyl carboxylase. *Blood* 96:973–978.

107. Berkner, K.L. 2005. The vitamin K-dependent carboxylase. *Annu Rev Nutr* 25:127–149.

108. Schmidt-Krey, I., W. Haase, V.P. Mutucumarana, D.W. Stafford, and W. Kuhlbrandt. 2007. Two-dimensional crystallization of human vitamin K-dependent gamma-glutamyl carboxylase. *J Struct Biol* 157:437–442.

109. Tie, J.K., M.Y. Zheng, K.L. Hsiao, L. Perera, D.W. Stafford, and D.L. Straight. 2008. Transmembrane domain interactions and residue proline 378 are essential for proper structure, especially disulfide bond formation, in the human vitamin K-dependent gamma-glutamyl carboxylase. *Biochemistry* 47:6301–6310.

110. Presnell, S.R. and D.W. Stafford. 2002. The vitamin K-dependent carboxylase. *Thromb Haemostas* 87:937–946.

111. Berkner, K.L. 2008. Vitamin K-dependent carboxylation. In *Vitamin K*, ed. G. Litwack, 131–156. New York: Academic Press.
112. Rishavy, M.A., B.N. Pudota, K.W. Hallgren, W. Qian, A.V. Yakubenko, J.-H. Song, K.W. Runge, and K.L. Berkner. 2004. A new model for vitamin K-dependent carboxylation: The catalytic base that deprotonates vitamin K hydroquinone is not Cys but an activated amine. *Proc Natl Acad Sci USA* 101:13732–13737.
113. Rishavy, M.A., K.W. Hallgren, A.V. Yakubenko, R.L. Shtofman, K.W. Runge, and K.L. Berkner. 2006. Bronsted analysis reveals Lys218 as the carboxylase active site base that deprotonates vitamin K hydroquinone to initiate vitamin K-dependent protein carboxylation. *Biochemistry* 45:13239–13248.
114. Rishavy, M.A. and K.L. Berkner. 2008. Insight into the coupling mechanism of the vitamin K-dependent carboxylase: Mutation of histidine 160 disrupts glutamic acid carbanion formation and efficient coupling of vitamin K epoxidation to glutamic acid carboxylation. *Biochemistry* 47:9836–9846.
115. Sun, Y.-M., D.-Y. Jin, R.M. Camire, and D.W. Stafford. 2005. Vitamin K epoxide reductase significantly improves carboxylation in a cell line overexpressing factor X. *Blood* 106:3811–3815.
116. Wajih, N., S.M. Hutson, J. Owen, and R. Wallin. 2005. Increased production of functional recombinant human clotting factor IX by baby hamster kidney cells engineered to overexpress VKORC1, the vitamin K 2,3-epoxide-reducing enzyme of the vitamin K cycle. *J Biol Chem* 280:31603–31607.
117. Hallgren, K.W., W. Qian, A.V. Yakubenko, K.W. Runge, and K.L. Berkner. 2006. r-VKORC1 expression in factor IX BHK cells increases the extent of factor IX carboxylation but is limited by saturation of another carboxylation component or by a shift in the rate-limiting step. *Biochemistry* 45:5587–5598.
118. Wajih, N., D.C. Sane, S.M. Hutson, and R. Wallin. 2004. The inhibitory effect of calumenin on the vitamin K-dependent gamma-carboxylation system. *J Biol Chem* 279:25276–25283.
119. Wajih, N., S.M. Hutson, and R. Wallin. 2006. siRNA silencing of calumenin enhances functional factor IX production. *Blood* 108:3757–3760.
120. Shah, D.V., J.K. Tews, A.E. Harper, and J.W. Suttie. 1978. Metabolism and transport of gamma-carboxyglutamic acid. *Biochim Biophys Acta* 539:209–217.
121. Matschiner, J.T., R.G. Bell, J.M. Amelotti, and T.E. Knauer. 1970. Isolation and characterization of a new metabolite of phylloquinone in the rat. *Biochim Biophys Acta* 201:309–315.
122. Bell, R.G. and J.T. Matschiner. 1972. Warfarin and the inhibition of vitamin K activity by an oxide metabolite. *Nature* 237:32–33.
123. Bell, R.G. and J.T. Matschiner. 1970. Vitamin K activity of phylloquinone oxide. *Arch Biochem Biophys* 141:473–476.
124. Sadowski, J.A. and J.W. Suttie. 1974. Mechanism of action of coumarins. Significance of vitamin K epoxide. *Biochemistry* 13:3696–3699.
125. Boyle, C.M. 1960. Case of apparent resistance of *Rattus norvegicus berkenhout* to anticoagulant poisons. *Nature* 188:517.
126. Lund, M. 1964. Resistance to warfarin in the common rat. *Nature* 203:778.
127. Zimmerman, A. and J.T. Matschiner. 1974. Biochemical basis of hereditary resistance to warfarin in the rat. *Biochem Pharmacol* 23:1033–1040.
128. Fasco, M.J., P.C. Preusch, E. Hildebrandt, and J.W. Suttie. 1983. Formation of hydroxy vitamin K by vitamin K epoxide reductase of warfarin-resistant rats. *J Biol Chem* 258:4372–4380.
129. Hildebrandt, E.F. and J.W. Suttie. 1982. Mechanism of coumarin action: Sensitivity of vitamin K metabolizing enzymes of normal and warfarin-resistant rat liver. *Biochemistry* 21:2406–2411.

130. Wallin, R., S.D. Patrick, and L.F. Martin. 1989. Vitamin K_1 reduction in human liver. *Biochem J* 260:879–884.

131. Fasco, M.J. and L.M. Principe. 1982. Vitamin K_1 hydroquinone formation catalyzed by DT-diaphorase. *Biochem Biophys Res Commun* 104:187–192.

132. Gong, X., R. Gutala, and A.K. Jaiswal. 2008. Quinone oxidoreductases and vitamin K metabolism. In *Vitamin K*, ed. G. Litwack, 85–101. New York: Academic Press.

133. Tie, J.-K. and D.W. Stafford. 2008. Structure and function of vitamin K epoxide reductase. In *Vitamin K*, ed. G. Litwack, 103–130. Academic Press: New York.

134. Hazelett, S.E. and P.C. Preusch. 1988. Tissue distribution and warfarin sensitivity of vitamin K epoxide reductase. *Biochem Pharmacol* 37:929–934.

135. Wilson, C.R., J.-M. Sauer, G.P. Carlson, R. Wallin, and M.P. Ward. 2003. Species comparison of vitamin K_1 2,3-epoxide reductase activity in vitro: Kinetics and warfarin inhibition. *Toxicology* 189:191–198.

136. Wallin, R. and S.M. Hutson. 2004. Warfarin and the vitamin K-dependent gamma-carboxylation system. *Trends Mol Med* 10:299–302.

137. Chu, P.-H., T.-Y. Huang, J. Williams, and D.W. Stafford. 2006. Purified vitamin K epoxide reductase alone is sufficient for conversion of vitamin K epoxide to vitamin K and vitamin K to vitamin KH_2. *Proc Natl Acad Sci USA* 103:19308–19313.

138. Rost, S., A. Frogin, V. Ivaskevicius, E. Conzelmann, K. Hortnagel, H.-J. Pelz, K. Lappegard, E. Seifried, I. Scharrer, E.G.D. Tuddenham, C.R. Muller, T.M. Strom, and J. Oldenburg. 2004. Mutations in VKORC1 cause warfarin resistance and multiple coagulation factor deficiency type 2. *Nature* 427:537–541.

139. Li, T., C.-Y. Chang, D.-Y. Jin, P.-J. Lin, A. Khvorova, and D.W. Stafford. 2004. Identification of the gene for vitamin K epoxide reductase. *Nature* 427:541–544.

140. Robertson, H.M. 2004. Genes encoding vitamin-K epoxide reductase are present in *Drosophila* and trypanosomatid protists. *Genetics* 168:1077–1080.

141. Tie, J.-K., C.V. Nicchitta, G. von Heijne, and D.W. Stafford. 2005. Membrane topology mapping of vitamin K epoxide reductase by in vitro translation/cotranslocation. *J Biol Chem* 280:16410–16416.

142. Lee, J.J. and M.J. Fasco. 1984. Metabolism of vitamin K and vitamin K 2,3-epoxide via interaction with a common disulfide. *Biochemistry* 23:2246–2252.

143. Gardill, S.L. and J.W. Suttie. 1990. Vitamin K epoxide and quinone reductase activities: Evidence for reduction by a common enzyme. *Biochem Pharmacol* 40:1055–1061.

144. Fasco, M.J., E.F. Hildebrandt, and J.W. Suttie. 1982. Evidence that warfarin anticoagulant action involves two distinct reductase activities. *J Biol Chem* 257:11210–11212.

145. Rost, S., A. Fregin, M. Hunerberg, C.G. Bevans, C.R. Muller, and J. Oldenburg. 2005. Site-directed mutagenesis of coumarin-type anticoagulant-sensitive VKORC1: Evidence that highly conserved amino acids define structural requirements for enzymatic activity and inhibition by warfarin. *Thromb Haemost* 94:780–786.

146. Jin, D.Y., J.K. Tie, and D.W. Stafford. 2007. The conversion of vitamin K epoxide to vitamin K quinone and vitamin K quinone to vitamin K hydroquinone uses the same active site cysteines. *Biochemistry* 46:7279–7283.

147. Johan, L., M. van Haarlem, B.A. Soute, and C. Vermeer. 1987. Vitamin K-dependent carboxylase. Possible role for thioredoxin in the reduction of vitamin K metabolites in liver. *FEBS Lett* 222:353–357.

148. Silverman, R.B. and D.L. Nandi. 1988. Reduced thioredoxin: A possible physiological cofactor for vitamin K epoxide reductase. Further support for an active site disulfide. *Biochem Biophys Res Commun* 155:1248–1254.

149. Preusch, P.C. 1992. Is thioredoxin the physiological vitamin K epoxide reducing agent? *FEBS Lett* 305:257–259.

150. Soute, B.A.M., M.M.C.L. Groenen-van Dooren, A. Holmgren, J. Lundstrom, and C. Vermeer. 1992. Stimulation of the dithiol-dependent reductases in the vitamin K cycle by the thioredoxin system. *Biochem J* 281:255–259.

151. Wajih, N., S.M. Hutson, and R. Wallin. 2007. Disulfide-dependent protein folding is linked to operation of the vitamin K cycle in the endoplasmic reticulum. *J Biol Chem* 282:2626–2635.

152. Oldenburg, J., C.G. Bevans, C.R. Muller, and M. Watzka. 2006. Vitamin K epoxide reductase complex subunit 1 (VKORC1): The key protein of the vitamin K cycle. *Antioxidants & Redox Signaling* 8:347–353.

153. Oldenburg, J., M. Watzka, S. Rost, and C.R. Muller. 2007. VKORC1: Molecular target of coumarins. *J Thromb Haemost* 5(Suppl 1):1–6.

154. Silverman, R.B. 1981. Chemical model studies for the mechanism of vitamin K epoxide reductase. *J Am Chem Soc* 103:5939–5941.

155. Preusch, P.C. and J.W. Suttie. 1983. A chemical model for the mechanism of vitamin K epoxide reductase. *J Org Chem* 48:3301–3305.

156. Deerfield D. II, C.H. Davis, T. Wymore, D.W. Stafford, and L.G. Pedersen. 2006. Quantum chemical study of the mechanism of action of vitamin K epoxide reductase (VKOR). *Int J Quantum Chem* 106:2944–2952.

157. Davis, C.H., D. Deerfield II, T. Wymore, D.W. Stafford, and L.G. Pedersen. 2007. A quantum chemical study of the mechanism of action of vitamin K epoxide reductase (VKOR) II. Transition states. *J Mol Graph Model* 26:401–408.

158. Gebauer, M. 2007. Synthesis and structure-activity relationships of novel warfarin derivatives. *Bioorg Med Chem* 15:2414–2420.

159. Wallin, R., D.C. Sane, and S.M. Hutson. 2003. Vitamin K 2,3-epoxide reductase and the vitamin K-dependent gamma-carboxylation system. *Thrombosis Res* 108:221–226.

5 Vitamin K-Dependent Proteins

5.1 HOW EXTENSIVE ARE VITAMIN K-DEPENDENT PROTEINS?

The number of clearly defined vitamin K-dependent proteins is not large (Table 5.1), but new proteins continue to be found. Following the discovery of Gla residues in 1974, it was quickly shown that this posttranslational modification was present in the other previously known vitamin K-dependent proteins (F VII, F IX, and F X) and subsequently in the other plasma proteins involved in some aspect of hemostasis. The first vitamin K-dependent protein not related to blood coagulation, osteocalcin, was discovered by 1976, and within 10 years of the discovery of Gla this modified Glu residue was found in a toxic peptide present in the venom of the *Conus* snail. Although Gla residues have not been found in plants or in single-celled organisms, new vitamin K-dependent proteins or peptides continue to be characterized, and it is likely that these reports will continue.

5.2 VITAMIN K-DEPENDENT CLOTTING FACTORS

5.2.1 ROLE OF VITAMIN K-DEPENDENT PROTEINS IN HEMOSTASIS

The vitamin K-dependent plasma clotting factors are components of a complex system of proteins whose function is that of normal hemostasis, the absence of either a hemorrhagic or thrombotic event. Prothrombin was a recognized plasma protein at the time that vitamin K was discovered, and it was demonstrated [1,2] that the activity of a crude prothrombin preparation was decreased when it was obtained from the plasma of a vitamin K-deficient chick. Initially, it was widely believed that the defect in the plasma of animals fed vitamin K-deficient diets was due solely to a lack of plasma prothrombin. However, the "whole blood clotting times" and the one-stage "Quick prothrombin time" assays used at that time were not specific for prothrombin and any crude preparation of prothrombin would also have contained other vitamin K-dependent clotting factors. It is not surprising, therefore, that it was some time before it was established that an increased concentration of prothrombin alone would not cure the coagulation defect resulting from a lack of vitamin K. A real understanding of the various factors involved in regulating the generation of thrombin from prothrombin did not begin until the early 1950s; and during the next 5 to 10 years factor VII [3,4], factor X [5], and factor IX [6,7] were discovered and subsequently shown to be dependent on vitamin K for their synthesis. The concentration of these proteins in plasma differs substantially; prothrombin is present

TABLE 5.1

Identified Vitamin K-Dependent Proteins

Hemostasis Related Plasma Proteins	Proteins Isolated from Bone
Prothrombin (F II)	Osteocalcin
Factor VII	Matrix Gla protein
Factor IX	–
Factor X	**Other Characterized Proteins**
Protein C	Gas6
Protein S	Periostin
Protein Z	Vitamin K-dependent carboxylase
	Transthyretin
	Gla-Rich Protein
Transmembrane Proteins	**Poisonous Venom**
Proline-rich Gla Protein-1	Many *Conus* peptides
Proline-rich Gla Protein-2	Some snake venoms
Transmembrane Gla Protein-3	**Proteins Produced by Urochordates**
Transmembrane Gla Protein-4	*C. intestinalis* proteins
	H. roretzi protein

at a concentration of about 100 μg/ml, factors IX and X at less than 10 μg/ml, and factor VII at less than 1 μg/ml.

These proteins were discovered by clinicians as altered gene products responsible for rare genetic diseases. That is, investigators discovered that normal plasma would cure a clotting defect in the plasma of a patient with a previously undescribed clotting disorder. As might be expected, different research groups independently discovered and named the same factor, causing a great deal of confusion in the literature. In an effort to unify the literature, a standing International Committee for the Nomenclature of Blood Clotting Factors was established in 1954. Actions of this group during a meeting in 1958 [8] led to the current practice [9] of using Roman numerals to designate the majority of the factors involved in blood coagulation. The very interesting historical developments involved in the identification of the proteins making up the complex system of blood coagulation have been reviewed in some detail [10–12]. Some of the more common terms previously associated with the vitamin K-dependent clotting factors are indicated in Table 5.2.

The four procoagulant proteins listed in Table 5.2, which were discovered by the mid-1950s, had been collectively called the "vitamin K-dependent clotting factors" for 25 years before Stenflo [13] discovered a fifth vitamin K-dependent plasma protein, now called protein C. This discovery followed the realization that the distinguishing feature of vitamin K-dependent proteins was the presence of γ-carboxyglutamyl residues formed by a posttranslational modification during their synthesis (see Chapter 4). The protein was identified as a contaminant following chromatography of a crude preparation of bovine prothrombin on DEAE-sephadex. The protein in peak C from this column was shown to contain γ-carboxyglutamic acid residues

TABLE 5.2

Synonyms and Former Terminology Used for the Historical "Vitamin K-Dependent Clotting Factors"

Factor	Other Nomenclature
II	Prothrombin
VII	Proconvertin, serum prothrombin conversion accelerator (SPCA), stable factor, autoprothrombin I
IX	Plasma thromboplastin component (PTC), Christmas factor, antihemophilic factor B, platelet cofactor II, autoprothrombin II
X	Stuart-Prower factor

Note: Fibrinogen (F-I) and calcium (F-IV) are no longer designated by Roman numerals. F-III and F-VI have been found not to designate specific proteins. F-V, F-VIII, and factors XI, XII, and XIII have functions related to coagulation but are not vitamin K-dependent.

and to be immunochemically distinct from the known vitamin K-dependent proteins. A sixth vitamin K-dependent plasma protein, protein S (discovered in Seattle) was identified by DiScipio and Davie [14] in much the same manner during the isolation of human factor IX and factor X. In an attempt to subfractionate a factor X preparation, Mattock and Esnouf [15] isolated a protein first thought to be a single-chain form of factor X, which was subsequently shown [16] to be a new protein and called protein Z.

The basis for an understanding of the roles of the multitude of factors that appeared to be involved in the ultimate conversion of circulating fibrinogen to a fibrin clot came with the understanding that many of the clotting factors were protease zymogens that could be activated by other specific proteases. These activated factors could activate still other zymogens by a complex series of reactions that were independently termed a "waterfall sequence" by Davie and Ratnoff [17] or an "enzyme cascade—functioning as a biochemical amplifier" by Macfarlane [18] in the early 1960s. These early theories of the activation of prothrombin to form the active fibrinogen-cleaving protease, thrombin, were correct in their basic hypothesis but obviously lacked a great deal of the complexity currently known to be involved. The key step in the ultimate formation of the fibrin clot is the generation of thrombin from prothrombin by the activated form of factor X (factor Xa). The other two classical vitamin K-dependent clotting factors, factors VII and IX, are involved in the activation of factor X. The enzymology of these events has been well described [19], and the history of our current understanding of these hemostatic events has been reviewed [20].

The remaining vitamin K-dependent plasma proteins are not procoagulant zymogens, but do have important hemostatic actions. Protein C in plasma is activated by endothelial cell contact [21], and it has been demonstrated that a specific membrane protein, thrombomodulin, is responsible for the activation of protein C by thrombin [22]. Activated protein C can inactivate factor Va [23,24] and factor VIIIa [25], and this protein therefore plays an inhibitory rather than a procoagulant role in the overall balance of events [26]. Protein S has been demonstrated [24] to influence the rate of in vitro inactivation of factor Va by activated protein C, and it was later demonstrated [27] that activated protein C and protein S form a specific complex [28] on a phospholipid surface. Protein C partially exists in plasma as a high-molecular-weight complex with the complement component, C4b-binding protein [29]. Plasma also contains a protein S-binding protein that modulates the rate of factor Va inactivation by protein S and activated protein C [30]. These two proteins are key factors in limiting the extent of thrombosis that will occur when clotting is initiated [31–33]. The role of protein Z in coagulation was not apparent for some time, but it has now been demonstrated that its interaction with a protein Z-dependent protease inhibitor [34] can regulate coagulation [35] and that genetic alterations in these two proteins can influence thrombotic risk [36–38]. The involvement of vitamin K-dependent proteins in hemostasis is only a portion of a very complex system of vascular biology. A simplified view of the action of these proteins in the generation of a fibrin clot is shown in figure 5.1. A number of recent extensive reviews of this process are available [39–42]. The data to support the action of these proteins in generating a thrombus has been largely obtained by in vitro studies, although it is now clear that cellular involvement is important when thrombotic events occur in vivo [43–45].

5.2.2 Pathway of Prothrombin Activation

The complex series of reactions illustrated in Figure 5.1 culminates in the generation of an active serine protease, thrombin, which is able to carry out the conversion of circulating fibrinogen to a fibrin clot. The activation of prothrombin is catalyzed by the activated form of factor X (X_a) and occurs in a complex (the prothrombinase complex) composed of prothrombin, factor X_a, factor V_a, an acidic phospholipid surface, and Ca^{++} [46,47]. The activation of factor X by factor IX in the presence of factor VIII_a, and the action of factor VII_a to convert factor X to factor X_a in the presence of tissue factor have similar properties. The activation of prothrombin has been most extensively studied, both as a model for these types of interactions and in an effort to understand the enzymology involved in the rapid generation of thrombin from its zymogen.

Early studies concentrated on the identification of the peptide cleavage products that resulted from the action of factor X_a on prothrombin. These studies were carried out in a number of laboratories, utilized mainly SDS-PAGE techniques to follow the time course of proteolysis of prothrombin, and have been adequately reviewed [19,48]. These studies identified the factor X_a-dependent cleavage sites and were complicated by the fact that the end product of the action of the complex was thrombin, which could also cleave some of the products generated. It was subsequently established [49,50] that only fragment 1–2 and the transient intermediate, prethrombin 2, resulted from the action of factor X_a; and the other products that could be seen on SDS gels, fragment-1, fragment-2, and another intermediate, prethrombin 1, were the result of the action of thrombin (Figure 5.2). Although these studies were important in establishing the pathway of coagulation factor zymogen activation, interest eventually shifted to efforts to understand very complex Ca^{++}-dependent interactions of substrates, proteases, and cofactors on a membrane surface that both promote and

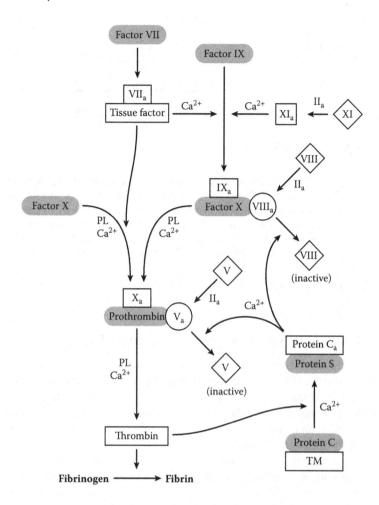

FIGURE 5.1 Action of the plasma proteins involved in the formation of a fibrin clot. The vitamin K-dependent procoagulants (grey ovals) are zymogens of the serine proteases; pro-thrombin, F-VII, F-IX, and F-X. Coagulation is initiated when they are converted to their active (subscript a) forms. This process can be initiated by an "extrinsic" pathway when vascular injury exposes the transmembrane protein, tissue factor, to blood. This cascade effect results in the rapid activation of prothrombin to thrombin and the subsequent conversion of soluble fibrinogen to the insoluble fibrin clot. The generation of thrombin involves an active protease (X_a), a second vitamin K-dependent protein substrate (prothrombin), and an additional plasma protein cofactor (factor V_a) (circles) to form a Ca^{2+}-mediated association with a phospholipid surface. When bound to tissue factor, factor VII is activated to VII_a which activates factor X to X_a and forms the prothrombinase complex, which generates thrombin. The formation of activated F-X can also occur through an "intrinsic" pathway involving thrombin activation of F-XI and subsequently F-IX to form a complex with factor VII_a, factor X, and a phospholipid surface. Two other vitamin K-dependent proteins participate in hemostatic control as anticoagulants, not procoagulants. Protein C is activated by thrombin (II_a) in the presence of an endothelial cell protein called thrombomodulin (TM). Protein C is then able to function in a complex with protein S to inactivate V_a and VIII_a and to limit clot formation.

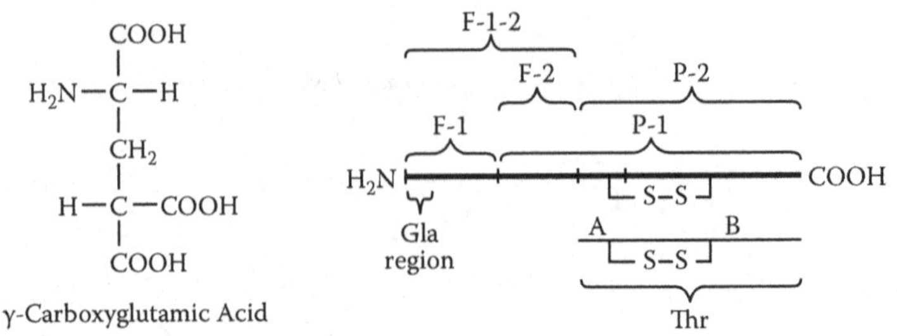

COOH
|
H₂N—C—H
|
CH₂
|
H—C—COOH
|
COOH

γ-Carboxyglutamic Acid

F-1-2
F-2   P-2
F-1   P-1
H₂N ⎡   ⎤ COOH
                 S–S
Gla   A   B
region   S–S
                    Thr

FIGURE 5.2 Structure of γ-carboxyglutamic acid (Gla) and a diagramatic representation of the prothrombin molecule. Specific proteolysis of prothrombin by factor X_a and thrombin will cleave prothrombin into the specific large peptides shown: fragment 1 (F-1), fragment 2 (F-2), fragment 1-2 (F-1-2), prethrombin 1 (P-1), prethrombin 2 (P-2), and thrombin (thr). The Gla residues in bovine prothrombin are located at residues 7, 8, 15, 17, 20, 21, 26, 27, 30, and 33, and they occupy homologous positions in the other vitamin K-dependent plasma proteins.

retard clot formation. The current understanding of these interactions has been well reviewed [39–42,51–54].

5.2.3 STRUCTURE OF VITAMIN K-DEPENDENT CLOTTING FACTORS

The vitamin K-dependent plasma proteins are a group of structurally related glycoproteins that represent less than 0.5% of the total plasma protein pool. Their distinguishing feature is the presence of from 9 to 13 γ-carboxyglutamate (Gla) residues in an amino-terminal domain. The majority of these proteins are zymogen forms of a serine protease, and a number contain a second posttranslational modified amino acid residue, γ-hydroxyaspartate.

The presence of the Gla domain and the structural homology of these proteins proved to be both an advantage and disadvantage in efforts to purify the vitamin K-dependent proteins. Early attempts to purify the most abundant of these proteins, prothrombin, by the classical techniques of protein fractionation were aided by the observation that this protein would strongly adsorb to a number of insoluble Ba and Mg salts, and by the late 1930s, it was possible to obtain a prothrombin preparation from oxalated bovine plasma [55] that may well have contained 25% to 50% prothrombin. Modification and extension of classical techniques of protein purification subsequently enabled investigators to obtain preparations of prothrombin that were "pure" by the standards of protein chemistry available in the late 1940s and early 1950s. The close homology of different members of this class of proteins assured, however, that these preparations were contaminated to varying degrees with the other vitamin K-dependent clotting factors. The development of protein chromatography techniques in the 1950s and 1960s eventually led to the isolation of not only prothrombin but also the other vitamin K-dependent proteins. These preparations were pure enough to be used in studies of the enzymatic activity of the clotting factors and could be used for amino acid sequencing. Specific references to the purification of the various vitamin K-dependent clotting factors are available in comprehensive reviews [19,56] and procedures for the isolation of these proteins by conventional techniques are readily available [57]. Methods utilizing immunoaffinity columns have been described [58], and the methods used to obtain the various vitamin K-dependent plasma proteins for therapeutic purposes have been reviewed [59]. Reversed-phase HPLC has also been used [60] for both identification and purification of vitamin K-dependent plasma proteins.

Early partial amino acid sequence data indicated a great deal of homology in the amino-terminal, Gla-containing region of the vitamin K-dependent proteins, and the complete amino acid sequence of prothrombin was determined by Magnusson and coworkers [61]. Because of the small quantities of material available, determination of the primary sequence of the other vitamin K-dependent proteins represented a formidable task in protein chemistry. Beginning in the early 1980s it became clear that the primary sequence of these proteins could be more easily obtained by utilizing the tools of moelcular biology than through protein sequencing. Our current understanding of the amino acid sequence of the vitamin K-dependent proteins is, therefore, based on both direct peptide sequencing and, particularly in the case of the human forms, an analysis of the cDNA structure. These data, presented in Table 5.3, indicate the close structural homology of the amino–terminal, Gla-containing region

---

TABLE 5.3

Amino Acid Sequence of the "Gla" Domain of the Human Plasma Vitamin K-Dependent Proteins Involved in Hemostasis

Protein									Sequence							
+1									+10							
F-II	Ala	Asn	Thr	-	Phe	Leu	**Gla**	**Gla**	Val	Arg	Lys	Gly	Asn	Leu	**Gla**	Arg
F-X	Ala	Asn	Ser	-	Phe	Leu	**Gla**	**Gla**	Met	Lys	Lys	Gly	His	Leu	**Gla**	Arg
F-IX	Tyr	Asn	Ser	Gly	Lys	Leu	**Gla**	**Gla**	Phe	Val	Gln	Gly	Asn	Leu	**Gla**	Arg
F-VII	Ala	Asn	Ala	-	Phe	Leu	**Gla**	**Gla**	Leu	Arg	Pro	Gly	Ser	Leu	**Gla**	Arg
P-C	Ala	Asn	Ser	-	Phe	Leu	**Gla**	**Gla**	Leu	Arg	His	Ser	Ser	Leu	**Gla**	Arg
P-S	Ala	Asn	Ser	-	Leu	Leu	**Gla**	**Gla**	Thr	Lys	Gln	Gly	Asn	Leu	**Gla**	Arg
+20									+30							
F-II	**Gla**	Cys	Val	**Gla**	**Gla**	Thr	Cys	Ser	Tyr	**Gla**	**Gla**	Ala	Phe	**Gla**	Ala	Leu
F-X	**Gla**	Cys	Met	**Gla**	**Gla**	Thr	Cys	Ser	Tyr	**Gla**	**Gla**	Ala	Arg	**Gla**	Val	Phe
F-IX	**Gla**	Cys	Met	**Gla**	**Gla**	Lys	Cys	Ser	Phe	**Gla**	**Gla**	Ala	Arg	**Gla**	Val	Phe
F-VII	**Gla**	Cys	Lys	**Gla**	**Gla**	Gln	Cys	Ser	Phe	**Gla**	**Gla**	Ala	Arg	**Gla**	Ile	Phe
P-C	**Gla**	Cys	Ile	**Gla**	**Gla**	Ile	Cys	Asp	Phe	**Gla**	**Gla**	Ala	Lys	**Gla**	Ile	Phe
P-S	**Gla**	Cys	Ile	**Gla**	**Gla**	Leu	Cys	Asn	Lys	**Gla**	**Gla**	Ala	Arg	**Gla**	Val	Phe
+40																
F-II	**Gla**	Ser	Ser	Thr	Ala	Thr	Asp	Val	Phe	Trp	Ala	Lys	Tyr			
F-X	**Gla**	Asp	Ser	Asp	Lys	Thr	Asn	**Gla**	Phe	Trp	Asn	Lys	Tyr			
F-IX	**Gla**	Asn	Thr	**Gla**	Arg	Thr	Thr	**Gla**	Phe	Trp	Lys	Gln	Tyr			
F-VII	Lys	Asp	Ala	**Gla**	Arg	Thr	Lys	Leu	Phe	Trp	Ile	Ser	Tyr			
P-C	Gln	Asn	Val	Asp	Asp	Thr	Leu	Ala	Phe	Trp	Ser	Lys	His			
P-S	**Gla**	Asn	Asp	Pro	**Gla**	Thr	Asp	Tyr	Phe	Tyr	Pro	Lys	Tyr			

of these proteins. In addition to a homologous Gla domain, prothrombin, factor X, factor IX, factor VII, and protein C share a serine protease domain containing the reactive serine and neighboring histidine and aspartate residues first identified in pancreatic digestive enzymes such as trypsin, chymotrypsin, and elastase. This serine protease homology is shared with the non-vitamin K-dependent proteins of the plasma coagulation system, kallikrein, and factors XI and XII, as well as plasmin and plasmin activators of the fibrin lytic systems [62]. Protein Z contains a pseudo (inactive) serine protease domain.

The availability of the complete sequence of the primary gene product of all of the vitamin K-dependent proteins has provided information on sequence homologies which were not previously apparent. Prothrombin contains two "Kringle" domains. These looped sequences, named [61] for their resemblance to the Danish pastry (Figure 5.3), are also found in the zymogen of the major enzyme of fibrinolysis, plasminogen and its activators, urokinase, and tissue plasminogen activator, but not in the other vitamin K-dependent clotting factors. With the exception of prothrombin, the plasma vitamin K-dependent clotting factors also contain one or more epidermal growth factor (EGF) precursor-like domains, and protein S contains a thrombin sensitive region (TSR) and a sex hormone binding globulin (SHGB) domain [63]. The basic structural composition of the vitamin K-dependent plasma proteins is illustrated in Figure 5.4. A second posttranslational modification of vitamin K-dependent proteins, the β-hydroxylation of aspartyl residues, was first described in protein C [64] and factor X [65]. It was subsequently shown [66] that both β-hydroxyaspartate and β-hydroxyasparagine are found in the EGF domains of protein S and that this posttranslational modification is also involved in the Ca^{++}-binding properties of these proteins [67,68]. The plasma coagulation factors have complex structures and in addition to γ-carboxylation of Glu residues and β-hydroxylation of Asp and Asn, they are subject to O and N glycosylation, Tyr sulfation, and Ser phosphorylation [69].

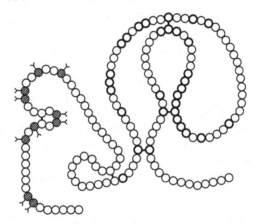

FIGURE 5.3 Structural relationship of the Gla domain and first Kringle domain of prothrombin.

The physiological importance of the vitamin K-dependent plasma proteins and their purification by the early 1960s resulted in efforts to obtain their tertiary structure by x-ray crystallography. The proteins are relatively large, contain a significant

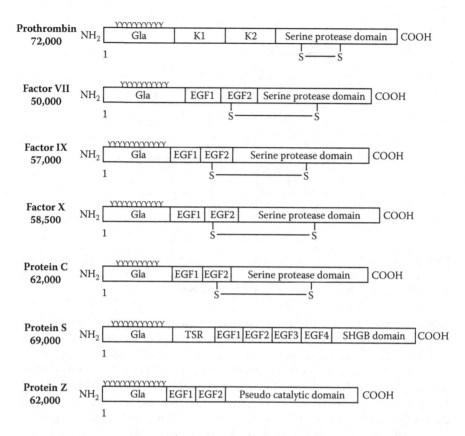

FIGURE 5.4 Structural domains of the vitamin K-dependent plasma procoagulants and thrombus inhibitors. All of the proteins contain an amino-terminal Gla domain followed by Kringle domains (K) in the case of prothrombin, or epidermal growth factor-like domains (EGF) in the other proteins. Protein S also contains a thrombin sensitive region (TSR) and a sex hormone binding globulin domain (SHGB). For additional detail, see Reference [266].

amount of carbohydrate, and strongly defracting crystals were difficult to obtain. Initial efforts centered on prothrombin were directed toward obtaining the structure of fragment 1 (residues 1–156) of bovine prothrombin. A low-resolution model [70], which did not allow the detailed location of individual amino acids, was obtained by 1982, and Park and Tulinsky [71] subsequently obtained a 2.8-Å resolution structure of this amino–terminal, Kringle-containing fragment. Additional studies have generated structures of this fragment that have been crystallized in the presence of Ca^{++} ions and show the location of the Gla residue to a resolution of 2.25 Å [72,73]. These structures (Figure 5.5) show a concentration of the Gla residues on a single face of the molecule and indicate that calcium ions are needed to stabilize this configuration of the structure. Although the original efforts to obtain high-resolution structures of the vitamin K-dependent plasma proteins were centered on prothrombin, crystal structures of factor VII, factor IX, factor X, and protein S are now available [74,75].

As structural information obtained through cDNA sequencing became available, it was revealed that the primary gene product of the vitamin K-dependent proteins

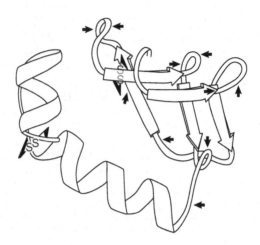

FIGURE 5.5 Ribbon drawing of the folding conformation of the Gla domain of prothrombin fragment 1. Gla residues which are present at residues 7, 8, 15, 17, 20, 21, 26, 27, 30, 33 are identified by an arrow. For details see Reference [73].

contains a basic amino acid-rich "propeptide" between the signal peptide region of the primary gene product and the amino-terminal end of the plasma form of the protein. These observations suggest that this homologous amino-terminal extension, which is cleaved prior to secretion into plasma, might play an important role in the recognition of these proteins by the microsomal carboxylase. The physiological importance of this region was soon confirmed by the demonstration that effective carboxylation of constructs of factor IX [76] or protein C [77] expressed in mammalian cell lines is dependent on the presence of a native propeptide region. It has also been shown [78] that a 20-residue peptide containing the octadeca propeptide of human factor X strongly stimulates the activity of the rat liver vitamin K-dependent carboxylase toward a low-molecular-weight peptide substrate, suggesting that this region of the vitamin K-dependent protein serves both a regulatory and recognition function. Relatively minor alterations in the propeptide structure of the various vitamin K-dependent proteins have a major influence on their affinity for the carboxylase (see Chapter 4) and can influence the utilization of the substrate pool available to this enzyme.

The genes for prothrombin [79,80], factor IX [81,82], factor X [83], factor VII [84,85], and protein C [86,87] have been characterized by DNA sequence analysis, and the similarities of their structures have been reviewed [88,89]. The relationship between factors VII, IX, X, and protein C are much closer than the relationship of this group to prothrombin. Although they all share strong similarities in the exon coding for the Gla and preproleader regions, they definitely diverge to two families downstream of the Gla exon. Not only does prothrombin contain three exons coding for the two Kringle regions rather than the EGF coding exons, but differences exist in the remainder of the gene. The serine protease (thrombin) region of prothrombin is coded for by five different exons which do not share homology in terms of intron sites with the factor IX family.

5.2.4 ASSAYS FOR VITAMIN K-DEPENDENT CLOTTING FACTORS

The first attempts to quantify a decrease in activity of one or more of the vitamin K-dependent clotting factors utilized what would now be called a "whole blood clotting time." Blood was drawn into a clean glass tube or porcelain dish, and the time required to clot was measured. The results were variable and greatly dependent on how the blood was drawn. By the mid-1930s [90] it was realized that plasma would not clot if Ca^{++} was complexed with an organic acid such as oxalate and that the time required for a clot to form after the addition of calcium to plasma could be standardized if a lung or brain extract (thromboplastin) which provided phospholipids and tissue factor was added. This assay was largely developed by Armand Quick [2,91] at the Marquette University Medical School and came to be called the "prothrombin time" or "Quick prothrombin time." Variations of this assay have been developed, and commercial reagent kits are available. Because of the presence of tissue extract, factor IX is bypassed, and the assay responds to the level of prothrombin and factors VII and X. Of these, factor VII has the shortest half-life, and its concentration decreases earliest when vitamin K action is impaired. It is likely therefore that these one-stage prothrombin assays often measure the level of factor VII rather than prothrombin. The classic "two-stage" prothrombin assay [92] was developed in the Brinkhaus laboratory at the University of Iowa, and is more specific for prothrombin. In this assay, thrombin is generated from prothrombin in one tube, and a portion of this tube is added to fibrinogen in a second tube to measure the amount of thrombin. As the procedure is somewhat tedious, it has seldom been used to assess vitamin K status. A number of snake venom preparations will liberate thrombin from prothrombin and have been used [93–95] to develop one-stage clotting assays that are more specific for prothrombin. The venoms in these preparations do not require that prothrombin be present in a calcium-dependent phospholipid complex for activation, and they will therefore activate the descarboxyprothrombin formed in vitamin K-deficient animals. For this reason they cannot be used to monitor a vitamin K deficiency.

These classical methods depend on measurements of the rate of formation of a fibrin clot as an endpoint; and, as there is not a linear relationship between the amount of prothrombin in plasma and the change in clotting rate, they are rather insensitive. Because of this relative lack of sensitivity, these historical clotting factor assays have had little value in determining vitamin K status. These assays are, however, used to monitor the large population of patients receiving oral anticoagulant therapy (see Chapter 7). As the actual clotting time measured by a Quick prothrombin time varies substantially with the sensitivity of the thromboplastin preparation used, the clotting times are converted to an International Normalized Ratio (INR) which corrects for this variation. These assays have historically required a blood draw and a laboratory-based assay, but in many cases [96] they now utilize portable coagulometers which use only a finger prick of blood taken by visiting nurses or by patients in their own homes. As the vitamin K-dependent clotting factors are serine proteases, chromogenic substrates can also be used to assay their activity. These assays, when utilized to assay prothrombin activity, actually measure the concentration of thrombin that has been generated from prothrombin by various methods [94]. There is a very comprehensive history of blood

coagulation written by Owen [12] which details the development of assays for prothrombin and for the other vitamin K-dependent clotting factors, and a historical
review of the development of assays for the measurement of thrombin generation
has also been recently published by Hemker [97].

5.2.5   Genetic Variants of Vitamin K-Dependent Clotting Factors

The pathway of thrombin generation from prothrombin followed by the formation
of a fibrin clot and the activation of platelets are the keys to normal hemostasis, the
lack of a thrombotic or hemorrhagic event. The bleeding risk associated with classical hemophilia (hemophilia A) is due to the lack of production of normal amounts
of F VIII or to the secretion of a genetically altered, less active form of this non-
vitamin K-dependent clotting factor. About 15% of patients with hemophilia suf-
fer from the loss of activity of the vitamin K-dependent protein F IX (hemophilia
B). As the genes for both proteins are on the X chromosome, with few exceptions,
only males are affected. Treatment of hemophilia utilizes concentrates of F VIII or
F IX which are obtained by purification from plasma, or recombinant technology.
Another relatively common bleeding disorder, von Willibrand disease, is caused by
decreased amounts or genetic variants of von Willibrand's factor, another plasma
protein not requiring vitamin K for its synthesis. This factor is required for normal
platelet adhesion to collagen and for transport of F VIII. The disease is treated with
plasma concentrates of von Willebrand's factor.

Some type of venous thrombosis affects a substantial fraction (~0.1%) of the
population each year, and these events are triggered by acquired (disease related)
factors or by genetic risk. A recent report [98] has identified nearly 1,000 mutations in the vitamin K-dependent plasma proteins, and many of them do represent
an altered phenotype. The most common risk factor for thrombotic event is a single
point mutation of the F V gene which decreases the ability of vitamin K-dependent
protein C to inactivate F V [32] and to shut down the normal thrombotic pathway.
Inherited deficiencies of the vitamin K-dependent clotting factors which would lead
to bleeding episodes other than F IX (hemophilia B) are relatively rare (Table 5.4)
but have been identified [99-101]. Deficiencies of F II (prothrombin), F VII, and F
X have been reported at a prevalence of from 1:500,000 to 1:2,000,000, and protein
C and protein S mutations have also been shown to impact the homeostatic balance. Although the vitamin K-dependent protein Z is not directly involved in the
generation of thrombin, a serpin that inhibits activated F X and F IX is dependent
on protein Z for its activity. Genetic alterations of this protein Z-dependent protease
inhibitor have been shown to increase the risk for venous thrombosis [36,38,102].

Mice heterozygous for a null mutation of the vitamin K-dependent carboxylase
appear normal and exhibit normal activities of the vitamin K-dependent clotting
factors [103]. However, the homozygous offspring resulting from intercrossing these
mice yields a phenotype characterized by embryonic loss of most fetuses and loss of
the others due to intraabdominal hemorrhage shortly after birth. Single point mutations of the carboxylase would also be expected in some cases to result in a combined deficiency of all of the vitamin K-dependent clotting factors, and a very small
number of patients with this disorder have been reported [104,105]. The severity

TABLE 5.4
Relative Frequency of Inherited Deficiencies of Vitamin K-Dependent Clotting Factors

Factor	Estimated Frequency
F VIII[a]	1:10,000
F IX[b]	1:50,000
F VII	1:500,000
F II	1:2,000,000
F X	1:1,000,000

[a] Hemophilia A (not vitamin K-dependent).
[b] Hemophilia B.
Source: Adapted from Reference [99].

of the clotting defect associated with this disorder varies widely and in some cases administration of large amounts of vitamin K will partially correct the symptoms. The first reported case of this combined deficiency [106,107] was subsequently shown to be the result of a mutated carboxylase, as were most of the cases that have been described. However, a defect in the vitamin K epoxide reductase has also been found to result in a similar phenotype [104,108]. As the gene structure of the vitamin K-dependent carboxylase is known, the specific location of the mutation responsible for the lowered clotting factor activity can be identified, and recombinant forms of the carboxylase can be produced in mammalian cell cultures and their activity studied to determine the basis for the lack of activity. There are substantial variations in the specific site of mutations studied, and although the three-dimensional structure of the carboxylase is not yet known, binding to the propeptide region of the substrate, binding of the reduced vitamin K substrate, or alterations in the catalytic action of the carboxylase have all been suggested as the molecular basis for the observed phenotypes [109–112]. A single point mutation of the carboxylase of Rambouillet sheep has also been identified [113] as the cause of a multi-clotting factor deficiency responsible for the death of newborn lambs through hemorrhage.

Patients being treated for hemophilia with plasma-derived F VIII or F IX concentrations often develop antibodies to these proteins, which inhibit the activity of the infused proteins and have an increased risk of viral transmission. An alternative therapy for hemophilia is the use of recombinant F VIII or F IX produced by mammalian cell culture techniques [114,115], and adverse events related to their use have been decreased through changes in the formulation of the products [116,117]. Two other vitamin K-dependent proteins have also been used as therapeutic drugs. The recombinant form of activated F VII (rVIIa) has been used as replacement therapy for the rare cases of F VII deficiency [118] and has been shown to be effective in treating hemophilia A and B patients who developed high levels of antibodies toward F IX or F VIII [119–121]. This preparation has also been found to be effective in nonhemophilia patients with various other bleeding disorders [122,123] and in treating severely injured trauma patients [124]. The other vitamin K-dependent protein that has been used therapeutically is rPC. During the generation of thrombin the activated form of protein C decreases the thrombotic response by cleaving and inactivating F V and F VIII. Protein C also has an anti-inflammatory action [125,126], and it has been used to treat patients with severe sepsis [127–129].

The lifetime need for therapy by hemophilia patients has led to serious attempts to develop a gene therapy approach to treating this disease. Gene transfer has been successfully demonstrated in animal models such as factor IX knockout mice or dogs with spontaneous hemophilia A or B, and sustained expression of these clotting factors at a level of 5% to 10% of normal have been demonstrated. A limited number of trials with small numbers of human subjects have failed to demonstrate specific expression of these proteins or only transient expression [130–132]. Although the potential for gene therapy is great, many obstacles remain before this approach will reach clinical practice [133,134].

5.2.6 Abnormal (des-γ-Carboxy) Vitamin K-Dependent Clotting Factors

The unique structural feature of the vitamin K-dependent clotting factors is the presence of γ-carboxyglutamyl residues. The eventual discovery of this amino acid (see Chapter 4) was based on the observation that, at least in some species, blockage of this posttranslational modification resulted in the secretion of a protein that lacked or had decreased biological activity. In 1963 Hemker [135] utilized a complex clotting assay to first postulate the existence of a biologically inactive prothrombin in the plasma of human patients receiving anticoagulant therapy. A few years later, a protein that was antigenically similar to prothrombin but lacked biological activity was demonstrated in the plasma of anticoagulant-treated patients by Ganrot and Nilehn [136], and a biologicaly inactive "abnormal prothrombin" species in these patients was detected through the use of staphylocoagulase to generate thrombin by the Josso group [137]. A form of prothrombin lacking biological activity was soon demonstrated in the plasma of anticoagulant-treated bovine by Stenflo [138], but substantial amounts of this protein were not found in every species following anticoagulant treatment. Only a small amount of an inactive form of rat prothrombin can be found in anticoagulant-treated or vitamin K-deficient rats [139], and it has been reported [93] that this protein appeared to be missing in plasma from anticoagulant-treated mice, hamsters, guinea pigs, rabbits, and dogs.

The basis for the secretion of incompletely carboxylated clotting factors in some species and not in others appears to be a function of the structure of the proteins, and their rate of degradation within the endoplasmic reticulum, rather than some underlying difference in the way these proteins are processed in different species. In cultured rat hepatoma cells, prothrombin secretion is decreased by 90% in the presence of warfarin, and the intracellular uncarboxylated precursor pool is rapidly degraded [140]. When rat prothrombin is stably transfected into warfarin-treated human hepatoma cells, undercarboxylated human prothrombin is secreted into the media, but rat prothrombin is not [141], indicating that whether or not under-γ-carboxylated prothrombin is secreted or degraded is related to a structural difference in the two proteins. Subsequent studies [142] have demonstrated that it is the small differences in the amino acid sequence of the first of the two Kringle domains of rat and human prothrombin that determine if the protein will be degraded within the endoplasmic reticulum or be secreted.

In addition to the reports of biologically inactive forms of prothrombin in bovine and human plasma after anticoagulant treatment, there is evidence of similar inactive forms of the other vitamin K-dependent clotting factors. Hemker, Muller, and Loeliger [143] first identified these proteins as "Proteins Induced by Vitamin K Absence or Antagonists (PIVKA)," and they have been referred to by many investigators as PIVKA-II (abnormal prothrombin), PIVKA-X (abnormal factor X), etc. The functional defect in these proteins is the inability of prothrombin lacking Gla residues to participate in a calcium-mediated interaction with a negatively charged phospholipid surface during the generation of thrombin [144] and the response observed is related to the degree of under-γ-carboxylation [145]. Multiple forms of the abnormal prothrombin exist in the plasma of the anticoagulant-treated bovine and by utilizing a technique of differential absorption to barium citrate, barium oxalate, or alumina gel, it has been possible to isolate plasma prothrombin preparations that contain 7, 5, 2, or 1 Gla residues per mole [146]. The amount of these inactive forms of plasma prothrombin can be measured by comparing the amount of thrombin generated by physiological activation to that generated by specific snake venoms, or by electrophoresis-immunofixation, or immunoassay [147]. Commercial kits that can be used to assay PIVKA-II by the latter method are now available, and the epitopes lacking the Gla sites needed for a positive reaction have been identified [148].

Current interest in these partially carboxylated forms of the vitamin K-dependent proteins lies in their use as a sensitive assay to detect a mild deficiency of vitamin K (see Chapter 8) or as a marker for hepatocellular carcinoma (HCC). The available data suggest that the commercial kits available to immunochemically measure serum des-γ-carboxy-prothrombin (DCP) provide a more sensitive and specific measure to differentiate patients with HCC from those with cirrhosis or chronic hepatitis than does measurement of another widely used marker, α-fetoprotein [149–151]. There is some evidence that a decrease in expression of the carboxylase itself may also play a role in the secretion of DCP in patients with hepatocellular carcinoma [152–154]. It has been established that DCP is also produced by apparently normal hepatocytes surrounding the tumor [155,156], and DCP has been shown to be an autologous mitogen for cultured HCC [157,158]. The impact of these findings on the development of HCC has, however, not been established.

5.3 VITAMIN K-DEPENDENT PROTEINS FOUND IN SKELETAL TISSUE

5.3.1 OSTEOCALCIN

The first report of the presence of Gla residues in proteins other than the vitamin K-dependent clotting factors was the discovery of this amino acid in a protein solubilized from chick bones by Hauschka, Lian, and Gallup [159]. A similar protein was independently demonstrated to be present in bones from a number of vertebrates by Price and colleagues [160], and this group subsequently sequenced [161] the bovine form of the protein. Much of the early research in this area was carried out by groups led by Lian, Price, or Hauschka, and extensive reviews of the early progress in this field are available [162–165]. Depending on the laboratory of the author, early publications referred to the protein as bone Gla protein (BGP) or osteocalcin, but the latter is the term most used at the present time.

Following the determination of the structure of bovine osteocalcin, this protein was isolated and sequenced from a number of other vertebrates (for citations of primary literature, see [163, 166,167]. The osteocalcins identified from various species were small, 49 or 50 amino acid residue proteins with 3 Gla residues and a short disulfide loop between residues 23 and 29 (Figure 5.6). The high degree of homology present in vertebrates extends to the osteocalcin of swordfish [168] which diverged from terrestrial vertebrates about 400 million years ago. Because of interest in the evolution of calcified tissue, the full or partial sequences of the osteocalcin from 28 species are available [169]. The search has extended to osteocalcin obtained from Neanderthal fossils [170], which is identical to that of modern humans. The Gla residues are typically located at positions 17, 21, and 24, although it appears that human osteocalcin is often under-γ-carboxylated at position 17 [171] and that in a teleost fish an additional Gla residue is present [166]. Osteocalcin is present in relatively high amounts in most vertebral species, where it represents 15% to 20% of the noncollagenous bone protein [164], although it is much lower in human skeletal tissue. Osteocalcin is also found in dentine, and although it can be found in areas of ectopic calcification, there is no evidence to suggest that it is produced in any soft tissue. It is a weak Ca^{++}-binding protein, but has a high affinity for hydroxyapatite. These properties are lost when Gla-deficient osteocalcin is produced in a vitamin K-deficient animal or when the Gla residues are decarboxylated to leave Glu residues at these positions within the molecule [172]. Early attempts to determine the three-dimensional structure of the protein through spectral analysis [173] indicated that the interaction with calcium led to the formation of a "Gla helix" in the central portion of the molecule where all of the Gla residues were on the same face of the α-helix with a spacing between them that was similar to the interatomic lattice spacing of calcium in the

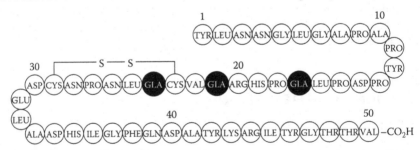

FIGURE 5.6   Amino acid structure of mature osteocalcin.

hydroxyapatite crystal. More recent studies utilizing NMR [174] and x-ray crystal structure analysis [166,175] have confirmed and extended previous models to show a charged protein surface utilizing the Gla residues to coordinate five Ca^{++} atoms in a spatial orientation that is complementary to the calcium ions in the hydroxyapatite crystal lattice.

Although osteocalcin is the second most abundant protein in bone, it has been difficult to clearly define its function. Because of its interaction with Ca^{++} in solution and its affinity for hydroxyapatite, the initial assumption appeared to be that it was in some way related to a promotion of calcification. Synthesis of osteocalcin by osteoblasts is stimulated by $1,25\text{-}(OH)_2D_3$ [176,177], and osteocalcin that lacks Gla residues does not accumulate in bone. In an attempt to produce animals with a very low content of skeletal osteocalcin, Price and colleagues [178,179] developed a rat protocol utilizing a high dose of the anticoagulant warfarin that prevented osteocalcin γ-carboxylation along with sufficient vitamin K to allow the hepatic synthesis of sufficient active clotting factors to prevent hemorrhage. This response suggests that the vitamin K quinone reductase which can drive Gla production in liver is not active in the osteoblast. Weanling rats placed on this feeding protocol for six weeks had only 2% as much osteocalcin in bone as the controls, but the length, weight, or total mineral content of the bones was indistinguishable from the controls. However, by eight months of age, a fusion of the tibia growth plate, which does not normally calcify, was evident in the warfarin-treated rats. These studies suggest that the role of osteocalcin is not to promote matrix calcification, but rather to in some manner control the process. This view is supported by the demonstration in the Karsenty laboratory [180] that the phenotype of an osteocalcin "knockout" mouse is marked by higher bone mass and the deposition of bone that has improved functional qualities. The molecular basis for this response has not yet been established.

Osteocalcin is also found in plasma and can be quantitated by radioimmunoassay [181]. Circulating osteocalcin is thought to be that fraction of the synthesized protein that does not associate with the hydroxyapatite of newly mineralized sites in an amount that decreases from childhood to maturity. It can be easily measured by radioimmunoassay, and commercial kits to assay its concentration are available. The absolute values reported tend to vary with differences in epitope specificity [182], which vary with the manufacturer of the kit. As its secretion by osteoblasts would suggest, osteocalcin concentrations are elevated in those metabolic bone diseases that are characterized by increased bone turnover, such as Paget disease, bone metastases, and hyperparathyroidism [163,164,183]. Its value as a marker of potential osteoporotic fracture is less sound. The extent of under-γ-carboxylation of osteocalcin has been widely used (see Chapter 7) as an indicator of vitamin K status [184]. There are commercial kits available that measure the amount of des-γ-carboxyosteocalcin immunochemically, but most reports define the fraction of the total osteocalcin that will not bind to hydroxyapatite as des-γ-carboxyosteocalcin. This is an approach with considerable problems [185].

5.3.2 MATRIX GLA PROTEIN

Osteocalcin is readily solubilized when bone powder is extracted in the presence of chelating agents, but early studies of this protein indicated that it was not the only protein present in bone [186,187], and that substantial amounts of non-osteocalcin Gla were also found in cartilage. The second protein tended to self-associate in solution and could only be solubilized in 4 to 6 M guanidine hydrochloride or other denaturing agents. This protein was isolated [188] and sequenced [189] from bovine bone by Price and colleagues and was named matrix Gla protein (MGP). It contains Gla residues at positions 2, 37, 41, 48, and 52 (Figure 5.7) of the 79 amino acid residues of human and bovine protein. As MGP is secreted by both vascular smooth muscle cells and chondrocytes, it is much more widely distributed in the body than osteocalcin. The structures of MGP from a large number of vertebrates, including mammals, amphibians, and cartilagenous and bony fish are available through direct sequencing, cloning, or genome searches [169]. The structure of MGP has many similarities to osteocalcin, and current studies of the evolution of these vitamin K-dependent proteins [169] suggest that the genes for MGP and osteocalcin originated before the evolution of jawless and jawed fish, with MGP appearing as cartilagenous structures emerged. Osteocalcin was apparently derived from MGP and appeared with the development of bony structures. Although initially isolated from bone, MGP has been shown to be expressed in various tissues with a high level of expression in vascular smooth muscle cells.

As with osteocalcin, the metabolic role of MGP has been difficult to clearly define. The demonstration by the Karsenty laboratory [190,191] that mice lacking the gene for MGP developed a spontaneous calcification of arteries and cartilage established its role in regulating the calcification process. The importance of MGP in regulation of mineralization has also been indicated by the finding that Keutel syndrome, a rare human autosomal recessive condition that leads to midfacial hypoplasia and ectopic abnormal calcification, is associated with mutations in the MGP gene [192,193]. Vascular calcification appears to be a passive event that will occur in the absence of functional inhibitors [194], and it

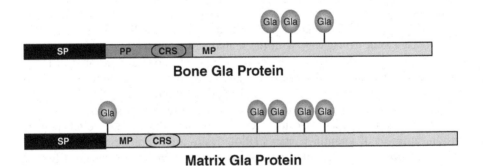

FIGURE 5.7 Structural organization of osteocalcin (BGP) and matrix Gla protein (MGP). The signal peptide (SP), propeptide (PP), mature protein (MP), and the carboxylase recognition site (CRS) are indicated. For details see Reference [169].

has been possible to demonstrate calcification of the elastic lamellae in arteries and heart valves in a rat model utilizing high doses of warfarin and sufficient vitamin K to prevent hemorrhage [195]. In addition to the presence of Gla residues, the ability of MGP to decrease the calcification of monolayer cultures of human vascular smooth muscle cells is also dependent on phosphorylation of specific serine residues in the amino-terminal region of the protein [196]. It has also been shown that in a rat model where the extent of γ-carboxylation of MGP was decreased by warfarin administration, aortic calcification was enhanced [197] but the degree of calcification regressed when warfarin was subsequently removed from the ration and the amount of dietary vitamin K was increased. Some MGP does circulate in serum, but raising the serum level of MGP through increased liver expression of MGP does not influence extracellular matrix mineralization such as is seen in atherosclerotic lesions [198]. Restoration of MGP expression in arteries of MGP knockout mice will, however, rescue the arterial mineralization of that phenotype. Although the role of MGP in preventing ectopic calcification is well established, the mechanism or mechanisms involved in this response are less definitive.

A number of possible roles for MGP have been summarized [199,200]. One early view was that by binding Ca^{++} in the form of small crystals in tissues, these crystals could be removed from the tissue site to prevent further mineralization. Clear evidence for this role is not available, and more current studies have shown that MGP is able to bind to and inactivate bone morphogenic protein-2 (BMP-2) and BMP-4 [201–203]. This response would be expected to prevent or reduce the osteo-inductive effects of bone morphogenic proteins on the vessel wall. Both the ability of MGP to bind to matrix components vitronectin and elastin and its possible influence on apoptosis of vascular smooth muscle cells have also been suggested as possible MGP-related events that might be involved in ectopic calcification. There are a number of genes that are known to be involved in extracellular matrix mineralization [204], and it appears that MGP may be involved in a number of situations leading to ectopic calcification. Pseudoxanthroma elasticum is a multisystem heritable disorder that leads to ectopic mineralization of soft connective tissues. Utilization of a transgenetic mouse model has shown that this mutation leads to a decrease in serum MGP, a substantial increase in the extent of undercarboxylated MGP, and an increase in connective tissue calcification [205]. The data obtained from these cellular and animal model studies has resulted in a great deal of interest in the possible impact of low intakes of vitamin K in the human population to cardiovascular disease. The results of these studies [206] have not provided consistent support for this hypothesis. They are discussed in Chapter 7.

5.4 VITAMIN K-DEPENDENT PROTEINS AND PEPTIDES IN VENOMS

5.4.1 CONUS SNAIL VENOMS

Following the discovery of the vitamin K coagulation factors, osteocalcin and MGP, a number of Gla-containing peptides were discovered in an unlikely source. The venom of the predatory cone snail (genus *Conus*) contains a very large number of physiologically active peptides which are unique in their extent of posttranslational modification and differ in their mode of lethal action. Most are proteolytically generated from propeptides, contain a disulfide bridge, and contain a number of modified amino acids, including hydroxyproline, hydroxy-valine, hydroxylysine, bromotryptophan, and sulfotyrosine. Many also contain epimerized amino acids and have amidated C-terminal residues [207]. Gla resi-dues were first identified in these toxic peptides by Olivera in a peptide called conatoxin-G [208] and have subsequently been demonstrated (Table 5.5) in venom obtained from a number of *Conus* species [207,209–211]. A large num-ber of Gla-containing peptides have been characterized by the Olivera and Furie laboratories, and these efforts have been recently reviewed by Bandyopadhyay [212]. The physiological role of the Gla residues appears not to be related to the molecular interactions between the mature folded peptide and its physiologi-cal target, but rather in promoting the biologically relevant disulfide configura-tion needed to form the active peptide through the action of protein disulfide

---

TABLE 5.5

Examples of Gla-Containing Peptides from Various Families of the *Conus* Snail

Conantokin	
Conantokin-G (Con-G)	GEγγLQγNQγLIRγKSN#
Conantokin-T	GEγγYQKMLγNLRγAEVKKNA#
Superfamily-T	
GlaMrIII	FCCRTQγVCCγAIKN#
GlaMrIV	CCITFγSCCγFDL
Superfamily-O	
Gla(1)-TxVI	MWGγCKDGLTTCLOPS-γCCSγDCγGS-CTMU
Gla(3)-TxVI	LCODYTγOCSHAH-γCCSUNCYNGHTCTG
de7a	ACKOKNNLCAITγMAγCCSGFCLIYRCS#
TxVIIA	CGGYSTYC-γ-VDS-γ-CCSDNCVRSYCTLF#
Tx-Rapid runner	CKTYSKYC-γADS-γCCTγQCVRSYCTLF#
Superfamily-A	
Vcla	GCCSDORCNYDHPγIC#
GID	IRDγCCSNPACRVNNOHVC
G-Scratcher	
	KFLSGGFKγIVCHRYCAKGIAKEFCNCPD#

Note: γ = Gla residues; # = C-terminal amidation; for an extended list of Gla-containing peptides isolated from *Conus* snails see a recent review of this research by Brandyopadhyay [212].

isomerase within the high Ca^{++} lumen of the endoplasmic reticulum [213]. The vitamin K-dependent carboxylase from the *Conus* snail has been shown to have similar properties to the mammalian enzyme [214], and the precursor form of the conotoxin substrates contains an amino-terminal "propeptide" sequence that promotes specificity by recognizing the carboxylase (see Chapter 4). However, the precursor of a Gla-containing conotoxin with a carboxy-terminal rather than an amino-terminal recognition site has been identified [215], and a large (~30 kDa) secretory protein from another *Conus* species has been shown to contain a single Gla residue and no obvious γ-carboxylation recognition site [216]. The number of physiologically active peptides produced by and localized in the venom of the *Conus* snail is very large and the subset of these which are subjected to a vitamin K-dependent modification continues to enlarge as additional examples are characterized [217,218].

5.4.2 SNAKE VENOMS

Proteins containing Gla residues have also been found in the venom of poisonous snakes. These proteins were shown to have functional and physiochemical properties similar to the activated form of coagulation factor X and were subsequently demonstrated to contain Gla residues [219,220]. More detailed studies have shown that the primary structure of these proteins (Table 5.6), including the Gla domain, is very similar to factor X [221,222]. The presence of Gla-containing proteins as toxic components of snake venoms is not widespread, and a screening of the venom from 21 snake species with a monoclonal antibody specific for protein-bound Gla residues found a positive response in only four species, all from a single subfamily [223].

TABLE 5.6

Examples of Gla-Containing Vitamin K-Dependent Proteins from Urochordates and Snakes

Source	Peptide or Amino-Terminal Protein Sequence
	Urochordates
C. intestinalis Ci-Gla 1	KNSWHHFγγAQQGNIγRγCIγγVCSWγγARγA-
Ci-Gla 2	ANSWLRFγγFQPGNIγRγCγγγRCSRγγARγA-
Ci-Gla 3	ANSGF-γγFAKGNFγQγCVγγICNYγγLRγV-
Ci-Gla 4	SNRGFVLγγFSPGNQγRγCVγγICNYγγAFγIS-
H. roretzi Gla-RTK	ANTASHFγγIQQGNIγRγCYγγLCSFγγARγV-
	Snakes
Tiger snake venom	SNSLFγγIRPGNIγRγCIγγKCSKγγARγV-
Human FX_a	ANSFLγγMKKGHLγRγCMγγTCSYγγARγV-

Note: γ = γ-carboxyglutamate; for details see References [222,252,253].

5.5   OTHER VITAMIN K-DEPENDENT PROTEINS

5.5.1   Gas6

In addition to those vitamin K-dependent proteins involved in hemostasis or present in bone, other circulating mammalian proteins have been found to be vitamin K-dependent. A number of genes are known to be involved in the upregulation of mammalian cells that are undergoing growth arrest, and the first of these identified was called the "growth arrest specific gene 6" [224]. The protein product of this gene (Gas6) was subsequently shown to be Gla-containing, vitamin K-dependent, and over 40% homologous to protein S [225] (Figure 5.8). Both proteins contain a Gla domain typical of the other vitamin K-dependent clotting factors, followed by four epidermal growth factor (EGF)-like repeats and a C-terminal domain that is homologous to a sex hormone binding globulin (SHBG) domain [226–228]. The action of growth factors is mediated through their interaction with a receptor tyrosine kinase (RTK). These are transmembrane proteins that interact extracellularly with a wide variety of ligands to trigger signal transduction within the cell by activating tyrosine kinase activity [229]. There are a large number of RTKs, and they have been divided into 20 distinct subfamilies based on amino acid sequence identities and structural similarities in the extracellular region of the receptor. The first demonstration of a physiological role for Gas6 was as a ligand for the Axl subfamily of RTKs [230] which also includes Sky and Mer.

Activation of these tyrosine kinases can lead to a large number of responses, and Gas6 has been reported to be related to a wide range of cellular alterations. These cover changes that would be protective in the face of cellular stress, stimulation of cell migration, or cell–cell adhesion, promotion of foam cell formation, phygocytosis of apoptotic cells, and the proliferation of vascular smooth muscle cells. In some cases, similar responses can be seen with protein S, but at a substantially higher concentration. The various responses to Gas6 that have been demonstrated in cellular systems or in animal models have been reviewed extensively [226,228,231–233]. A specific portion of the SHBG region of both Gas6 and protein S has been shown to be the site on the molecule that is needed to bind to the RTK receptors [234,235]. The Gla domain is not directly involved in this interaction, but the interaction of the Gla domain of Gas6 with phosphatidylserine-containing phospholipid membranes clearly points to its function. Studies utilizing cultured cells [236–238] or animal models [239] carried out in the presence of warfarin have shown that the anticipated Gas6 response is lacking, and that the Gla domain is essential to maintain the activity of native Gas6.

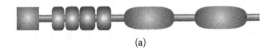

(a)

FQVFγγAKQGHLγRγCVγLCSRγγARγVFγNDPγTDYFY–

(b)

FIGURE 5.8   Structural aspects of Gas6. (a) Schematic representation of the Gas6 molecule with an amino-terminal Gla domain followed by a sequence of four epidermal growth factor-like domains and two laminin A chains, which are similar to a sex hormone binding globulin. (b) Amino acid sequence of the Gla domain of Gas6.

5.5.2 TRANSMEMBRANE GLA PROTEINS

Two proline-rich Gla proteins (PRGP-1, PRGP-2) were initially discovered [240] as transmembrane proteins with an extracellular amino-terminal domain that is rich in Gla residues and closely related to the Gla domain of prothrombin (Table 5.7). Two other members of this transmembrane Gla protein family (TMG-3 and TMG-4) were subsequently cloned [241]. The specifics of the role of these apparent cell-surface receptors are not yet known, but the structures of the proteins suggest that they might be involved in signal transduction in response to extracellular phosphatidylserine exposures. One of these proteins, PRGP-2, has been demonstrated to be located on the cell surface with the Gla domain, which binds to a known extracellularly exposed transcriptional coactivator [242].

TABLE 5.7
Gla Domains of Vitamin K-Dependent Transmembrane Proteins

Proline-rich Gla Protein-1	ANGF-FγγIRQGNIγRγCKγγFCTFγγARγAFγNNγKTKγFWST-
Proline-rich Gla Protein-2	ANHWDLγLLTPGNLγRgCLγγRCSWγγARγYFγDNTLTERFWES-
Transmembrane Gla Protein-3	AN--EFLγγLRQGTIγRγCMγγICSYγVKγVFγNKγKTMγFW-
Transmembrane Gla Protein-4	LLYNRFDLγLFTPGNLγRγCNγγLγNYγγARγIFVDγDKIAFW-

5.5.3 PERIOSTIN

A third Gla-containing protein synthesized in bone has been identified more recently [243]. The protein was found when the proteins secreted by bone marrow-derived mesenchymal stromal cells (MSCs) were subjected to a proteomics search. The proteins were separated by two-dimensional SDS-PAGE, screened by an anti-Gla immunoplot, and identified by tandem mass spectrometry. The mass spectral analysis of the trypsin digest of the proteins of interest yielded sufficient sequence data to identify the Gla-containing protein as a previously known protein, periostin, an extracellular matrix associated protein known to promote cell migration and angiogenesis [244–246]. The protein is composed of four fascilin-like [247] domains each containing a number of Gla residues and a region homologous to known carboxylase recognition sites. The metabolic role of periostin is not known, but it has been found [243] to associate with the calcified matrix produced by osteoblasts and to be deposited on bone nodules produced in vitro. It has also been found that periostin null mice were grossly normal at birth but that ~15% of the null mice died before weaning and the remaining were severely growth retarded [244]. These mice also showed severe enamel defects and developed a phenotype associated with early onset periodontal disease. The need for periostin to be fully γ-carboxylated to show its protective effect on these responses has not been demonstrated.

5.5.4 VITAMIN K-DEPENDENT CARBOXYLASE

The carboxylase itself has been shown by Berkner [248] to be a substrate for the carboxylase, and the enzyme present in cells from vitamin K-replete animals was shown to be carboxylated at three sites. The effect of this modification on the activity or specificity of the carboxylase is not yet known. Carboxylation does appear to increase the rate of turnover of this protein in cultured cells, but the effect of this posttranslational modification on the rate of release of substrates from the enzyme or the control of processivity during the carboxylation of multi Gla proteins has not been determined.

5.5.5 TRANSTHYRETIN

The plasma retinol and thyroxin-binding protein transthyretin has recently been reported [249] to be a Gla-containing protein. A single Gla residue of this 127 amino acid protein was identified following two-dimensional electrophoresis and tandem mass spectrum analysis of a protease-generated peptide of this protein. The role of this vitamin K-dependent modification of transthyretin is not known.

5.5.6 GLA-RICH PROTEIN

A recent report by Price [250] has described a previously unknown Gla containing protein found in calcified cartilage. This protein which has been named Gla-rich protein (GRP) has been identified in numerous mammals, amphibians, reptiles, and fish. There is no significant sequence homology between GRP and the Gla region of other vitamin K-dependent proteins. The metabolic role of the protein has not been identified.

5.5.7 OTHER GLA-CONTAINING PROTEINS

Proteins containing Gla domains have now been demonstrated to be present in invertebrates. Genomic screening of puffer fish [251] has identified orthologs of clotting factors VII and IX, and a novel Gla protein has been identified [252] in a tunicate, *Halocynthia roretzi*. This protein, called Gla-RTK, has a Gla domain typical of the vitamin K-dependent clotting factors, a transmembrane domain, and a receptor tyrosine kinase domain (Table 5.6). The Gla and receptor tyrosine kinase domains are highly homologous to the receptive domains of Gas6 and Axl, but the function of this gene product is not yet known. The sequencing of cDNAs from another chordate, the sea squirt (*C. intestinalis*), has identified four proteins with typical Gla domains, including Gla-RTK [253]. These findings are of particular interest in regard to the evolutionary development of the vitamin K-dependent carboxylation reaction as a posttranslational protein modification. As the evolutionary emergence of the urochordates occurred tens of millions of years before the emergence of vertebrates, it is clear that these Gla-containing proteins had currently unknown functions and that use of this domain was later adopted to function in the complex pathway of vertebral hemostasis. Although much of the current knowledge of these putative proteins is based on genetic analysis, a 16-amino-acid peptide derived from a protein related to insulin has been identified in the sea slug and shown by the techniques of modern mass spectrometry to contain a single Gla residue [254].

5.5.8 POSSIBLE GLA PROTEINS

Following the discovery of osteocalcin in the mid-1970s and matrix Gla protein in the mid-1980s, there were a number of reports of the discovery of Gla-containing proteins in other mineralized tissues or in pathologically calcified tissues. These proteins were not extensively characterized, and their relationship to osteocalcin or matrix Gla protein or to fragments of these proteins is not clear. A protein shown to inhibit calcium oxalate crystal growth in human urine [255] has been isolated from bovine kidney tissue and characterized [256] as a 14,000 kDa Gla-containing glycoprotein which is present in four isoforms, but little additional data are available.

A calcium-binding protein has been identified in organ cultures of the chorioallantoic membrane (CAM) of chick embryos, and it has been demonstrated that the ability of this protein to transfer calcium from the shell to the embryo was dependent on vitamin K [257]. This protein was purified and characterized as a high-molecular-weight (M_r = ~100,000) protein with specific calcium-binding sites and a number of Gla residues [258]. Following homogenization of the CAM, the microsomal fraction was shown to support a vitamin K-dependent incorporation of $^{14}CO_2$ into proteins present in the microsomal preparation, and fixed CO_2 was shown to be in Gla residues [259]. When the protein was subjected to denaturation in SDS and dithiothreitol and subjected to gel electrophoresis it migrated as a single band of 22,000 to 25,000 molecular weight, suggesting that the native protein was composed of four subunits of equal size. The amino acid sequence or location of the Gla residues has not been reported.

There have also been reports of specific Gla-containing proteins in liver mitochondria [260], kidney [261], spermatozoa, and a number of other sources [262,263]. Data sufficient to characterize them as unique Gla-containing proteins were never obtained, and there is little evidence of attempts to determine if they were specific vitamin K-dependent proteins by utilizing Gla-specific antibodies or modern proteomics techniques.

5.6 CURRENT STATUS OF RESEARCH EFFORTS

The number of firmly established vitamin K-dependent proteins is not large but has been found to be rather diverse. Some of the earlier claims of additional proteins lacked sufficient data to be included in a list of known Gla proteins, but it is possible that a reassessment of these proteins with newer techniques might yield a definitive claim. There has been no uniformity in the metabolic role promoted by the known Gla proteins, and it appears that the role of the posttranslational modification of a Glu residue is to bring two proteins together or to bring them adjacent on a phospholipids-containing membrane. Attempts to find proteins with Gla residues in single-celled organisms or in plants have failed, but as negative attempts do not get published, it is difficult to determine how much effort has been put into this direction.

The early efforts to find new vitamin K-dependent proteins through the genomic search for homology to a known Gla domain or to a carboxylase recognition site had some success, but it is now clear that there are multiple types of these proteins and that it is not easy to determine what homologies should be sought. It seems very interesting that the two most recent Gla-containing proteins that have been discovered, periostin and transthyretin, were proteins with a known metabolic role that had been studied for some time before they were known to be vitamin K-dependent. In both cases, application of mass-spectrometry proteomics was involved. With the large expansion of proteomics research in recent years, there appears to be a real possibility that some additional Gla proteins will be found by this approach. The vitamin K-dependent carboxylase is present in *Drosophila*, and this enzyme will carboxylate Glu-containing substrates. However, no Gla-containing proteins have been found in this organism. Whether Gla-containing products of this enzyme exist within *Drosophila* and have not been found or if they are not present is not known. It is also possible that the active carbanion generated by the carboxylase is used for a different purpose which might or might not modify the structure of some protein. If so, it is unlikely that an individual modified protein will be found until the product of the new reaction being performed is identified.

It does seem likely that additional Gla-containing proteins will continue to be identified. It is also likely that they will not be found by restricting the amount of vitamin K in the diet of humans or laboratory animals. The lack of the observation of adverse side effects in the huge population of warfarin-treated patients would suggest that if there are vitamin K-dependent proteins not yet identified, the amount of the presumed Gla-containing form needed is very small. The only Gla-containing proteins that have been discovered in this manner were the plasma clotting factors.

REFERENCES

1. Dam, H., F. Schonheyder, and E. Tage-Hansen. 1936. Studies on the mode of action of vitamin K. *Biochem J* 30:1075–1079.
2. Quick, A.J. 1937. The coagulation defect in sweet clover disease and in the hemorrhagic chick disease of dietary origin. A consideration of the source of prothrombin. *Am J Physiol* 118:260–271.
3. Owen, Jr, C.A., T.B. Magath, and J.L. Bollman. 1951. Prothrombin conversion factors in blood coagulation. *Am J Physiol* 166:1–11.
4. Koller, F., A. Loeliger, and F. Duckert. 1951. Experiments on a new clotting factor (factor VII). *Acta Haematol* 6:1–18.
5. Hougie, C., E.M. Barrow, and J.B. Graham 1957. Stuart clotting defect. I. Segregation of an hereditary hemorrhagic state from the heterogeneous group heretofore called "stable factor" (SPCA, proconvertin, factor VII) deficiency. *J Clin Invest* 36:485–496.

6. Aggeler, P.M., S.G. White, M.B. Glendening, E.W. Page, T.B. Leake, and G. Bates. 1952. Plasma thromboplastin component (PTC) deficiency: A new disease resembling hemophilia. *Proc Soc Exp Biol Med* 79:692–694.

7. Biggs, R., A.S. Douglas, R.G. Macfarlane, J.V. Dacie, W.R. Pitney, C. Merskey, and J.R. O'Brien. 1952. Christmas disease. A condition previously mistaken for haemophilia. *Brit Med J* ii:1378–1382.

8. Monroe, D.M., M. Hoffman, and H.R. Roberts. 2007. Fathers of modern coagulation. *Thromb Haemost* 98:3–5.

9. Wright, I.S., 1962. Nomenclature of blood clotting factors. *Thrombos Diathes haemorrh* 7:381–388.

10. Giangrande, P.L.F. 2003. Six characters in search of an author: The history of the nomenclature of coagulation factors. *Brit J Haematol* 121:703–712.

11. Roberts, H.R. 2007. Memories of a senior scientist. Contributions to the evolution of knowledge about hereditary hemorrhagic disorders. *Cell Mol Life Sci* 64:517–521.

12. Owen, Jr, C.A. 2001. In *A History of Blood Coagulation*, ed. W.L. Nichols and E.J.W. Bowie. Rochester, MN: Mayo Foundation for Medical Education & Research.

13. Stenflo, J. 1976. A new vitamin K-dependent protein. Purification from bovine plasma and preliminary characterization. *J Biol Chem* 251:355–363.

14. DiScipio, R.G. and E.W. Davie. 1979. Characterization of protein S, a gamma-carboxyglutamic acid containing protein from bovine and human plasma. *Biochemistry* 18:899–904.

15. Mattock, P. and M.P. Esnouf. 1973. A form of bovine factor X with a single polypeptide chain. *Nature New Biol* 242:90–92.

16. Prowse, C.V. and M.P. Esnouf. 1977. The isolation of a new warfarin-sensitive protein from bovine plasma. *Biochem Soc Trans* 5:255–256.

17. Davie, E.W. and O.D. Ratnoff. 1964. Waterfall sequence for intrinsic blood clotting. *Science* 145:1310–1312.

18. Macfarlane, R.G. 1964. Haematology. An enzyme cascade in the blood clotting mechanism, and its function as a biochemical amplifier. *Nature* 202:498–499.

19. Jackson, C.M. and Y. Nemerson. 1980. Blood coagulation. *Annu Rev Biochem* 49:765–811.

20. Davie, E.W. 2003. A brief historical review of the waterfall/cascade of blood coagulation. *J Biol Chem* 278:50819–50832.

21. Owen, W.G. and C.T. Esmon. 1981. Functional properties of an endothelial cell cofactor for thrombin-catalyzed activation of protein C. *J Biol Chem* 256:5532–5535.

22. Esmon, N.L., W.G. Owen, and C.T. Esmon. 1982. Isolation of a membrane-bound cofactor for thrombin-catalyzed activation of protein C. *J Biol Chem* 257:859–864.

23. Kisiel, W., W.M. Canfield, L.H. Ericsson, and E.W. Davie. 1977. Anticoagulant properties of bovine plasma protein C following activation by thrombin. *Biochemistry* 16:5824–5831.

24. Walker, F.J., P.W. Sexton, and C.T. Esmon. 1979. The inhibition of blood coagulation by activated protein C through the selective inactivation of activated factor V. *Biochim Biophys Acta* 571:333–342.

25. Vehar, G.A. and E.W. Davie. 1980. Preparation and properties of bovine factor VIII (antihemophilic factor). *Biochemistry* 19:401–410.

26. Clouse, L.H. and P.C. Comp. 1986. The regulation of hemostasis: The protein C system. *New Engl J Med* 314:1298–1304.

27. Walker, F.J. 1981. Regulation of activated protein C by protein S: The role of phospholipid in factor Va inactivation. *J Biol Chem* 256:11128–11131.

28. Preston, R.J.S., E. Ajzner, C. Razzari, S. Karageorgi, S. Dua, B. Dahlback, and D.A. Lane. 2006. Multifunctional specificity of the protein C/activated protein C Gla domain. *J Biol Chem* 281:28850–28857.

29. Dahlback, B. and J. Stenflo. 1981. High molecular weight complex in human plasma between vitamin K-dependent protein S and complement component C4b-binding protein. *Proc Natl Acad Sci USA* 78:2512–2516.
30. Walker, F.J. 1986. Identification of a new protein involved in the regulation of the anticoagulant activity of activated protein C. Protein S-binding protein. *J Biol Chem* 261:10941–10944.
31. Dahlback, B. and B.O. Villoutreix. 2005. The anticoagulant protein C pathway. *FEBS Lett* 579:3310–3316.
32. Dahlback, B. 2005. Blood coagulation and its regulation by anticoagulant pathways: Genetic pathogenesis of bleeding and thrombotic diseases. *J Int Med* 257:209–223.
33. Dahlback, B. and B.O. Villoutreix. 2005. Regulation of blood coagulation by the protein C anticoagulant pathway. *Arterioscler Thromb Vasc Biol* 25:1311–1320.
34. Han, Y., R. Fiehler, and G.J. Broze, Jr. 1998. Isolation of a protein Z-dependent plasma protease inhibitor. *Proc Natl Acad Sci USA* 95:9250–9255.
35. Broze, G.J., Jr. 2001. Protein Z-dependent regulation of coagulation. *Thromb Haemostas* 86:8–13.
36. Al-Shanqeeti, A., A. van Hylckma Vlieg, E. Bentorp, F.R. Rosendaal, and G.J. Broze, Jr. 2005. Protein Z and protein Z-dependent protease inhibitor. Determinants of levels and risk of venous thrombosis. *Thromb Haemostas* 93:411–413.
37. Yin, Z.-F., Z.-F. Huang, J. Cui, R. Fiehler, N. Lasky, D. Ginsburg, and G.J. Broze, Jr. 2000. Prothrombotic phenotype of protein Z deficiency. *Proc Natl Acad Sci USA* 97:6734–6738.
38. Van de Water, N., T. Tan, F. Ashton, A. O'Grady, T. Day, P. Browett, P. Ockelford, and P. Harper. 2004. Mutations within the protein Z-dependent protease inhibitor gene are associated with venous thromboembolic disease: A new form of thrombophilia. *Brit J Haematol* 127:190–194.
39. Spronk, H.M.H., J.W.P. Govers-Riemslag, and H. ten Cate. 2003. The blood coagulation system as a molecular machine. *BioEssays* 25:1220–1228.
40. Schenone, M., B.C. Furie, and B. Furie. 2004. The blood coagulation cascade. *Current Opinion Hematol* 11:272–277.
41. Brummel-Ziedins, K., C.Y. Vossen, F.R. Rosendaal, K. Umezaki, and K.G. Mann. 2005. The plasma hemostatic proteome: Thrombin generation in healthy individuals. *J Thromb Haemost* 3:1472–1481.
42. Dahlback, B. 2000. Blood coagulation. *Lancet* 355:1627–1632.
43. Hoffman, M. and D.M. Monroe. 2007. Coagulation 2006: A modern view of hemostasis. *Hematol Oncol Clin North Am* 21:1–11.
44. Furie, B. and B.C. Furie. 2007. In vivo thrombus formation. *J Thromb Haemost* 5(Suppl 1):12–17.
45. Orfeo, T., K.E. Brummel-Ziedins, M. Gissel, S. Butenas, and K.G. Mann. 2008. The nature of the stable blood clot procoagulant activities. *J Biol Chem* 283:9776–9786.
46. Mann, K.G. and M.P. Esnouf. 1985. Prothrombinase molecular assembly. In *Hemostasis and Thrombosis*, ed. E.J.W. Bowie and A.A. Sharp, 148–172. London: Butterworths.
47. Mann, K.G. 1987. The assembly of blood clotting complexes on membranes. *Trends Biochem Sci* 12:229–233.
48. Suttie, J.W. and C.M. Jackson. 1977. Prothrombin structure, activation, and biosynthesis. *Physiol Rev* 57:1–70.
49. Stenn, K.S. and E.R. Blout. 1972. Mechanism of bovine prothrombin activation by an insoluble preparation of bovine factor Xa (thrombokinase). *Biochemistry* 11:4502–4515.
50. Esmon, C.T., W.G. Owen, and C.M. Jackson. 1974. A plausible mechanism for prothrombin activation by factor X, factor V, phospholipid, and calcium ions. *J Biol Chem* 249:8045–8047.

51. Nelsestuen, G.L., A.M. Shah, and S.B. Harvey. 2000. Vitamin K-dependent proteins. *Vitamins and Hormones* 58:355–389.
52. Mann, K.G. 2003. Thrombin formation. *Chest* 124:4S–10S.
53. Stassen, J.M., J. Arnout, and H. Deckmyn. 2004. The hemostatic system. *Curr Med Chem* 11:2245–2260.
54. Frederick, R., L. Pochet, C. Charlier, and B. Masereel. 2005. Modulators of the coagulation cascade: Focus and recent advances in inhibitors of tissue factor, factor VIIa and their complex. *Curr Med Chem* 12:397–417.
55. Seegers, W.H., H.P. Smith, E.D. Warner, and K.M. Brinkhous. 1938. The purification of prothrombin. *J Biol Chem* 123:751–754.
56. Davie, E.W. and K. Fujikawa. 1975. Basic mechanisms in blood coagulation. *Annu Rev Biochem* 44:799–829.
57. Lorand, L. 1976. Section II. Blood clotting enzymes. A. Enzymes of blood coagulation. *Meth Enzymol* 45 (Part B):31–177.
58. Jenny, R., W. Church, B. Odegaard, R. Litwiller, and K. Mann. 1986. Purification of six human vitamin K-dependent proteins in a single chromatographic step using immunoaffinity columns. *Prep Biochem* 16:227–245.
59. Josic, D., L. Hoffer, and A. Buchacher. 2003. Preparation of vitamin K-dependent proteins, such as clotting factors II, VII, IX, and X and clotting inhibitor protein C. *J Chromatogr B*, 790:183–197.
60. Litwiller, R.D., R.J. Jenny, and K.G. Mann. 1986. Identification and isolation of vitamin K-dependent proteins by HPLC. *Analyt Biochem* 158:355–360.
61. Magnusson, S., T.E. Petersen, L. Sottrup-Jensen, and H. Claeys. 1975. Complete primary structure of prothrombin: Isolation, structure and reactivity of ten carboxylated glutamic acid residues and regulation of prothrombin activation by thrombin. In *Proteases and Biological Control,* 123–149. Cold Spring Harbor Conf. on Cell Proliferation. New York: Cold Spring Harbor.
62. Walz, D.A., D. Hewett-Emmett, and M.C. Guillin. 1986. Amino acid sequences and molecular homology of the vitamin K-dependent clotting factors. In *Prothrombin and Other Vitamin K Proteins,* 125–160. Boca Raton, FL: CRC Press.
63. Dahlback, B., A. Lundwall, and J. Stenflo. 1986. Primary structure of bovine vitamin K-dependent protein S. *Proc Natl Acad Sci USA* 83:4199–4203.
64. Drakenberg, T., P. Fernlund, P. Roepstorff, and J. Stenflo. 1983. Beta-hydroxyaspartic acid in vitamin K-dependent protein C. *Proc Natl Acad Sci USA* 80:1802–1806.
65. McMullen, B.A., K. Fujikawa, and W. Kisiel. 1983. The occurrence of beta-hydroxyaspartic acid in the vitamin K-dependent blood coagulation zymogens. *Biochem Biophys Res Commun* 115:8–14.
66. Stenflo, J., A. Lundwall, and B. Dahlback. 1987. Beta-hydroxyasparagine in domains homologous to the epidermal growth factor precursor in vitamin K-dependent protein S. *Proc Natl Acad Sci USA* 84:368–372.
67. Persson, E., M. Selander, S. Linse, T. Drakenberg, A.K. Ohlin, and J. Stenflo. 1989. Calcium binding to the isolated beta-hydroxyaspartic acid-containing epidermal growth factor-like domain of bovine factor X. *J Biol Chem* 264:16897–16904.
68. Dahlback, B., B. Hildebrand, and S. Linse. 1990. Novel type of very high affinity calcium-binding sites in beta-hydroxy-asparagine-containing epidermal growth factor-like domains in vitamin K-dependent protein S. *J Biol Chem* 265:18481–18489.
69. Hansson, K. and J. Stenflo. 2005. Post-translational modifications in proteins involved in blood coagulation. *J Thromb Haemostas* 3:2633–2648.
70. Olsson, G., L. Andersen, O. Lindqvist, L. Sjolin, S. Magnusson, T.E. Petersen, and L. Sottrup-Jensen. 1982. A low resolution model of fragment 1 from bovine prothrombin. *FEBS Lett* 145:317–322.

71. Park, C.H. and A. Tulinsky. 1986. Three dimensional structure of the Kringle sequence: Structure of prothrombin fragment 1. *Biochemistry* 25:3977–3982.

72. Seshadri, T.P., A. Tulinsky, E. Skrzypczak-Jankun, and C.H. Park. 1991. Structure of bovine prothrombin fragment 1 refined at 2–25 Å resolution. *J Mol Biol* 220:481–494.

73. Soriano-Garcia, M., C.H. Park, A. Tulinsky, K.G. Ravichandran, and E. Skrzypczak-Jankun. 1989. Structure of Ca^{2+} prothrombin fragment 1 including the conformation of the Gla domain. *Biochemistry* 28:6805–6810.

74. Bode, W., H. Brandstetter, T. Mather, and M.T. Stubbs. 1997. Comparative analysis of haemostatic proteinases: Structural aspects of thrombin, factor Xa, factor IXa and protein C. *Thromb Haemost* 78:501–511.

75. Banner, D.W. 1997. The factor VIIa/tissue factor complex. *Thromb Haemost* 78:512–515.

76. Jorgensen, M.J., A.B. Cantor, B.C. Furie, C.L. Brown, C.B. Shoemaker, and B. Furie. 1987. Recognition site directing vitamin K-dependent gamma-carboxylation residues on the propeptide of factor IX. *Cell* 48:185–191.

77. Foster, D.C., M.S. Rudinski, B.G. Schach, K.L. Berkner, A.A. Kumar, F.S. Hagen, C. Sprecher, M. Insley, and E.W. Davie. 1987. Propeptide of human protein C is necessary for gamma-carboxylation. *Biochemistry* 26:7003–7011.

78. Knobloch, J.E. and J.W. Suttie. 1987. Vitamin K-dependent carboxylase. Control of enzyme activity by the "propeptide" region of factor X. *J Biol Chem* 262: 15334–15337.

79. Degen, S.J.F., R.T.A. MacGillivray, and E.W. Davie. 1983. Characterization of the complementary deoxyribonucleic acid and gene coding for human prothrombin. *Biochemistry* 22:2087–2097.

80. Irwin, D.M., K.G. Ahern, G.D. Pearson, and R.T.A. MacGillivray. 1985. Characterization of the bovine prothrombin gene. *Biochemistry* 24:6854–6861.

81. Anson, D.S., K.H. Choo, D.J.G. Rees, F. Gianelli, K. Gould, J.A. Huddleston, and G.G. Brownlee. 1984. Gene structure of human anti-haemophilic factor IX. *EMBO J* 3:1053–1064.

82. Yoshitake, S., B.G. Schach, D.C. Foster, E.W. Davie, and K. Kurachi. 1985. Nucleotide sequence of the gene for human factor IX (antihemophilic factor B). *Biochemistry* 24:3736–3750.

83. Leytus, S.P., D.C. Foster, K. Kurachi, and E.W. Davie. 1986. Gene for human factor X: A blood coagulation factor whose gene organization is essentially identical with that of factor IX and protein C. *Biochemistry* 25:5098–6012.

84. O'Hara, P.J., F.J. Grant, B.A. Haldeman, C.L. Gray, M.Y. Insley, F.S. Hagen, and M.J. Murray. 1987. Nucleotide sequence of the gene coding for human factor VII, a vitamin K-dependent protein participating in blood coagulation. *Proc Natl Acad Sci USA* 84:5158–5162.

85. Hagen, F.S., C.L. Gray, P. O'Hara, F.J. Grant, G.C. Saari, R.G. Woodbury, C.E. Hart, M. Insley, W. Kisiel, K. Kurachi, and E.W. Davie. 1986. Characterization of a cDNA coding for human factor VII. *Proc Natl Acad Sci USA* 83:2412–2416.

86. Foster, D.C., S. Yoshitake, and E.W. Davie. 1985. The nucleotide sequence of the gene for human protein C. *Proc Natl Acad Sci USA* 82:4673–4677.

87. Plutzky, J., J. Hoskins, G.L. Long, and G.R. Crabtree. 1986. Evolution and organization of the human protein C gene. *Proc Natl Acad Sci USA* 83:546–550.

88. Kurachi, K. and S.H. Chen. 1987. Human genes for factor IX and other vitamin K dependent blood proteins. In *Advances in Experimental Medicine and Biology* 214, *The New Dimensions of Warfarin Prophylaxis*, 67–81. New York: Springer.

89. Fung, M.R. and R.T.A. MacGillivray. 1988. Organization of the genes coding for the vitamin K-dependent clotting factors. In *Current Advances in Vitamin K Research*, ed. J.W. Suttie, 143–151. New York: Elsevier Science Publishing Co.

90. Brinkhous, K.M. 1940. Plasma prothrombin; vitamin K. *Medicine* 19:329–416.
91. Quick, A.J. 1936. On various properties of thromboplastin (aqueous tissue extracts). *Am J Physiol* 114:282–296.
92. Warner, E.D., K.M. Brinkhous, and H.P. Smith. 1936. A quantitative study on blood clotting: prothrombin fluctuations under experimental conditions. *Am J Physiol* 114:667–675.
93. Carlisle, T.L., D.V. Shah, R. Schlegel, and J.W. Suttie. 1975. Plasma abnormal prothrombin and microsomal prothrombin precursor in various species. *Proc Soc Exp Biol Med* 148:140–144.
94. Kirchhof, B.R.J., C. Vermeer, and H.C. Hemker. 1978. The determination of prothrombin using synthetic chromogenic substrates; choice of a suitable activator. *Thrombosis Res* 13:219–232.
95. Denson, K.W.E., R. Borrett, and R. Biggs. 1971. The specific assay of prothrombin using the Taipan snake venom. *Brit J Haematol* 21:219–226.
96. Jackson, S.L., L.R. Bereznicki, G.M. Peterson, K.A. Marsden, D.M.L. Jupe, E. Tegg, J.H. Vial, and R.I. Kimber. 2004. Accuracy, reproducibility and clinical utility of the CoaguChek S portable international normalized ratio monitor in an outpatient anticoagulation clinic. *Clin Lab Haem* 26:49–55.
97. Hemker, H.C. 2008. Recollections on thrombin generation. *J Thromb Haemost* 6:219–226.
98. Saunders, R.E. and S.J. Perkins. 2008. CoagMDB: A database analysis of missense mutations within four conserved domains in five vitamin K-dependent coagulation serine proteases using a text-mining tool. *Hum Mutat* 29:333–344.
99. Peyvandi, F., S. Duga, S. Akhavan, and P.M. Mannucci. 2002. Rare coagulation deficiencies. *Haemophilia* 8:308–321.
100. Endler, G. and C. Mannhalter. 2003. Polymorphisms in coagulation factor genes and their impact on arterial and venous thrombosis. *Clin Chim Acta* 330:31–55.
101. Bick, R. 2003. Prothrombin G20210A mutation, antithrombin, heparin cofactor II, protein C, and protein S defects. *Hematol Oncol Clin North Am* 17:9–36.
102. Corral, J., R. Gonzalez-Conejero, J.M. Soria, J.R. Gonzalez-Porras, E. Perez-Ceballos, R. Lecumberri, V. Roldan, J.C. Souto, A. Minano, D. Hernandez-Espinosa, I. Alberca, J. Fontcubert, and V. Vicente. 2006. A nonsense polymorphism in the protein Z-dependent protease inhibitor increases the risk for venous thrombosis. *Blood* 108:177–183.
103. Zhu, A., H. Sun, R.M. Raymond, Jr, B.C. Furie, B. Furie, M. Bronstein, R.J. Kaufman, R. Westrick, and D. Ginsburg. 2007. Fatal hemorrhage in mice lacking gamma-glutamyl carboxylase. *Blood* 109:5270–5275.
104. Oldenburg, J., B. von Brederlow, A. Fregin, S. Rost, W. Wolz, W. Eberl, S. Eber, E. Lenz, R. Schwaab, H.H. Brackmann, W. Effenberger, U. Harbrecht, L.J. Schurgers, C. Vermeer, and C.R. 2000. Muller. Congenital deficiency of vitamin K dependent coagulation factors in two families presents as a genetic defect of the vitamin K-epoxide-reductase-complex. *Thromb Haemostas* 84:937–941.
105. Zhang, B. and D. Ginsburg. 2004. Familial multiple coagulation factor deficiencies: New biologic insight from rare genetic bleeding disorders. *J Thromb Haemostas* 2:1564–1572.
106. McMillan, C.W. and H.R. Roberts. 1966. Congenital combined deficiency of coagulation factors II, VII, IX and X. *New Engl J Med* 274:1313–1315.
107. Chung, K.S., A. Bezeaud, J.C. Goldsmith, C.W. McMillan, D. Menache, and H.R. Roberts. 1979. Congenital deficiency of blood clotting factors II, VII, IX, and X. *Blood* 53:776–787.
108. Pauli, R.M., J.B. Lian, D.F. Mosher, and J.W. Suttie. 1987. Association of congenital deficiency of multiple vitamin K-dependent coagulation factors and the phenotype of the warfarin embryopathy: Clues to the mechanism of teratogenicity of coumarin derivatives. *Am J Hum Genet* 41:566–582.

109. Rost, S., A. Fregin, D. Koch, M. Compes, C.R. Muller, and J. Oldenburg. 2004. Compound heterozygous mutations in the gamma-glutamyl carboxylase gene cause combined deficiency of all vitamin K-dependent blood coagulation factors. *Brit J Haematol* 126:546–549.
110. Soute, B.A.M., D.-Y. Jin, H.M.H. Spronk, V.P. Mutucumarana, P.-J. Lin, T.M. Hackeng, D.W. Stafford, and C. Vermeer. 2004. Characteristics of recombinant W501S mutated human gamma-glutamyl carboxylase. *J Thromb Haemostas* 2:597–604.
111. Darghouth, D., K.W. Hallgren, R.L. Shtofman, A. Mrad, Y. Gharbi, A. Maherzi, R. Kastally, S. LeRicousse, K.L. Berkner, and J.-P. Rosa. 2006. Compound heterozygosity of novel missense mutations in the gamma-glutamyl-carboxylase gene causes hereditary combined vitamin K-dependent coagulation factor deficiency. *Blood* 208:1925–1931.
112. Rost, S., C. Geisen, A. Fregin, E. Seifried, C.R. Muller, and J. Oldenburg. 2006. Founder mutation Arg485Pro led to recurrent compound heterozygous GGCX genotypes in two German patients with VKCFD type 1. *Blood Coagulation and Fibrinolysis* 17:503–507.
113. Johnson, J.S., W.S. Laegreid, R.J. Basaraba, and D.C. Baker. 2006. Truncated gamma-glutamyl carboxylase in rambouillet sheep. *Vet Pathol* 43:430–437.
114. Fukutake, K. 2006. Current status of hemophilia patients and recombinant coagulation factor concentrates in Japan. *Sem Thromb Hemostas* 26:29–32.
115. Schlesinger, K.W. and M.V. Ragni. 2002. Safety of the new generation recombinant factor concentrates. *Expert Opin Drug Saf* 1:213–223.
116. Frampton, J.E. and A.J. Wagstaff. 2008. Sucrose-formulated octocog alfa: A review of its use in patients with haemophilia A. *Drugs* 68:839–853.
117. Rothschild, C., I. Scharrer, H.H. Brackmann, N. Steitjes, M. Vicariot, M.F. Torchet, and W. Effenberger. 2002. European data of a clinical trial with a sucrose formulated recombinant factor VIII in previously treated haemophilia A patients. *Haemophilia* 8(Suppl 2):10–14.
118. Ziedins, K.B., G.E. Rivard, R.L. Pouliot, S. Butenas, M. Gissel, B. Parhami-Seren, and K.G. Mann. 2004. Factor VIIa replacement therapy in factor VII deficiency. *J Thromb Haemostas* 2:1735–1744.
119. Hedner, U. 2006. Mechanism of action, development and clinical experience of recombinant FVIIa. *J Biotechnology* 124:747–757.
120. Konkle, B.A., L.S. Ebbesen, E. Erhardtsen, R.P. Bianco, T. Lissitchkov, L. Rusen, and M.A. Serban. 2007. Randomized prospective clinical trial of recombinant factor VIIa for secondary prophylaxis in hemophilia patients with inhibitors. *J Thromb Haemost* 5:1904–1913.
121. Hoots, W.K., L.S. Ebbesen, B.A. Konkle, G.K. Auerswald, H.R. Roberts, J. Weatherall, J.M. Ferran, and R.C. Ljung. 2008. Secondary prophylaxis with recombinant activated factor VII improves health-related quality of life of haemophilia patients with inhibitors. *Haemophilia* 14:466–475.
122. Siddiqui, M.A.A. and L.J. Scott. 2005. Recombinant factor VIIa (Eptacog alfa): A review of its use in congenital or acquired haemophilia and other congenital bleeding disorders. *Drugs* 65:1161–1177.
123. Roberts, H.R., D.M. Monroe, and G.C. White. 2004. The use of recombinant factor VIIa in the treatment of bleeding disorders. *Blood* 104:3858–3864.
124. Horton, J.D., K.J. DeZee, and M. Wagner. 2008. Use of rFVIIa in the trauma setting: Practice patterns in United States trauma centers. *Am Surg* 74:413–417.
125. Esmon, C.T. 2005. The interactions between inflammation and coagulation. *Brit J Haematol* 131:417–430.
126. Esmon, C.T. 2006. Inflammation and the activated protein C anticoagulant pathway. *Sem Thromb Hemostas* 32(S1):49–60.

127. Fourrier, F. 2004. Recombinant human activated protein C in the treatment of severe sepsis: An evidence-based review. *Crit Care Med* 32:S534–S541.
128. Baillie, J.K. 2007. Activated protein C: Controversy and hope in the treatment of sepsis. *Curr Opin Investig Drugs* 8:933–938.
129. John, J., A. Awab, D. Norman, T. Dernaika, and G.T. Kinasewitz. 2007. Activated protein C improves survival in severe sepsis patients with elevated troponin. *Intensive Care Med* 33:2122–2128.
130. Vandendriesche, T., D. Collen, and M.K.L. Chuah. 2003. Gene therapy for the hemophilias. *J Thromb Haemostas* 1:1550–1558.
131. Lozier, J. 2004. Gene therapy of the hemophilias. *Semin Hematol* 41:287–296.
132. Lillicrap, D., T. Vandendriessche, and K. High. 2006. Cellular and genetic therapies for haemophilia. *Haemophilia* 12(Suppl 3):36–41.
133. High, K.A. 2003. Gene transfer as an approach to treating hemophilia. *Sem Thromb Hemostas* 29:107–119.
134. Murphy, S.L. and K.A. High. 2008. Gene therapy for haemophilia. *Br J Haematol* 140:479–487.
135. Hemker, H.C., J.J. Veltkamp, A. Hensen, and E.A. Loeliger. 1963. Nature of prothrombin biosynthesis: Preprothrombinaemia in vitamin K- deficiency. *Nature* 200:589–590.
136. Ganrot, P.O. and J.E. Nilehn. 1968. Plasma prothrombin during treatment with dicumarol. II. Demonstration of an abnormal prothrombin fraction. *Scand J Clin Lab Invest* 22:23–28.
137. Josso, F., J.M. Lavergne, M. Gouault, O. Prou-Wartelle, and J.P. Soulier. 1968. Differents états moléculaires du facteur II (prothrombine). Leur étude a l'aide de la staphylocoagulase et d'anticorps anti-facteur II. *Thrombos Diathes haemorrh* 20:88–98.
138. Stenflo, J. 1970. Dicoumarol-induced prothrombin in bovine plasma. *Acta Chem Scand* 24:3762–3763.
139. Shah, D.V., J.C. Swanson, and J.W. Suttie. 1984. Abnormal prothrombin in the vitamin K-deficient rat. *Thrombosis Res* 35:451–458.
140. Zhang, P. and J.W. Suttie. 1992. Prothrombin biosynthesis in H-35 rat hepatoma cells: Effects of vitamin K and warfarin on transcription and translation. *FASEB J* 6:A1939.
141. Wu, W., J.D. Bancroft, and J.W. Suttie. 1996. Differential effects of warfarin on the intracellular processing of vitamin K-dependent proteins. *Thromb Haemostas,* 76:46–52.
142. Wu, W., J.D. Bancroft, and J.W. Suttie. 1997. Structural features of the Kringle domain determine the intracellular degradation of under-gamma-carboxylated prothrombin: Studies of chimeric rat/human prothrombin. *Proc Natl Acad Sci USA* 94:13654–13660.
143. Hemker, H.C., A.D. Muller, and E.A. Loeliger. 1970. Two types of prothrombin in vitamin K deficiency. *Thrombos Diathes haemorrh* 23:633–637.
144. Esmon, C.T., J.W. Suttie, and C.M. Jackson. 1975. The functional significance of vitamin K action. Difference in phospholipid binding between normal and abnormal prothrombin. *J Biol Chem* 250:4095–4099.
145. Malhotra, O.P., M.E. Nehseim, and K.G. Mann. 1985. The kinetics of activation of normal and gamma-carboxyglutamic acid-deficient prothrombins. *J Biol Chem* 260:279–287.
146. Malhotra, O.P. Dicoumarol-induced prothrombins. 1981. *Ann NY Acad Sci* 370:426–437.
147. Widdershoven, J., P. van Munster, R.A. De Abreu, H. Bosman, T. van Lith, M. van der Putten-van Meyel, K. Motohara, and I. Matsuda. 1987. Four methods compared for measuring des-carboxy-prothrombin (PIVKA-II). *Clin Chem* 33:2074–2078.
148. Naraki, T., N. Kohno, H. Saito, Y. Fujimoto, T. Ohhira, T. Morita, and Y. Kohgo. 2002. Gamma-carboxyglutamic acid content of hepatocellular carcinoma-associated des-gamma-carboxy prothrombin. *Biochim Biophys Acta* 1586:287–298.

149. Marrero, J.A., G.L. Su, W. Wei, D. Emick, H.S. Conjeevaram, R.J. Fontana, and A.S. Lok. 2003. Des-gamma carboxyprothrombin can differentiate hepatocellular carcinoma from nonmalignant chronic liver disease in American patients. *Hepatology* 37:1114–1121.

150. Okuda, H., T. Nakanishi, K. Takatsu, A. Saito, N. Hayashi, K. Takasaki, K. Takenami, M. Yamamoto, and M. Nakano. 2000. Serum levels of des-gamma-carboxy prothrombin measured using the revised enzyme immunoassay kit with increased sensitivity in relation to clinicopathologic features of solitary hepatocellular carcinoma. *Cancer* 88:544–549.

151. Hakamada, K., N. Kimura, T. Miura, H. Morohashi, K. Ishido, M. Nara, Y. Toyoki, S. Narumi, and M. Sasaki. 2008. Des-gamma-carboxy prothrombins an important prognostic indicator in patients with small hepatocellular carcinoma. *World J Gastroenterol* 14:1370–1377.

152. Shah, D.V., J.A. Engelke, and J.W. Suttie. 1987. Abnormal prothrombin in the plasma of rats carrying hepatic tumors. *Blood* 69:850–854.

153. Shah, D.V., P. Zhang, J.A. Engelke, A.U. Bach, and J.W. Suttie. 1993. Vitamin K-dependent carboxylase activity, prothrombin mRNA, and prothrombin production in two cultured rat hepatoma cell lines. *Thrombosis Res* 70:365–373.

154. Huisse, M.-G., M. Leclercq, J. Belghiti, J.-F. Flejou, J.W. Suttie, A. Bezeaud, D.W. Stafford, and M.-C. Guillin. 1994. Mechanism of the abnormal vitamin K-dependent gamma-carboxylation process in human hepatocellular carcinomas. *Cancer* 74:1533–1541.

155. Tang, W., K. Miki, N. Kokudo, Y. Sugawara, H. Imamura, M. Minagawa, L.-W. Yuan, S. Ohnishi, and M. Makuuchi. 2003. Des-gamma-carboxy prothrombin in cancer and non-cancer liver tissue of patients with hepatocellular carcinoma. *Int J Oncol* 22:969–975.

156. Tang, W., N. Kokudo, Y. Sugawara, Q. Guo, H. Imamura, K. Sano, H. Kanako, X. Qu, M. Nakata, and M. Makuuchi. 2005. Des-gamma-caraboxyprothrombin expression in cancer and/or non-cancer liver tissues: Association with survival of patients with resectable hepatocellular carcinoma. *Oncology Reports* 13:25–30.

157. Suzuki, M., H. Shiraha, T. Fujikawa, N. Takaoka, N. Ueda, Y. Nakanishi, K. Koike, A. Takaki, and Y. Shiratori. 2005. Des-gamma-carboxy prothrombin is a potential autologous growth factor for hepatocellular carcinoma. *J Biol Chem* 280:6409–6415.

158. Fujikawa, T., H. Shiraha, N. Ueda, N. Takaoka, Y. Nakanishi, N. Matsuo, S. Tanaka, S.I. Nishina, M. Suzuki, A. Takaki, K. Sakaguchi, and Y. Shiratori. 2007. Des-gamma-carboxy prothrombin-promoted vascular endothelial cell proliferation and migration. *J Biol Chem* 282:8741–8748.

159. Hauschka, P.V., J.B. Lian, and P.M. Gallop. 1975. Direct identification of the calcium-binding amino acid gamma-carboxyglutamate, in mineralized tissue. *Proc Natl Acad Sci USA* 72:3925–3929.

160. Price, P.A., A.S. Otsuka, J.W. Poser, J. Kristaponis, and N. Raman. 1976. Characterization of a gamma-carboxyglutamic acid-containing protein from bone. *Proc Natl Acad Sci USA* 73:1447–1451.

161. Price, P.A., J.W. Poser, and N. Raman. 1976. Primary structure of the gamma-carboxyglutamic acid-containing protein from bovine bone. *Proc Natl Acad Sci USA* 73:3374–3375.

162. Hauschka, P.V. 1986. Osteocalcin: The vitamin K-dependent Ca^{2+}-binding protein of bone matrix. *Haemostasis* 16:258–272.

163. Hauschka, P.V., J.B. Lian, D.E.C. Cole, and C.M. Gundberg. 1989. Osteocalcin and matrix Gla protein: Vitamin K-dependent proteins in bone. *Physiol Rev* 69:990–1047.

164. Price, P.A. 1985. Vitamin K-dependent formation of bone Gla protein (osteocalcin) and its function. *Vitamins and Hormones* 42:65–108.

165. Price, P.A. 1988. Role of vitamin K-dependent proteins in bone metabolism. *Annu Rev Nutr* 8:565–583.

166. Frazao, C., D.C. Simes, R. Coelho, D. Alves, P.A. Williamson, P.A. Price, M.L. Cancela, and M.A. Carrondo. 2005. Structural evidence of a fourth Gla residue in fish osteocalcin: Biological implications. *Biochemistry* 44:1234–1242.

167. Nishimoto, S.K., J.H. Waite, M. Nishimoto, and R.W. Kriwacki. 2003. Structure, activity, and distribution of fish osteocalcin. *J Biol Chem* 278:11843–11848.

168. Price, P.A., A.S. Otsuka, and J.W. Poser. 1977. Comparison of gamma-carboxyglutamic acid-containing proteins from bovine and swordfish bone: Primary structure and Ca^{++} binding. In *Calcium-Binding Proteins and Calcium Function*, 333–337. New York: Elsevier.

169. Laize, V., P. Martel, C.S.B. Viegas, P.A. Price, and M.L. Cancela. 2005. Evolution of matrix and bone gamma-carboxyglutamic acid proeins in vertebrates. *J Biol Chem* 290:26659–26668.

170. Nielsen-Marsh, C.M., M.P. Richards, P.V. Hauschka, J.E. Thomas-Oates, E. Trinkaus, P.B. Petitt, I. Karavanic, H. Poinar, and M.J. Collins. 2005. Osteocalcin protein sequences of Neanderthals and modern primates. *PNAS* 102:4408–4413.

171. Cairns, J.R. and P.A. Price. 1994. Direct demonstration that the vitamin K-dependent bone Gla protein is incompletely gamma-carboxylated in humans. *J Bone Miner Res* 9:1989–1997.

172. Poser, J.W. and P.A. Price. 1979. A method for decarboxylation of gamma-carboxyglutamic acid in proteins. Properties of the decarboxylated gamma-carboxyglutamic acid protein from calf bone. *J Biol Chem* 254:431–436.

173. Hauschka, P.V. and S.A. Carr. 1982. Calcium-dependent alpha-helical structure in osteocalcin. *Biochemistry* 21:2538–2547.

174. Dowd, T.L., J.F. Rosen, L. Li, and C.M. Gundberg. 2003. The three-dimensional structure of bovine calcium ion-bound osteocalcin using ^{1}H NMR spectroscopy. *Biochemistry* 42:7769–7779.

175. Hoang, Q.Q., F. Sicheri, A.J. Howard, and D.S. Yang. 2003. Bone recognition mechanism of porcine osteocalcin from crystal structure. *Nature* 425:977–980.

176. Gundberg, C.M., D.E.C. Cole, J.B. Lian, T.M. Reade, and P.M. Gallop. 1983. Serum osteocalcin in the treatment of inherited rickets with 1,25-dihydroxyvitamin D_3. *J Clin Endocrinol Metab* 56:1063–1067.

177. Price, P.A. and S.A. Baukol. 1981. 1,25-Dihydroxyvitamin D_3 increases serum levels of the vitamin K-dependent bone protein. *Biochem Biophys Res Commun* 99:928–935.

178. Price, P.A. and M.K. Williamson. 1981. Effects of warfarin on bone. Studies on the vitamin K-dependent protein of rat bone. *J Biol Chem* 256:12754–12759.

179. Price, P.A., M.K. Williamson, T. Haba, R.B. Dell, and W.S.S. Jee. 1982. Excessive mineralization with growth plate closure in rats on chronic warfarin treatment. *Proc Natl Acad Sci USA* 79:7734–7738.

180. Ducy, P., C. Desbois, B. Boyce, G. Pinero, B. Story, C. Dunstan, E. Smith, J. Bonadio, S. Goldstein, C.M. Gundberg, A. Bradley, and G. Karsenty. 1996. Increased bone formation in osteocalcin-deficient mice. *Nature* 382:448–452.

181. Price, P.A. and S.K. Nishimoto. 1980. Radioimmunoassay for the vitamin K-dependent protein of bone and its discovery in plasma. *Proc Natl Acad Sci USA* 77:2234–2238.

182. Garnero, P., M. Grimaux, P. Seguin, and P.D. Delmas. 1994. Characterization of immunoreactive forms of human osteocalcin generated in vivo and in vitro. *J Bone Miner Res* 9:255–264.

183. Szulc, P. and P.D. Delmas. 2001. Biochemical markers of bone turnover in men. *Calcif Tiss Int* 69:229–234.

184. Sokoll, L.J., M.E. O'Brien, M.E. Camilo, and J.A. Sadowski. 1995. Undercarboxylated osteocalcin and development of a method to determine vitamin K status. *Clin Chem* 41:1121–1128.

185. Gundberg, C.M., S.D. Nieman, S. Abrams, and H. Rosen. 1998. Vitamin K status and bone health: An analysis of methods for determination of undercarboxylated osteocalcin. *J Clin Endocrinol Metab* 83:3258–3266.

186. Hauschka, P.V., J. Frenke, R. DeMuth, and C.M. Gundberg. 1983. Presence of osteocalcin and related higher molecular weight 4-carboxyglutamic acid-containing proteins in developing bone. *J Biol Chem* 258:176–182.
187. Price, P.A., J.W. Lothringer, and S.K. Nishimoto. 1980. Absence of the vitamin K-dependent bone protein in fetal rat mineral. Evidence for another gamma-carboxyglutamic acid-containing component in bone. *J Biol Chem* 255:2938–2942.
188. Price, P.A., M.R. Urist, and Y. Otawara. 1983. Matrix Gla protein, a new gamma-carboxyglutamic acid-containing protein which is associated with the organic matrix of bone. *Biochem Biophys Res Commun* 117:765–771.
189. Price, P.A. and M.K. Williamson. 1985. Primary structure of bovine matrix Gla protein, a new vitamin K-dependent bone protein. *J Biol Chem* 260:14971–14975.
190. Luo, G., P. Ducy, M.D. McKee, G.J. Pinero, E. Loyer, R.R. Behringer, and G. Karsenty. 1997. Spontaneous calcification of arteries and cartilage in mice lacking matrix Gla protein. *Nature* 386:78–81.
191. El-Maadawy, S., M.T. Kaartinen, T. Schinke, M. Murshed, G. Karsenty, and M.D. McKee. 2003. Cartilage formation and calcification in arteries of mice lacking matrix Gla protein. *Connective Tissue Research* 44(Suppl):272–278.
192. Munroe, P.B., R.O. Olgunturk, J.-P. Fryns, L. Van Maldergem, F. Ziereisen, B. Yuksel, R.M. Gardiner, and E. Chung. 1999. Mutations in the gene encoding the human matrix Gla protein cause Keutel syndrome (Letter). *Nature Genet* 21:142–144.
193. Hur, D.J., G.V. Raymond, S.G. Kahler, D.L. Riegert-Johnson, B.A. Cohen, and S.A. Boyadjiev. 2005. A novel MGP mutation in a consanguineous family: Review of the clinical and molecular characteristics of Keutel syndrome. *Am J Med Genet* 135A:36–40.
194. Schinke, T. and G. Karsenty. 2000. Vascular calcification: A passive process in need of inhibitors. *Nephrol Dial Transplant* 15:1272–1274.
195. Price, P.A., S.A. Faus, and M.K. Williamson. 1998. Warfarin causes rapid calcification of the elastic lamellae in rat arteries and heart valves. *Arterioscler Thromb Vasc Biol* 18:1400–1407.
196. Schurgers, L.J., H.M.H. Spronk, J.N. Skepper, T.M. Hackeng, C.M. Shanahan, C. Vermeer, P.L. Weissberg, and D. Proudfoot. 2007. Post-translational modifications regulate matrix Gla protein function: Importance for inhibition of vascular smooth muscle cell calcification. *J Thromb Haemostas* 5:2503–2511.
197. Schurgers, L.J., H.M.H. Spronk, B.A.M. Soute, P.M. Schiffers, J.G.R. DeMey, and C. Vermeer. 2007. Regression of warfarin-induced medial elastocalcinosis by high intake of vitamin K in rats. *Blood* 109:2823–2831.
198. Murshed, M., T. Schinke, M.D. McKee, and G. Karsenty. 2004. Extracellular matrix mineralization is regulated locally; different roles of two Gla-containing proteins. *J Cell Biol* 165:625–630.
199. Ducy, P. and G. Karsenty. 1996, Skeletal Gla proteins: Gene structure, regulation of expression, and function. In *Principles of Bone Biology*, ed. J.P. Bilezikian, 183–195. San Diego: Academic Press.
200. Proudfoot, D. and C.M. Shanahan. 2006. Molecular mechanisms mediating vascular calcification: Role of matrix Gla protein. *Nephrology* 11:455–461.
201. Yao, Y., A.F. Zebboudj, E. Shao, M. Perez, and K. Bostrom. 2006. Regulation of bone morphogenetic protein-4 by matrix Gla protein in vascular endothelial cells involves activin-like kinase receptor 1. *J Biol Chem* 28:33921–33930.
202. Zebboudj, A.F., M. Imura, and K. Bostrom. 2002. Matrix Gla protein, a regulatory protein for bone morphogenetic protein-2. *J Biol Chem* 277:4388–4394.
203. Sweatt, A., D.C. Sane, S.M. Hutson, and R. Wallin. 2002. Matrix Gla protein (MGP) and bone morphogenetic protein-2 in aortic calcified lesions of aging rats. *J Thromb Haemostas* 1:178–185.

204. Cario-Toumaniantz, C., C. Boularan, L. Schurgers, M. Heymann, M. Le Cunff, J. Leger, G. Loirand, and P. Pacaud. 2007. Identification of differentially expressed genes in human varicose veins: Involvement of matrix Gla protein in extracellular matrix remodeling. *J Vasc Res* 44:444–459.

205. Li, Q., Q. Jiang, L.J. Schurgers, and J. Uitto. 2007. Pseudoxanthoma elasticum: reduced gamma-glutamyl carboxylation of matrix gla protein in a mouse model (abcc6-/-). *Biochem Biophys Res Commun* 364:208–213.

206. Erkkila, A.T. and S.L. Booth. 2008. Vitamin K intake and atherosclerosis. *Curr Opin Lipidol* 19:39–42.

207. Buczek, O., G. Bulaj, and B.M. Olivera. 2005. Conotoxins and the posttranslational modification of secreted gene products. *Cell Mol Life Sci* 62:3067–3079.

208. McIntosh, J.M., B.M. Olivera, L.J. Cruz, and W.R. Gray. 1984. Gamma-carboxyglutamate in a neuroactive toxin. *J Biol Chem* 259:14343–14346.

209. Craig, A.C., P.K. Bandyopadhyay, and B.M. Olivera. 1999. Post-translationally modified neuropeptides from *Conus* venoms. *Eur J Biochem* 264:271–275.

210. Czerwiec, E., D.E. Kalume, P. Roepstorff, B. Hambe, B. Furie, B.C. Furie, and J. Stenflo. 2006. Novel gamma-carboxyglutamic acid-containing peptides from the venom of *Conus textile*. *FEBS J* 273:2779–2788.

211. Hansson, K., B. Furie, B.C. Furie, and J. Stenflo. 2004. Isolation and characterization of three novel Gla-containing *Conus marmoreus* venom peptides, one with a novel cysteine pattern. *Biochem Biophys Res Commun* 319:1081–1087.

212. Bandyopadhyay, P.K. 2008. Vitamin K-dependent gamma-glutamylcarboxylation: An ancient posttranslational modification. In *Vitamin K*, ed. G. Litwack, 157–185. New York: Academic Press.

213. Bulaj, G., O. Buczek, I. Goodsell, E.C. Jimenez, J. Kranski, J.S. Nielsen, J.E. Garrett, and B.M. Olivera. 2003. Efficient oxidative folding of conotoxins and the radiation of venomous cone snails. *Proc Natl Acad Sci USA* 100:14562–14568.

214. Czerwiec, E., G.S. Begley, M. Bronstein, J. Stenflo, K.L. Taylor, B.C. Furie, and B. Furie. 2002. Expression and characterization of recombinant vitamin K-dependent gamma-glutamyl carboxylase from an invertebrate, *Conus textile*. *Eur J Biochem* 269:6162–6172.

215. Brown, M.A., G.S. Begley, E. Czerwiec, L.M. Stenberg, M. Jacobs, D.E. Kalume, P. Roepstorff, J. Stenflo, B.C. Furie, and B. Furie. 2005. Precursors of novel Gla-containing conotoxins contain a carboxy-terminal recognition site that directs gamma-carboxylation. *Biochemistry* 44:9150–9159.

216. Clarke, P., S.J. Mitchell, R. Wynn, S. Sundaram, V. Speed, E. Gardener, D. Roeves, and M.J. Shearer. 2006. Vitamin K prophylaxis for preterm infants: A randomized, controlled trial of 3 regimens. *Pediatrics* 118:2524–2525.

217. Aguilar, M.B., K.S. Luna-Ramirez, D. Echeverria, A. Falcon, B.M. Olivera, E.P. Heimer de la Cotera, and M. Maillo. 2008. Conorfamide-Sr2, a gamma-carboxyglutamate-containing FMRF amide-related peptide from the venom of *Conus spurius* with activity in mice and mollusks. *Peptides* 29:186–195.

218. Zugasti-Cruz, A., M. Maillo, E. Lopez-Vera, A. Falcon, E.P. Heimer de la Cotera, B.M. Olivera, and M.B. Aguilar. 2006. Amino acid sequence and biological activity of a gamma-conotoxin-like peptide from the worm-hunting snail *Conus austini*. *Peptides* 27:506–511.

219. Tans, G., J.W.P. Govers-Riemslag, J.L.M.L.v. Rijn, and J. Rosing. 1985. Purification and properties of a prothrombin activator from the venom of *Notechis scutatus scutatus*. *J Biol Chem* 260:9366–9370.

220. Speijer, H., J.W.P. Govers-Riemslag, R.F.A. Zwaal, and J. Rosing. 1986. Prothrombin activation by an activator from the venom of *Oxyuranus scutellatus* (Taipan snake). *J Biol Chem* 261:13258–13267.

221. Brown, M.A., L.M. Stenberg, U. Persson, and J. Stenflo. 2000. Identification and puri-fication of vitamin K-dependent proteins and peptides with monoclonal antibodies spe-cific for gamma-carboxyglutamyl (Gla) residues. *J Biol Chem* 275:19795–19802.
222. Kini, R.M., V.S. Rao, and J.S. Joseph. 2001. Procoagulant proteins from snake venoms. *Haemostasis* 31:218–224.
223. Brown, M.A., B. Hambe, B. Furie, B.C. Furie, J. Stenflo, and L.M. Stenberg. 2002. Detection of vitamin K-dependent proteins in venoms with a monoclonal antibody spe-cific for gamma-carboxyglutamic acid. *Toxicon* 40:447–453.
224. Schneider, C., R.M. King, and L. Philipson. 1988. Genes specifically expressed at growth arrest of mammalian cells. *Cell* 54:787–793.
225. Manfioletti, G., C. Brancolini, G.C. Avanzi, and C. Schneider. 1993. The protein encoded by a growth arrest-specific gene (Gas6) is a new member of the vitamin K-dependent proteins related to protein S, a negative coregulator in the blood coagulation cascade. *Mol Cell Biol* 13:4976–4985.
226. Stenhoff, J., B. Dahlback, and S. Hafizi. 2004. Vitamin K-dependent Gas6 activates ERK kinase and stimulates growth of cardiac fibroblasts. *Biochem Biophys Res Commun* 319:871–878.
227. Cheung, A.Y., J.A. Engelke, M.C. Harbeck, and J.W. Suttie. 1988. Influence of the sub-strate propeptide region on the activity of the vitamin K-dependent carboxylase. *FASEB J* 2:A552.
228. Hafizi, S. and B. Dahlback. 2006. Gas6 and protein S. *FEBS J* 273:5231–5244.
229. Robinson, D.B., Y.M. Wu, and S.F. Lin. 2000. The protein tyrosine kinase family of the human genome. *Oncogene* 19:5548–5557.
230. Varnum, B.C., C. Young, G. Elliott, A. Garcia, T.D. Bartley, Y.-W. Fridell, R.W. Hunt, G. Trail, C. Clogston, R.J. Toso, D. Yanagihara, L. Bennett, M. Sylber, L.A. Merewether, A. Tseng, E. Escobar, E.T. Liu, and H.K. Yamane. 1995. Axl receptor tyrosine kinase stimulated by the vitamin K-dependent protein encoded by growth-arrest-specific gene 6. *Nature* 373:623–626.
231. Melaragno, M.G., Y.-W.C. Fridell, and B.C. Berk. 1999. The Gas6/Axl system. A novel regulator of vascular cell function. *TCM* 9:250–253.
232. Saxena, S.P., E.D. Israels, and L.G. Israels. 2001. Novel vitamin K-dependent pathways regulating cell survival. *Apoptosis* 6:57–68.
233. Bellido-Martin, L. and P. Garcia de Frutos. 2008. Vitamin K-dependent actions of Gas6. In *Vitamin K*, ed. G. Litwack, 185–209. New York: Academic Press.
234. Fisher, P.W., M. Brigham-Burke, S.J. Wu, J. Luo, J. Carton, K. Staquet, W. Gao, S.L. Jackson, D. Bethea, C.-H. Chen, B. Hu, J. Giles-Komar, and J. Yang. 2005. A novel site contributing to growth-arrest specific gene 6 binding to its receptors as revealed by a human monoclonal antibody. *Biochem J* 387(Pt 3):727–735.
235. Sasaki, T., P.G. Knyazev, N.J. Clout, Y. Cheburkin, W. Gohring, A. Ullrich, R. Timpl, and E. Hohenester. 2006. Structural basis for Gas6-Axl signalling. *EMBO J* 25:80–87.
236. Tanabe, K., K. Nagata, K. Ohashi, T. Nakano, H. Arita, and K. Mizuno. 1997. Roles of gamma-carboxylation and a sex hormone-binding globulin-like domain in receptor-binding and in biological activities of Gas6. *FEBS Lett* 408:306–310.
237. Hasanbasic, I., I. Rajotte, and M. Blostein. 2005. The role of gamma-carboxylation in the anti-apoptotic function of Gas6. *J Thromb Haemostas* 3:2790–2797.
238. Nakano, T., K. Kawamoto, J. Kishino, K. Nomura, K. Higashino, and H. Arita. 1997. Requirement of gamma-carboxyglutamic acid residues for the biological activity of Gas6. Contribution of endogenous Gas6 to the proliferation of vascular smooth muscle cells. *Biochem J* 323:387–392.
239. Yanagita, M., H. Arai, K. Ishii, T. Nakano, K. Ohashi, K. Mizuno, B. Varnum, A. Fukatsu, T. Doi, and T. Kita. 2001. Gas6 regulates mesangial cell proliferation through Axl in experimental glomerulonephritis. *Am J Pathol* 158:1423–1432.

240. Kulman, J.D., J.E. Harris, B.A. Haldeman, and E.W. Davie. 1997. Primary structure and tissue distribution of two novel proline-rich gamma-carboxyglutamic acid proteins. *Proc Natl Acad Sci USA* 94:9058–9062.

241. Kulman, J.D., J.E. Harris, L. Xie, and E.W. Davie. 2001. Identification of two novel transmembrane gamma-carboxyglutamic acid proteins expressed broadly in fetal and adult tissues. *Proc Natl Acad Sci USA* 98:1370–1375.

242. Kulman, J.D., J.E. Harris, L. Xie, and E.W. Davie. 2007. Proline-rich Gla protein 2 is a cell-surface vitamin K-dependent protein that binds to the transcriptional coactivator Yes-associated protein. *Proc Natl Acad Sci USA* 104:8767–8772.

243. Coutu, D.L., J.H. Wu, A. Monette, G.-E. Rivard, M.D. Blostein, and J. Galipeau. 2008. Periostin: A member of a novel family of vitamin K-dependent proteins is expressed by mesenchymal stromal cells. *J Biol Chem* 283:17991–18001.

244. Rios, H., S.V. Koushik, H. Wang, J. Wang, H.M. Zhou, A. Lindsley, R. Rogers, Z. Chen, M. Maeda, A. Kruzynska-Frejtag, J.Q. Feng, and S.J. Conway. 2005. Periostin null mice exhibit dwarfism, incisor enamel defects, and an early-onset periodontal disease-like phenotype. *Mol Cell Biol* 25:11131–11144.

245. Shao, R-X. and X. Guo. 2004. Human microvascular endothelial cells immortalized with human telomerase catalytic protein: A model for the study of in vitro angiogenesis. *Biochem Biophys Res Commun* 321:788–794.

246. Gillan, L., D. Matei, D.A. Fishman, C.S. Gerbin, B.Y. Karlan, and D.D. Chang. 2002. Periostin secreted by epithelial ovarian carcinoma is a ligand for alpha(V)beta(3) and alpha(V)beta(5) integrins and promotes cell motility. *Cancer Res* 62:5358–5364.

247. Wang, W.C., K. Zinn, and P.J. Bjorkman. 1993. Expression and structural studies of fasciclin I, an insect cell adhesion molecule. *J Biol Chem* 268:1448–1455.

248. Berkner, K. and B.N. Pudota. 1998. Vitamin K-dependent carboxylation of the carboxylase. *Proc Natl Acad Sci USA* 95:466–471.

249. Ruggeberg, S., P. Horn, X. Li, P. Vajkoczy, and T. Franz. 2008. Detection of a gamma-carboxy-glutamate as novel post-translational modification of human transthyretin. *Protein Pept Lett* 15:43–46.

250. Viegas, C.S.B., D.C. Simes, V. Laize, M.K. Williamson, P.A. Price, and M.L. Cancela. 2008. Gla-rich protein (GRP): A new vitamin K-dependent protein identified from sturgeon cartilage and highly conserved in vertebrates. *J Biol Chem* 283:36655–36664.

251. Jiang, Y. and R.F. Doolittle. 2003. The evolution of vertebrate blood coagulation as viewed from a comparison of puffer fish and sea squirt genomes. *Proc Natl Acad Sci USA* 100:7527–7532.

252. Wang, C.-P., K. Yagi, P.J. Lin, D.Y. Jin, K.W. Makabe, and D.W. Stafford. 2002. Identification of a gene encoding a typical gamma-carboxyglutamic acid domain in the tunicate *Halocynthia roretzi*. *J Thromb Haemostas* 1:118–123.

253. Kulman, J.D., J.E. Harris, N. Nakazawa, M. Ogasawara, M. Satake, and E.W. Davie. 2006. Vitamin K-dependent proteins in *Ciona intestinalis*, a basal chordate lacking a blood coagulation cascade. *Proc Natl Acad Sci USA* 103:15794–15799.

254. Jakubowski, J.A., N.G. Hatcher, F. Xie, and J.V. Sweedler. 2006. The first gamma-carboxyglutamate-containing neuropeptide. *Neurochem Int* 49:223–229.

255. Nakagawa, Y., V. Abram, F.J. Kezdy, E.T. Kaiser, and F.L. Coe. 1983. Purification and characterization of the principal inhibitor of calcium oxalate monohydrate crystal growth in human urine. *J Biol Chem* 258:12594–12600.

256. Mustafi, D. and Y. Nakagawa. 1994. Characterization of calcium-binding sites in the kidney stone inhibitor glycoprotein nephrocalcin with vanadyl ions: Electron paramagnetic resonance and electron nuclear double resonance spectroscopy. *Proc Natl Acad Sci USA* 91:11323–11327.

257. Tuan, R.S., W.A. Scott, and Z.A. Cohn. 1978. Calcium-binding protein of the chick chorioallantoic membrane. II. Vitamin K-dependent expression. *J Cell Biol* 77:752–761.

258. Tuan, R.S., W.A. Scott, and Z.A. Cohn. 1978. Purification and characterization of calcium-binding protein from chick chorioallantoic membrane. *J Biol Chem* 253:1011–1016.

259. Tuan, R.S. 1979. Vitamin K-dependent gamma-glutamyl carboxylase activity in the chick embryonic chorioallantoic membrane. *J Biol Chem* 254:1356–1364.

260. Matschiner, J.T. and J.M. Amelotti. 1968. Characterization of vitamin K from bovine liver. *J Lipid Res* 9:176–179.

261. Hauschka, P.V., P.A. Friedman, H.P. Traverso, and P.M. Gallop. 1976. Vitamin K-dependent gamma-carboxyglutamic acid formation by kidney microsomes in vitro. *Biochem Biophys Res Commun* 71:1207–1213.

262. Martius, C. 1956. Uber die intracellulare verteilung des vitamin K in verschiedenen organen des huhnes. *Biochem Z* 327:407–409.

263. Matschiner, J.T. and A.K. Willingham. 1974. Influence of sex hormones on vitamin K deficiency and epoxidation of vitamin K in the rat. *J Nutr* 104:660–665.

264. Suttie, J.W. 2001. Vitamin K. In *Handbook of Vitamins*, ed. R.B. Rucker, J.W. Suttie, D.B. McCormick, and L.J. Machlin, 115–164. New York: Marcel Dekker.

265. Lian, J.B., R.J. Levy, J.T. Levy, and P.A. Friedman. 1980. Other vitamin K dependent proteins. In *Calcium-Binding Proteins: Structure and Function,* 449–460. New York.

266. Mann, K.G., K. Brummel-Ziedins, T. Orfeo, and S. Butenas. 2006. Models of blood coagulation. *Blood Cell Mol Dis* 36:108–117.

6 Absorption, Storage, and Metabolism of Vitamin K

6.1 ABSORPTION, BIOAVAILABILITY, AND PLASMA TRANSPORT

6.1.1 UPTAKE FROM THE GUT

As with all nonpolar lipids, the absorption of vitamin K into the lymphatic system requires incorporation into mixed micelles composed of bile salts and the products of pancreatic enzyme lipolysis. Early studies utilizing radioactive phylloquinone followed the uptake of the vitamin into rat everted intestinal sacs, which indicated that the process was an energy-mediated process that was located predominantly in the small bowel [1,2], and this process was subsequently investigated in unanesthetized rats with cannulated bile and lymph ducts [3,4]. Absorption of phylloquinone from the intestine is via the lymphatic system and is therefore decreased in individuals with biliary insufficiency or various malabsorption syndromes. It has been found [5] that normal human subjects excrete less than 20% of a large (1 mg) dose of phylloquinone in the feces, but as much as 70% to 80% of the ingested phylloquinone has been shown to be excreted unaltered in the feces of patients with impaired fat absorption caused by obstructive jaundice, pancreatic insufficiency, or adult celiac disease.

Although the amount of menaquinones in a typical diet is very low, substantial amounts of long-chain menaquinones are present in the form of bacterial membranes in the lower bowel. There is, however, currently little understanding of the extent to which this source of vitamin K may be utilized [6]. A specific menaquinone, MK-9, has been shown to be absorbed by a passive diffusion non-energy-dependent process [7,8] by the use of everted rat colonic or ileal sacs, and this pathway has also been demonstrated in a live unanesthetized restrained rat model [9]. More recent studies [10] have shown that in the presence of bile, both MK-4 and MK-9 are absorbed by the lymphatic pathway from the rat jejunum. Although the extent of absorption has not been determined, oral administration of 1 mg of long-chain menaquinones to anticoagulated human subjects [11] has also been found to effectively decrease the extent of the acquired hypoprothrombinemia. This response demonstrates that the human digestive tract must be able to absorb these forms of the vitamin from the small intestine but does not address their absorption from the large pool of menaquinones present in the large bowel. However, a small but nutritionally significant portion of the intestinal content of vitamin K is located not in the large bowel but in a region where bile acid-mediated absorption could occur [12]. Menadione is used widely as a source of vitamin K in poultry and swine rations and in laboratory animal diets, but not in human diets. Menadione, lacking a hydrophobic side chain, does not have biological activity, but after absorption it can be alkylated to MK-4, a biologically active form of the vitamin. It has been demonstrated to be absorbed from both the small intestine and the colon by a passive process [13,14].

6.1.2 BIOAVAILABILITY OF VITAMIN K FROM FOODS

The substantial available literature dealing with the response of various markers of vitamin K status to alterations in vitamin K intake have seldom addressed the question of bioavailability of the vitamin. In most cases the assumption appears to be that vitamin K absorbed from foods would have the same impact on vitamin K status as supplemental vitamin K. This is unlikely, and the extent of absorption of the vitamin probably differs substantially between the rather limited number of vitamin K-rich food sources in a typical diet.

The bioavailability of vitamin K from different food sources has not been adequately studied, and the published data are somewhat variable. In a rather small study of healthy young adults, which utilized the area under the absorption curve (AUC) to measure bioavailability, phylloquinone (1 mg) was found to be absorbed only about 15% as well from spinach as from a detergent-solubilized preparation of phylloquinone (Konakion) when it was consumed with 25 g of butter [15], and less than 2% as well when butter was omitted (Figure 6.1). A second very similar study [16] indicated that phylloquinone (200 to 500 μg) in broccoli, spinach, or romaine lettuce, consumed with a diet containing 30% fat, was only about 15% to 20% as bioavailable as phylloquinone added to the meal as a tablet (Figure 6.2). These two studies, utilizing a standard bioavailability protocol, would suggest that those foods commonly reported as very good sources of vitamin K are rather poor sources of available vitamin. Other studies have suggested that the ability to absorb vitamin K from a food matrix is not that different than the absorption of the pure vitamin.

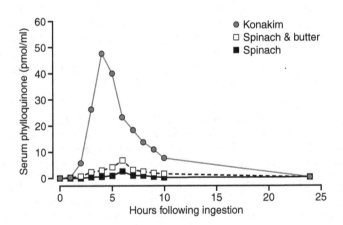

FIGURE 6.1 Serum phylloquinone concentrations following the oral administration of 1 mg phylloquinone to fasting subjects. The single dose contained Konakion, a detergent solubilized form of phylloquinone, boiled spinach, or boiled spinach + 25 g of butter. For details see Reference [15].

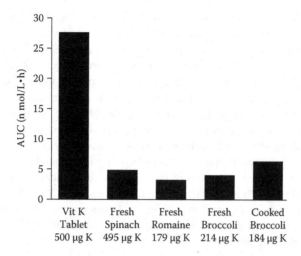

FIGURE 6.2 Absorption of phylloquinone as a tablet or as fresh or cooked vegetables. All subjects consumed a 400 kcal meal containing 27% of calories as fat with the phylloquinone source. For details, see Reference [16].

A study [17] in which subjects were fed an additional 300 µg of phylloquinone per day as phylloquinone-fortified corn oil or as microwaved broccoli in addition to a mixed diet containing 100 µg phylloquinone per day, found that the increase in fasting plasma phylloquinone in the subjects was about 70% as large in the group fed broccoli as in the fortified corn oil group. This difference was not statistically significant. In a follow up of this study [18] where the broccoli or fortified corn oil was consumed at lunch and dinner, the 24-h AUC for plasma phylloquinone was about doubled in the subjects given fortified corn oil compared to those given broccoli as a source of vitamin K. These data would suggest that phylloquinone in a food matrix is about 50% as available as the pure compound rather than the estimation of 20% or less seen in the earlier studies. The data currently available are not sufficient to make a reasonable estimation of the bioavailability of the vitamin K sources utilized in the large number of published studies that have related vitamin K intake to a change in a vitamin K responsive marker.

The ability to label phylloquinone with deuterium or ^{13}C during the growth of plants [19–21] will make it possible to determine the bioavailability of phylloquinone under conditions that more nearly duplicate the normal digestive process and should improve the current understanding of this key factor in assessing vitamin K status. The use of specifically labeled synthetic heavy isotopes of vitamin K appears to be a second approach to the determination of bioavailability. A recent study [22,23] assessed the absorption of 4 µg of ring-D_4-phylloquinone administered to 10 subjects in a gelatin capsule along with 0.5 ml of ground nut oil. A small meal was fed after 3 h and it was found that 13% ± 9% of the dose was absorbed by 6 h. The variation among subjects was large (range 2% to 26%), and the amount of vitamin K administered was rather low, but this report does demonstrate that there are methodologies available that should result in better estimates of vitamin K availability.

The impact of food preparation, cooked or raw, has not been adequately addressed, and the available data suggest that a simple calculation of vitamin K intake from a food composition database is not a good measure of available vitamin K in the diet. Although the majority of supplemental vitamin K consumed in North America and Europe is phylloquinone, supplemental MK-4 is commonly used in Asian countries, and its absorption is also dependent on dietary fat and appears to be less readily absorbed than phylloquinone [15]. Large amounts (three 15-mg tablets/day) of supplemental MK-4 are often consumed as a therapy for osteoporosis in many Asian countries, and the absorption of these pharmacological doses is also very dependent on fat intake. The absorption of a dose of MK-4 has been found [24] to be increased threefold when the caloric content of fat in an isocaloric meal taken with the tablet was increased from 11% to 43% of the meal. Some cheeses [25] and a fermented soybean product, natto, consumed mainly in the Japanese market, contain substantial amounts of long-chain menaquinones, and the large amounts of MK-7 in natto have led to its use as a supplement.

6.1.3 PLASMA TRANSPORT AND CELLULAR UPTAKE OF VITAMIN K

Following absorption, plasma phylloquinone is predominantly carried in the circulation by the triglyceride-rich lipoprotein fraction composed of very low density lipoproteins (VLDL) and chylomicrons [5]. The concentration of phylloquinone in the plasma of subjects consuming a fat-rich meal containing about 100 μg of added phylloquinone has been shown [26] to peak at 6 h, and the majority of the vitamin was associated with the triglyceride-rich lipoprotein fraction (Figure 6.3). Similar responses were seen when much higher, nonphysiological, amounts of phylloquinone (50 μg/kg) were ingested, and during the postprandial phase (12 h after feeding) of these studies, a substantial amount of the total plasma phylloquinone was carried on LDL (~14%) and HDL (~11%) particles.

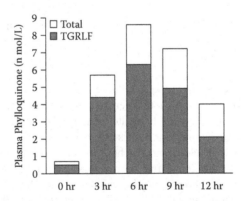

FIGURE 6.3 Plasma phylloquinone absorption from a fat-rich meal by adult subjects. The liquid diet contained 1.4 μg/kg of added phylloquinone, and the concentrations of phylloquinone in both total plasma and the triacylglycerol-rich lipoprotein fraction (TGRL) were obtained. For details, see Reference [26].

As would be expected from their association with lipoproteins, plasma phyllo-quinone concentrations are strongly correlated with plasma lipid levels [27–29]. The major route of entry of phylloquinone into tissues appears to be via clearance of chylomicron remnants by apolipoprotein E (apoE) receptors. The polymorphism of apoE has been found to influence the fasting plasma phylloquinone concentrations in patients undergoing hemodialysis therapy [27], and plasma phylloquinone concentra-tions have been shown to decrease according to the apoE genotype: apoE2 > apoE3 > apoE4 (Figure 6.4). This response would be consistent with the hepatic clearance of chylomicron remnants from the circulation, with apoE2 having the slowest rate of removal. However, studies [30] in other populations have not observed the same response to the apoE genotype. Lipoprotein receptors are also present in human osteoblasts [31], and removal of circulating phylloquinone by osteoblasts has been shown [32] to be modulated by the apoE genotype. The extent of γ-carboxylation of the vitamin K-dependent protein osteocalcin is reported [29] to be related to apoE genotypes, with subjects carrying the apoE2 genotype having circulating osteocalcin with the lower degree of carboxylation. Most of the information regarding the trans-port of vitamin K has dealt with phylloquinone, and there is evidence that not all vitamers are handled in the same manner. In a study [33] with human subjects con-suming 2 μmol each of phylloquinone, MK-4, and MK-9 added to corn oil, there were substantial differences in the peak time and amount of each vitamer, the time taken to reach baseline, and the postprandial distribution of the vitamers with cir-culating lipid fractions (Table 6.1). Phylloquinone reached the highest concentra-tion, although MK-4 peaked earlier, and the half life of MK-9, although its peak concentration was low, was much longer than the others. At 24 h after consumption, the majority of ingested phylloquinone was in the triglyceride-rich fraction while MK-4 was predominantly located in the HDL fraction, and MK-9 in the LDL frac-tion. These differences are a function of both the amount and the rate of absorption of each vitamer and the uptake of each vitamer by tissues. Until these variables are

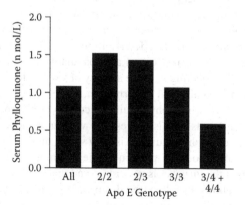

FIGURE 6.4 Relationship between ApoE lipoprotein genotype and serum phylloquinone concentration. Serum was obtained from 28 hemodialysis patients, 7 per genotype group, who were consuming a free choice diet. Significant difference (E2/2 + E2/3) vs. (E3/3) vs. (E3/4 + E4/4) = $p < 0.01$. For details, see Reference [27].

TABLE 6.1

Variation in Peak Serum Concentrations, Clearance Rate, and Predominant Lipoprotein Carrier of Three Different Forms of Vitamin K

Vitamer	Peak Concentration (nmol/L) (Major Fraction)	Postprandial Concentration (nmol/L)	
		8 h	24 h
Phylloquinone	46.8 @ 4 h (~60% TGRLF)	10.1 (~70% TGRLF)	2.6 (~75% TGRLF)
MK-4	18.1 @ 2 h (~40% TGRLF)	1.4 (~80% LDL)	0.4 (~65% HDL)
MK-9	5.6 @ 4 h (~75% TGRLF)	1.4 (~80% TGRLF)	1.5 (~60% LDL)

Note: Young adult males were given 2 μmol of each form of vitamin K dissolved in corn oil and sampled at timed intervals for total vitamin K concentration and for the distribution of each vitamer to triacylglycerol-rich lipoprotein fraction (TGRLF), high density lipoproteins (HDL), and low density lipoproteins (LDL). For details, see Reference [33].

much better understood, the impact of the variation of plasma vitamin concentration on vitamin K status cannot be clearly delineated. It appears from the discussion in some reports that a higher circulating concentration of vitamin K is thought of as an indicator of "better status," but if this is a function of a slower transfer from the circulation to functional cells, this may not be the case.

The interest in vitamin K supplementation has increased because of the substantial literature dealing with the possible role of vitamin K in skeletal and cardiovascular health (see Chapter 7); and MK-7, the vitamer present in high concentrations in the Japanese soybean product natto, has been studied as a possible supplement. This form of the vitamin clearly maintains a significantly higher plasma concentration following daily supplementation than does an equivalent amount of phylloquinone and has been reported to be more effective in terms of increasing the Gla form of osteocalcin and as an antagonist to oral anticoagulant therapy [34]. There has not been a great deal of data dealing with the activity of various forms of vitamin K, and these findings also need additional confirmation.

Neither the degree to which phylloquinone can be transferred from the liver to other organs nor the details of this process are well understood. It is clear that the total human body pool of phylloquinone is very small, and early studies using pharmacological doses of radioactive phylloquinone or amounts in the range of daily intakes indicated that the turnover is very rapid and that it is biphasic. A more recent study [23] with the ability to follow the disappearance of methyl-^{13}C-labeled phylloquinone found that the disposal kinetics of a 30-μg intravenous dose of phylloquinone were resolved into an early exponential with a half-life of 0.22 ± 0.14 h followed by a slower decay with a half-life of 2.66 ± 1.69 h. These values are similar to those obtained from the earlier studies [5,35,36]. There are only limited available data assessing the disappearance of small amounts (<1 μg) of infused ^{3}H-phylloquinone from human subjects, and these [37] suggest a body pool turnover of about 1.5 days and a body pool size of about 100 μg. Both the much slower turnover rate and a higher estimate of the total body pool in this study may reflect differences in the time points at which plasma was sampled. Other data, based on liver biopsies of patients fed diets very low in vitamin K prior to surgery [38], indicated that about two-thirds of hepatic phylloquinone was lost in 3 days. These findings are also consistent with a small-sized pool of phylloquinone that turns over very rapidly. It should be recognized that there may be pools of vitamin K in fat deposits or membranes that turn over very slowly and are not measured by the loss of the vitamin from the circulation. Details of the uptake of vitamin K into cells are not well understood. It has been shown that phylloquinone is taken up by normal rat hepatocytes against a saturable concentration gradient and that the rate and extent of the uptake is reduced when studied in rat hepatoma cell lines [39] rather than normal hepatocytes. Recent studies using ^{18}O-labeled forms of phylloquinone and MK-4 have shown that in cultured human cell lines (HepG2) MK-4 is more rapidly taken up and metabolized to the epoxide form than is phylloquinone [40]. The mechanisms involved in this discrimination of the two vitamins have not been elucidated, but a nuclear MK-4-binding protein, which also binds to phylloquinone, has been isolated from human osteoblasts [41]. Whether or not a similar vitamin K-binding protein is involved in transporting this lipophylic compound between various cellular membranes or across cellular membranes is not known.

6.2 UTILIZATION OF MENAQUINONES FROM THE GUT

Substantial amounts of vitamin K are present in the human gut in the form of long-chain menaquinones. Relatively few of the bacteria that comprise the normal intestinal flora are major producers of menaquinones, but obligate anaerobes of the *Bacteroide fragilis*, *Eubacterium*, *Propionibacterium*, and *Arachnia* groups are, as are facultative anaerobic organisms such as *E. coli* [42]. The specific menaquinone produced by various organisms differs considerably [43,44] and can be used as an aid in identifying these organisms. The amount of vitamin K in the gut can be quite large, and methods for the analysis of the extensive range of vitamers present have been described [45]. The total amount of various menaquinones found in intestinal tract contents from five adult colonoscopy patients has been reported [12] to range from 0.3 to 5.1 mg, with MK-9 and MK-10 being the major contributors. These totals do not include contributions from MK-11, which could not be accurately quantitated. The majority of the menaquinones were found in the distal colon, with much less observed in the ileum, and menaquinones were essentially lacking from the jejunum. In this study the total intestinal phylloquinone content was much less and ranged from 0.13 to 0.63 mg. Fecal long-chain menaquinones have been reported [46] to be present in substantial amounts in most formula-fed infants three days after birth, but in only about 15% of breast-fed infants. This difference persists for some time, and the stool content of the vitamers MK-4 to MK-10 of formula-fed infants was found to be three times that of breast-fed infants at one month of age [11]. This study also presents data showing the close relationship between fecal menaquinone content and the number of menaquinone-producing organisms in the stool.

Although the extent to which the large amount of menaquinones in the gut can be absorbed is not known [6,42], nutrition texts often indicate that they furnish a significant portion of the human requirement. Much of the data to support the view that menaquinones produced in the gut are important is based on the relatively high incidence of vitamin K-responsive, antibiotic-induced hypoprothrombinemia. As early as the late 1940s and early 1950s, antibiotic therapy was recognized as a potential contributing factor in the development of potentially serious hypoprothrombinemia, a vitamin K deficiency in hospitalized patients that is predominantly associated with antibiotic administration, which can contribute to morbidity and mortality. Numerous case reports of antibiotic-induced hypoprothrombinemia have been summarized [47,48], and these cases of hypoprothrombinemia are not limited to the use of a single antibiotic. Penicillin, semisynthetic penicillins, and cephalosporins have commonly been involved, but the use of aminoglycosides, trimethoprim, chloramphenicol, amphotericin B, erythromycin, and clindamycin have also been reported. These antibiotic-induced hypoprothrombinemias have historically been assumed to result from a decrease in the synthesis of menaquinones by gut organisms. The use of broad spectrum antibiotics has been shown to decrease hepatic menaquinone concentrations [49], but in nearly all of the available case reports of observed hypoprothrombinemia, evidence of decreased menaquinone synthesis in the presence of antibiotic treatment is lacking. There was increased concern in the early 1980s when the newer β-lactam antibiotics, in particular celphalosporin, cefamandole, or the related oxa-β-lactam, moxalactam, were associated with numerous hypoprothrombinemia responses. The initial reaction to these reports was to assume that these antibiotics inhibited menaquinone production, but this has not been clearly determined. It has been reported that these antibiotics, all of which contain an N-methylthiotetrazole (NMTT) side chain, decrease the numbers of fecal organisms producing menaquinones and subsequently the fecal menaquinone content in neutropenic patients [50]. However, controlled studies of the action of NMTT-containing antibiotics have not found this to be a consistent response [51]. It was found that patients receiving these antibiotics had increased concentrations of circulating vitamin K-2,3-epoxide [52] and that NMTT was an inhibitor of the epoxide reductase [53]. Additional studies conclusively demonstrate that antibiotics containing an NMTT side chain can cause an inhibition of the hepatic vitamin K epoxide reductase, resulting in a coumarin-like response. However, these antibiotics are very weak anticoagulants, and an adverse response is seen only in those patients with low vitamin K status [54,55].

The currently available data do not make it possible to determine the extent of menaquinone absorption from the gut, and although some patients receiving antibiotics do develop vitamin K responsive hypoprothrombinemias [6,42], they are a small fraction of this patient population. The difficulty in producing a clinically significant hypoprothrombinemia in an adult by dietary restriction of vitamin K (see Chapter 7) has also been seen as an indication that intestinal menaquinones must be furnishing the needed amount of vitamin K. This, of course, depends on how low the requirement for vitamin K is. Routine prothrombin time measurements are a very insensitive measure of vitamin K status (see Chapter 8), and much more sensitive markers are now available that may provide a better approach to determining the physiological role of gut menaquinones. The most direct approach would be to determine which of the tissue forms of vitamin K, dietary phylloquinone or bacterial menaquinones, was being utilized as a substrate for the vitamin K-dependent carboxylase. This approach has been utilized [56] with some success in experimental animals, but it will be a difficult technique to apply to human subjects. Newer developments that make it possible to routinely measure the metabolic degradation products of vitamin K [57] and the finding that both menaquinones and phylloquinone are metabolized to the same excretion product suggest a possible approach to this question. It is possible that bacterially synthesized, but not dietary vitamin K, could be labeled with a heavy isotope to provide a way to measure the relative amount of each form of the vitamin which is being degraded and secreted. The alternate approach would also seem feasible: synthetically produced, labeled phylloquinone could be used as the source of vitamin K in a low vitamin K diet, the decrease in specific activity of the degradation metabolites might provide the data for a calculation of the extent to which the dietary source has been diluted by menaquinones from the gut. These approaches would lead to calculation of the relative amount of phylloquinone and menaquinones that are turned over in a given period of time rather than a measure of use of each form, but it would provide much more information than is currently available. A definitive understanding of the amount of gut menaquinones utilized is probably not a real public health concern, but it is a very interesting nutritional question, and it is likely that efforts to solve it will continue.

6.3   VITAMIN K IN VARIOUS ORGANS AND TISSUES

The distribution of vitamin K in various body organs of the rat was first studied with radioactive forms of the vitamin by using both massive [58] and more physiological [59] amounts of phylloquinone. The liver was found to retain the majority of the vitamin at early time points, but the half-life in the liver appeared to be in the range of 10 to 15 h [59,60], and it was rapidly lost. Whole-body radiography [61] following administration of large amounts of radiolabeled phylloquinone detected high concentrations in liver, but also located substantial amounts in adrenal glands, lungs, bone marrow, kidneys, and lymph nodes. Initial interest in the distribution of vitamin K in animal tissues focused on the liver because of its role in clotting factor synthesis. Because of the small amounts of vitamin K present, it was difficult to determine which of the vitamers were present in tissues from different species. The limited data available have been compiled and reviewed by Matschiner [62]. These data (Table 6.2) were obtained largely by thin-layer chromatography, and indicate that phylloquinone is found in the liver of those species ingesting plant material and that, in addition to this, menaquinones containing 6 to 13 prenyl units in the alkyl chain are found in the liver of most species. Some of these long-chain vitamers identified were partially saturated. More recent studies utilized improved assay procedures to quantitate the tissue concentration of vitamin K and to gain an understanding of the distribution of the vitamin among various tissues. A study utilizing vitamin K-deficient adult male rats and comparing the results to rats supplemented with phylloquinone [63] is summarized in Table 6.3. Over a nine-day period consuming an essentially vitamin K-free diet, the tissue concentration of phylloquinone fell to very low levels and was selectively increased when adequate phylloquinone was added to the ration.

TABLE 6.2
Various Forms of Vitamin K in Liver

	Species of Liver Studied						
	Human[a]	Beef	Rabbit	Chicken	Pig	Dog	Horse
Vitamin content							
Total K_1 equivalent (µg/g)	0.06	1.2	–	–	0.4	0.6	0.2
Number of forms found	10	4	2	2	13	19	1
Form identified							
Phylloquinone	X	X	X	X	X		X
MK-6						X	
MK-7	X				X	X	
MK-8	X				X	X	
MK-9	X				X	X	
MK-10	X	X			X	X	
MK-11	X	X				X	
MK-12		X				X	
MK-13						X	

Note: The data are qualitative but indicate the presence of various vitamers (X). See [62] for references to original data for each species.

Source: Adapted from Reference [62].

TABLE 6.3
Phylloquinone and MK-4 Concentration in Tissues of Rats Fed a Vitamin K-Deficient Diet or this Diet Supplemented with Phylloquinone

	Phylloquinone (ng/g)		MK-4 (ng/g)	
Tissue	Deficient	Supplemented	Deficient	Supplemented
Liver	<1	90	<1	2
Muscle	<1	10	2	3
Kidney	<1	11	2	6
Heart	2	75	1	4
Lung	<1	4	<1	3
Brain	<1	2	9	22
Pancreas	2	20	130	250
Salivary	<1	18	65	150
Bone	2	38	4	10

Note: Male rats were fed a vitamin K-deficient diet or this diet supplemented with phylloquinone (4.2 µg/g) for 9 days. No MK-4 was added to the diet [63].

Considering the large muscle mass compared to other organs, the majority of tissue phylloquinone is located in liver, muscle, and heart tissue. Although the diet contained no MK-4, the pancreas, salivary glands, and brain of vitamin K-deficient rats contained substantial concentrations of MK-4, and these concentrations were doubled in rats fed phylloquinone. Small amounts of MK-4 were found in most of the other tissues and represent the conversion of phylloquinone to MK-4 (see Section 6.2).

Although dietary phylloquinone is predominantly targeted to the liver, analysis of a limited number of human liver specimens by HPLC has shown that phylloquinone represents only about 10% of the total vitamin K pool [6], and that a broad mixture (Table 6.4) of menaquinones is present. The predominant forms appear to be MK-7, MK-8, MK-10, and MK-11. These vitamers are not found in substantial quantities in most diets and must be derived from the gut. The tissue content of menaquinones appears to increase with age. The hepatic menaquinone content of five 24-month-old infants has been reported [64] to be approximately sixfold higher than that of three infants less than two weeks of age, and another study [65] has failed to find menaquinones in neonatal livers. Although the long-chain menaquinones are present in liver and are a potential source of vitamin K activity, efforts to determine the extent to which they are utilized have been unsuccessful. To some extent the presence of high concentrations of long-chain menaquinones in hepatic tissue is a function of the slow turnover of these vitamers, which has been demonstrated in both human subjects [38] and in an animal model [66]. A study conducted in rats [56] has demonstrated that the utilization of MK-9 as a substrate for the vitamin K-dependent carboxylase is only about 20% as extensive as phylloquinone when the two compounds are present in the liver in equal concentrations.

TABLE 6.4
Vitamin K Content of Human Liver

Vitamer	pmol/g Liver[a]			
	Study A	Study B	Study C	Study D
Phylloquinone	22 ± 5	18 ± 4	28 ± 4	17 ± 7
MK-5	12 ± 18	NR	NR	NR
MK-6	12 ± 13	NR	NR	4 ± 1
MK-7	57 ± 59	122 ± 61	34 ± 12	3 ± 1
MK-8	95 ± 157	11 ± 2	9 ± 2	7 ± 1
MK-9	2 ± 4	4 ± 2	2 ± 1	8 ± 2
MK-10	67 ± 71	96 ± 16	75 ± 10	23 ± 7
MK-11	90 ± 15	94 ± 36	99 ± 15	15 ± 6
MK-12	15 ± 13	21 ± 6	14 ± 2	NR
MK-13	5 ± 6	8 ± 3	5 ± 1	NR

[a] Values are mean ± SEM for 6 or 7 subjects in each study; A [110], B [111], C [38], and D [89]. NR, not reported. Values from studies A and B have been recalculated from data presented as ng/g liver. Studies A, B, and C are from Japanese populations where the consumption of natto, which contains high concentrations of MK-7, is prevalent.

There are aspects of the location of tissue vitamin K that may be related to specific functions of the vitamin not yet identified. There appears to be a relationship between the metabolism of sphingolipids and vitamin K, which has recently been reviewed [67]. It has been known for some time that some bacteria have an obligate requirement for growth that is related to a specific step in sphingolipid synthesis [68], and about 20 years later it was found that when young mice were fed a nonlethal amount of warfarin, the concentration of sulfatides and the main sulfatide synthesizing enzyme in rat brain were both decreased [69,70]. This response could be reversed by feeding the mice phylloquinone, and it was also found that brain sulfatide concentration and the activity of the galactocerebroside sulfotransferase could be altered by feeding mice varying amounts of vitamin K [71]. Although the mice in these studies were fed phylloquinone, the predominant form of vitamin K in the brain is MK-4, and an extensive study of sphingolipid concentration in different regions of the rat brain has shown that brain MK-4 concentration was positively correlated with the concentrations of sulfatides and sphingomyelin, but negatively correlated with gangliosides [72]. The mechanism by which vitamin K regulates the synthesis or turnover of these important complex lipids is not known. Studies conducted in an effort to delineate the specific role of vitamin K have been reviewed recently [67]. Although the currently available data do not point to a clear mechanism, the apparent requirement for MK-4 within the brain suggests that the brain does not maintain a concentration of phylloquinone that is sufficient to drive the need for γ-glutamyl carboxylation or that the role of MK-4 is not related to the action of the vitamin K-dependent carboxylase. A second apparent unique role of the vitamin is associated with the high concentration of MK-4 in the pancreas. There are lipid-rich components of pancreatic juice that have been shown [73] to contain caveolin, a membrane protein involved in cholesterol trafficking and endocytosis in cells. It has been shown that MK-4 is secreted from rat pancreas in vivo in amounts that are directly related to the secretion of caveolin and phospholipids [74]. Whether or not this very specific secretion of MK-4 into the gut might be related in some way to digestive zymogens secreted from the pancreas has not been determined.

Limited information regarding the subcellular distribution of vitamin K within various tissues is available. Early studies based on bioassays of isolated fractions of liver [75] indicated a wide distribution within subcellular organelles. Studies utilizing radioactive phylloquinone [76] indicated that more than 50% of the liver radioactivity was recovered in the microsomal fraction, and substantial amounts were found in the mitochondria and cellular debris fractions. The specific activity (picomoles vitamin K per milligram protein) of injected radioactive phylloquinone has been assessed [77], and only the mitochondrial and microsomal fractions had a specific activity that was enriched over that of the entire homogenate, with the highest activity in the microsomal fraction. A more detailed study [78] found the highest specific activity of radioactive phylloquinone to be in the Golgi and smooth microsomal membrane fractions, and the rate of vitamin loss from the cytosol has been shown to be more rapid than from membrane fractions as a deficiency develops [79]. The subcellular distribution of phylloquinone has now been studied with more recent analytical techniques [63], and the specific activity (nanograms phylloquinone/milligram protein) was found to be very low in the cytosolic fraction and rather similar in the mitochondrial and microsomal fractions of various tissue homogenates (Table 6.5). Only limited data on the cellular distribution of menaquinones are available, although MK-9 has been reported [56] to be preferentially localized in a mitochondrial rather than a microsomal subcellular fraction. Factors influencing intracellular distribution of the vitamin are not well understood, and only preliminary evidence of an intracellular vitamin K-binding protein that might facilitate intraorganelle movement has been presented [80].

TABLE 6.5
Intracellular Distribution of Phylloquinone in Rat Tissues

Tissue	ng/g Tissue Wet Wt.	ng/mg Protein in Homogenate			
		Total Tissue	Cytosol	Mitochondria	Microsomes
Liver	23.7	0.44	0.03	0.50	0.40
Heart	11.2	0.11	0.04	0.08	0.12
Pancreas	8.1	0.21	0.01	0.13	0.06
Kidney	2.9	0.07	0.01	0.10	0.04
Lung	1.4	0.07	0.02	0.15	0.09

Note: Rats were fed a chow ration (~2 µg phylloquinone/g) and tissue homogenates were separated by standard procedures to cytosol, mitochondria, and microsomal fractions.
Source: Modified from Reference [63].

6.4   TISSUE METABOLISM OF VITAMIN K

6.4.1   SYNTHESIS OF MENAQUINONE-4 FROM PHYLLOQUINONE

Although the majority of the menaquinones found in animal tissues are the product of bacterial menaquinone biosynthesis in the gut, very little MK-4 is produced by these organisms, but substantial amounts are present in some tissues and organs and can be formed by alternate pathways. Early studies by Martius [81], utilizing radioactive menadione administered to experimental animals, established that animal tissues could convert menadione to MK-4. Subsequent studies demonstrated that MK-4 could be generated by the in vitro incubation of rat or chick liver homogenates with menadione and geranylgeranyl pyrophosphate [82]. Although it has been shown [83,84] that the activity is located in microsomes and that other isoprenoid pyrophosphates can serve to alkylate menadione, the details of this enzymatic activity (Figure 6.5) have not been well characterized, nor has the enzyme been purified.

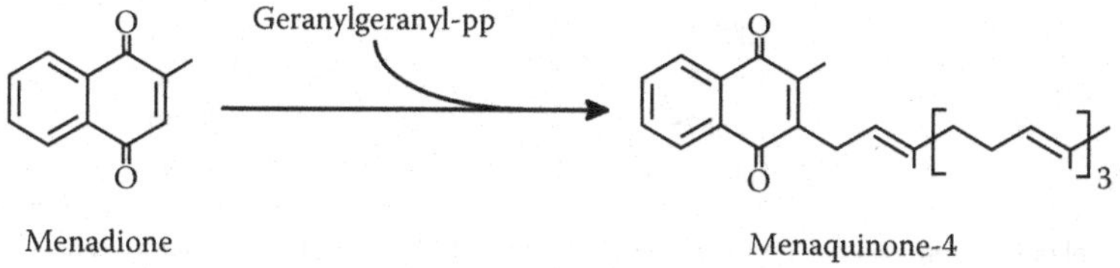

Menadione   Menaquinone-4

FIGURE 6.5   Prenylation of menadione to form menaquinone-4. This reaction can be demonstrated in a large number of cell types and is the metabolic conversion needed for menadione to become an active form of vitamin K.

Dietary intake of this menaquinone is very low, but due to supplementation of poultry rations with menadione as a vitamin K source, the major sources of vitamin K in chicken meat and eggs is MK-4.

The early studies of MK-4 synthesis also demonstrated that when birds were fed double-labeled phylloquinone, it was converted to tissue MK-4 by a process that required dealkylation of the phytyl side chain and subsequent realkylation of menadione with a geranylgeranyl side chain [85,86]. As the conversion was observed only when phylloquinone was administered orally, it was concluded that gut bacteria were generating menadione through the dealkylation of phylloquinone and that the menadione released was absorbed from the gut and realkylated in the liver. More recent studies [63,71,87,88] have demonstrated that the phylloquinone to MK-4 conversion is very extensive in extrahepatic tissues such as brain, pancreas, and salivary gland, and that its concentrations in those tissues exceed those of phylloquinone. The very high concentration of MK-4 relative to phylloquinone in specific tissues of rats (Tables 6.3 and 6.6) would suggest a specific function of MK-4 in those tissues, and distributions of MK-4 similar to those seen in rats have also been observed in human tissues [89]. Although an increase in dietary MK-4 will increase MK-4 concentrations in these tissues, it has been established that high tissue concentrations of MK-4 are more readily obtained in rats by phylloquinone supplementation than by supplementation with MK-4 [90].

The demonstration that gut bacteria are not needed for this conversion [91,92] has established that MK-4 is not formed by the alkylation of menadione produced by bacterial dealkylation of phylloquinone, and cultured kidney cells have been shown [91] to convert phylloquinone to MK-4 in a sterile incubation medium. This finding is consistent with the hypothesis that dealkylation of phylloquinone occurs within those cell types synthesizing large amounts of MK-4 and that menadione, or an initial cleavage product that is subsequently converted to menadione, is subsequently prenylated to form MK-4 (Figure 6.6). The dealkylation step in this conversion has

---

TABLE 6.6

Relative Phylloquinone and MK-4 Concentrations in Tissues of Rats Fed Phylloquinone as a Source of Vitamin K[a]

Tissue	Enrichment of MK-4	
	Phylloquinone:MK-4	Tissue:Liver Ratio
Liver	100:3	1
Heart	100:13	4
Kidney	100:25	8
Salivary Gland	100:575	190
Brain	100:875	290
Pancreas	100:5,600	1,870

[a] Values obtained from rats fed 1.5 µg phylloquinone/g diet [91] except for the pancreas data obtained from rats fed 6 µg phylloquinone/g diet [92]. The diets were not supplemented with menaquinone-4 or menadione.

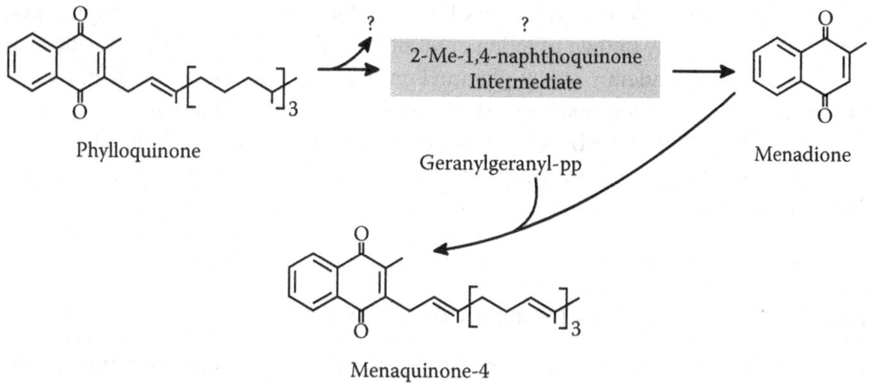

FIGURE 6.6 Cellular conversion of phylloquinone to menaquinone-4. The products of the initial dealkylation step have not been identified. There are data indicating that some of the long-chain menaquinones can also serve as the original substrate for the conversion.

been thought to require the double bond present in the first isoprenoid group of phylloquinone, as 2′,3′-dihydrophylloquinone has been reported to be incapable of being converted to MK-4 when administered orally [93,94]. This finding, however, is not supported by a comprehensive study [95] showing that rats fed equivalent amounts of phylloquinone or dihydrophylloquinone (~200 μg/kg diet) for 28 days had tissue MK-4 concentrations that were only marginally reduced in the rats fed dihydrophylloquinone. An alternate theory to the cellular conversion of phylloquinone to MK-4 [94] is that an unidentified enzyme within the intestinal wall is carrying out this first step of the process and that the menadione released is then transferred to and converted to MK-4 in the target tissues (Figure 6.5). This conclusion is based on the observation that urinary excretion of menadione was not observed when phylloquinone was administered to rats subcutaneously rather than orally. This response is, however, somewhat different than the results of a previous study [63] by the same group where substantial amounts of MK-4 were found in rat tissues following intravenous infusion of phylloquinone. These differences will require additional study. A more extensive study of the formation of MK-4 in cerebral tissue of mice [96] has also found that oral or enteral administration of phylloquinone that was deuterium-labeled in the naphthoquinone ring resulted in labeled MK-4 in cerebral tissue, but that this did not occur when the phylloquinone was administered parenterally or intracerebroventricularly. However, the same study demonstrated that incubation of cerebral slice cultures or embryonic primary cerebral cell cultures with phylloquinone resulted in the formation of MK-4. The authors suggest that there are two pathways to the synthesis of MK-4 in this tissue, prenylation of menadione, which had been generated in intestinal cells from phylloquinone or cleavage of phylloquinone to generate menadione within the target cells followed by prenylation. It is of interest that both the initial report of the generation of MK-4 from phylloquinone in cultured cells [91] and the more recent report of MK-4 formation in cultured cells [96] found that the preponderance of MK-4 generated in the cells was present as MK-4 epoxide. The preponderance of MK-4 formed by the alkylation of menadione by a number of investigators is, however, MK-4. As both phylloquinone and MK-4 are effective substrates for the only known function of vitamin K, the formation of Gla residues by the vitamin K-dependent gamma-glutamyl carboxylase, the metabolic significance of the apparent phylloquinone to MK-4 conversion is not yet apparent. The most likely role would be that MK-4 is a ligand for receptors that are involved with the control of metabolism within specific cells. At the present time there are no data to support this hypothesis.

6.4.2 Degradation and Excretion of Vitamin K

Initial studies utilizing relatively large doses of ^{14}C phylloquinone administered to rats [58] demonstrated that the major route of excretion was in the feces and that very little unmetabolized phylloquinone was present. Subsequent studies utilizing intravenously injected ^{3}H-phylloquinone (1 mg) in human subjects conducted by Shearer [35] established that urinary excretion was essentially complete after three days, and represented about 20% of the intravenous dose administered. Biliary excretion via the feces after five days represented about 35% of the dose. This split of the metabolites of vitamin between urine and feces does not appear to be heavily dependent on amount, as a second similar study utilizing a more physiological dose (45 μg of ^{3}H-phylloquinone) found that a single subject secreted 18% and 51% of the dose in urine and feces [5].

The most abundant cellular metabolite of phylloquinone is its 2,3-epoxide formed as a product of the action of the vitamin K-dependent carboxylase. This metabolite was discovered [97] during a follow-up of an observation [76] that warfarin treatment caused an increase in the amount of radioactive vitamin K in the liver. This increase was shown to be due to the presence of significant amounts of a metabolite more polar than phylloquinone that was isolated and characterized as phylloquinone-2, 3-epoxide. Further studies of this compound [98] revealed that about 10% of the vitamin K in the liver of a normal rat is present as the epoxide and that this can become the predominant form of the vitamin following treatment with coumarin anticoagulants. Although the total amount of a single dose of radioactive phylloquinone excreted in urine or feces was found not to be substantially altered by a therapeutic dose of warfarin, the amount found in urine was about doubled, and that in feces was decreased by approximately 50% [99,100]. This alteration presumably represents a difference in the rate and/or extent by which phylloquinone and phylloquinone-2, 3-epoxide are metabolized to secreted compounds. The current understanding of the nature of degradation products of phylloquinone formed following warfarin treatment has been well reviewed [5] and suggests that there are metabolites that are not simply 2,3-epoxides of the previously identified phylloquinone metabolites, but are the aglycones of metabolites that in some cases differ from those associated with phylloquinone degradation.

The first characterization of a urinary metabolite of vitamin K followed the demonstration [101] that the side chains of phylloquinone and MK-4 are shortened by the rat to 7 carbon atoms, yielding a terminal carboxylic acid group end that cyclized to form a γ-lactone from the remaining side chain of phylloquinone (Figure 6.7).

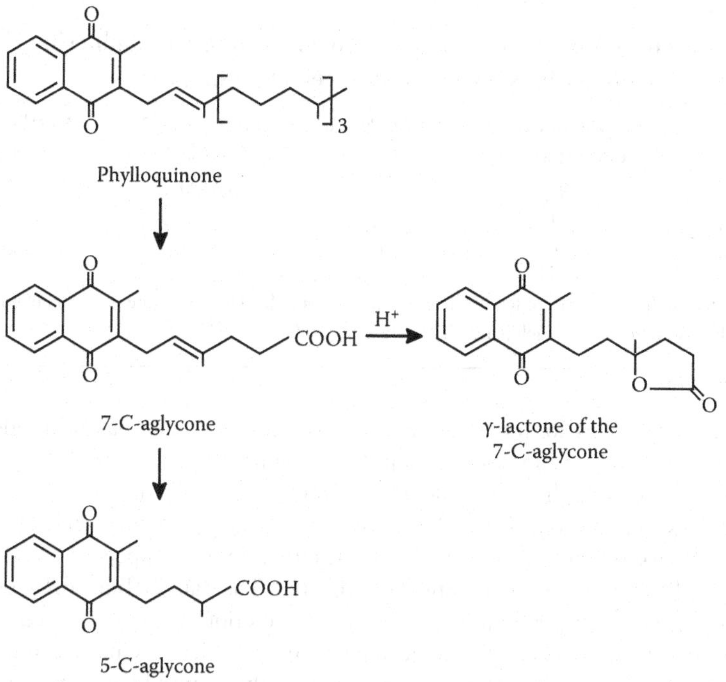

Phylloquinone

7-C-aglycone

γ-lactone of the
7-C-aglycone

5-C-aglycone

FIGURE 6.7   Structures of the two major urinary aglycones of phylloquinone and of the first identified urinary metabolite, the γ -lactone of the 7-C-aglycone. Long-chain menaquinones appear to be substrates for the same pathway of degradation.

Later studies in human subjects indicate that more than 80% of the radioactivity present in urine could be attributed to acidic conjugates derived from phylloquinone and that almost all could be specifically hydrolyzed by β-glucuronidase. Following removal of the conjugated sugar by acid hydrolysis, there are two main aglycone acidic metabolites [5] containing either seven of the side chain carbons ending in a carboxylic acid group (metabolite I), or a 5-carbon acidic chain II (metabolite II). The neutral γ-lactone originally identified appears to be an artifact formed during the acid hydrolysis of the conjugates. The same two major metabolites have been observed following the administration of MK-4 to rats [102]. The pathway of formation appears to be ω oxidation of the side chain by cytochrome P450 enzymes followed by β-oxidation to shorten the isoprenyl side chain. This is the same pathway utilized for the oxidation of the multiprenyl side chains of tocopherols and coenzyme Qs [103]. The initial ω oxidation of vitamin E is known to be self-regulated by the induction of cytochrome P450s via the nuclear receptor PXR [103], and both phylloquinone and particularly MK-4 will also activate this system.

Newer methodology [57] has made it possible to routinely measure the urinary concentration of these major metabolites of vitamin K. The response of these

TABLE 6.7

Urinary Excretion of Total C5 and C7 Phylloquinone Metabolites by Human Subjects Consuming Varying Amounts of Phylloquinone

Diet	Phylloquinone Intake (µg/day)	Intake Period (days)	Total C5 + C7 (µg/day)	Metabolites (molar %)
Control	93	5	5.5 ± 0.2	9.2
Depletion	11	15	3.5 ± 0.2	49.4
Repletion	206	10	10.6 ± 0.3	8.0

Note: Nine adult subjects were fed the designated diets, and the data shown are the data obtained from the last three days of each period. For details see Reference [112].

excreted metabolites to alterations in daily vitamin K intake has been addressed by using stored urine samples from a previous human study which investigated the impact of changes in phylloquinone or dihydrophylloquinone intake on bone formation and resorption [104]. It was found that the 5C-aglycone represents about 75% of the total excretion and that the daily urinary excretion appeared to be closely related to the amount of phylloquinone in the diet. The data in Table 6.7 present the relationship between phylloquinone intake on excretion of the combined 5C- and 7C-aglycone metabolites as the subjects consumed a relatively normal diet (95 µg phylloquinone/day), a depletion diet containing only 11 µg phylloquinone per day, and a repletion diet, which was the depletion diet with the addition of 206 µg of phylloquinone dissolved in corn oil and added to the muffins consumed at the breakfast meal. The results do suggest a relationship of metabolites to intake and the logarithm of the total urinary metabolite excretion at phylloquinone intakes of 11, 93, and 206 µg per day was found to be approximately linearly related to phylloquinone intake. Extrapolation of this relationship to a 0 intake of phylloquinone gave an estimate of about 3 µg per day of urinary aglycones, which the authors suggest may represent the utilization of menaquinones produced by intestinal organisms that have been transferred to tissues metabolizing the vitamin, or to the release of phylloquinone from tissue stores. In contrast to significant excretion of both aglycones from phylloquinone consumption, during 2′,3′-dihydrophylloquinone consumption, nearly 100% of the excretion was in the form of the 5C-aglycone. The possibility of a 7C-aglycone without the 2′,3′ double bond was suggested, but its existence has not been reported. This study represents a real advance in an understanding of vitamin K degradative metabolism, which could be a valuable indicator of vitamin K status. However, assumptions regarding the impact of increased phylloquinone intake on the ratio of urinary to biliary secretion and a better understanding of the bioavailability of phylloquinone from foods currently question the accuracy of the calculations, and they appear to be open to further study.

The most recent advance in the understanding of vitamin K metabolism is the report that a fraction of dietary phylloquinone is catabolized to menadione. Early studies using [105–108] radioactive menadione established that both urine and bile

TABLE 6.8

Excretion of Urinary Menadione Following Ingestion of Various Forms of Vitamin K

Form of Vitamin K	Amount (mg)	% of Dose Excreted as Menadione
Menadione ($n = 2$)	10	19.8 ± 3.6
Phylloquinone ($n = 3$)	10	3.5 ± 2.1
Menaquinone-4 ($n = 3$)	15	1.8 ± 0.8
Menaquinone-7 ($n = 1$)	1	~0.7

Note: The various forms of vitamin K were consumed in a single dose by adult male subjects, and the excretion of menadione followed hourly for 24 h. For details, see Reference [94].

contained menadione, as glucuronides and sulfate conjugates. When the urinary conjugates are treated with acid, free menadione is released; and it has now been found [94] that human subjects consuming milligram amounts of prenylated forms of vitamin K are excreting substantial amounts of menadione (Table 6.8). The metabolism to menadione occurs rapidly, and the peak excretion of menadione from phylloquinone occurred three hours after the dose was administered and dropped to very low levels within eight hours. Although the amounts of vitamin K consumed were substantially above the amount that could be consumed in a normal diet, analysis of archived samples from a previously published study [104] indicated that alterations of phylloquinone intake from a normal diet (~100 µg) to a restricted diet (~11 µg) to a repleted diet (~200 mg) resulted in urinary excretion of menadione that was positively related to the phylloquinone intake.

The available information does not make it possible to calculate an accurate estimate of the fraction of ingested phylloquinone that is subject to side-chain cleavage during its metabolic pathway. Both ingested MK-4 and MK-7 were shown to lead to menadione excretion, but at a lower level than phylloquinone. Menadione was not observed following the ingestion of $2',3'$-dihydrophylloquinone, nor was it observed when phylloquinone was administered subcutaneously. The authors of the study suggested that the extent of catabolism of phylloquinone to menadione might be in the range of 5% to 25%. It will be a difficult measurement to quantify, as the bioavailability of the vitamin and the distribution between urinary and biliary excretion are not known. The rate of cleavage may also be influenced by the amount of substrate, as a 10 mg dose of phylloquinone produced a urinary menadione excretion rate of 16 µg/mg of vitamin/24 h, while the deletion/repletion study produced a urinary menadione excretion rate of ~40 µg/mg of vitamin/24 h from an intake of 200 µg/day. Further studies will be needed to clearly define the importance of this metabolic pathway in vitamin K degradation (Figure 6.8). At this time, evidence of any further metabolism of the naphthoquinone ring itself, other than alkylation to MK-4, is lacking. Studies with hepatectomized rats [109] have, however, indicated that both extrahepatic and hepatic metabolism of menadione are involved in its removal from tissues.

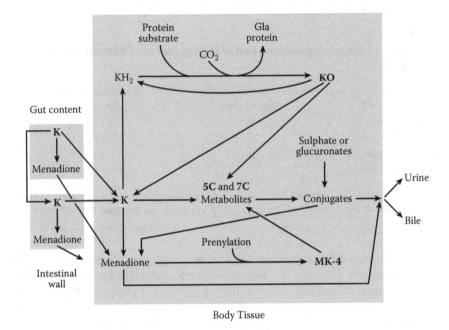

FIGURE 6.8 Known and postulated pathways for the metabolism and degradation of phylloquinone (K), reduced phylloquinone (KH_2), phylloquinone-2,3-epoxide (KO), and menaquinone-4 (MK-4).

6.5 CURRENT STATUS OF RESEARCH EFFORTS

The physiology of the absorption and plasma transport of vitamin K is reasonably well understood and in general seems to be similar to the pathway established for other hydrophobic metabolites. There has been substantial interest in the different rates of plasma clearance of phylloquinone, the major dietary source of the vitamin; menaquinone-4, a very minor dietary contributor; and long-chain menaquinones, which may contribute a significant amount of vitamin K to the diets of some people. Decreases in the rate of clearance lead to higher circulating concentrations of the vitamin, but provide no information regarding what is probably the most important factor, the movement of various vitamers into cells. Studies of the impact of a range of dietary intakes of various forms of vitamin K on a panel of markers of vitamin K status would be of interest and could be done in laboratory animals at a reasonable cost, but would probably be prohibitively expensive in a human subjects trial.

One area that should be focused on is the lack of reliable information on the bioavailability of vitamin K from various foods. The currently available data are not consistent, but would suggest that the phylloquinone present in a normal diet might be as low as 10% to 15% as available as a phylloquinone supplement or that it might be about 50% as available. Most discussions of the appropriate dietary intake of vitamin K utilize studies where vitamin K intake, either as food or a supplement, is varied and tend to focus on the intake of the vitamin without any attempt to assess how much is available to the subject. This presents a substantial problem. Better data on the bioavailability of vitamin K from the components of normal mixed foods diets would be very useful for groups attempting to establish dietary reference intakes (DRIs) for vitamin K, and, as only a few foods contain substantial amounts of the vitamin, these data could be obtained in a relatively short time. The ability to obtain vitamin K labeled with heavy isotopes should also aid in obtaining bioavailability data that would provide better information than is now available.

Probably the most interesting subject related to vitamin K is the question of what is the physiological role of menaquinone-4. Two well-established findings appear to point to one or more specific functions of this vitamer. One, animals have evolved a metabolic pathway to convert phylloquinone, and probably long-chain menaquino-nes, to MK-4; and two, very high concentrations of MK-4 are present in specific tis-sues. Although MK-4 is a good substrate for the vitamin K-dependent carboxylase, it is not needed for this role, and it would seem that it might be acting as a ligand for a receptor controlling metabolism in those tissues that concentrate this vitamer. Although an intriguing hypothesis, no evidence for this role is currently available. The pathway of the synthesis of MK-4 by animals is also an open question. It is clear that generation of menadione from phylloquinone in the intestinal wall is a pathway that could lead to MK-4 by the well-known pathway that results in the alkylation of menadione to MK-4. Two other studies have found that conversion of phylloquinone to MK-4 can be an intracellular process not requiring absorption of menadione. Although this pathway needs additional verification, it appears likely that both pathways may be involved in the formation of this unique form of vitamin K. A possible specific role of MK-4 in the brain and indications that an interaction with complex lipids is involved is also an area of research that would expand our current understanding of the possible function of vitamin K.

The major metabolic pathway leading to the degradation of vitamin K appears to have been identified, but the details regarding the control of and specificity of this ω-oxidation pathway are not established. The finding that a significant portion of dietary phylloquinone is subjected to side-chain cleavage to generate menadione is a very important advance in understanding the overall process of vitamin K metabo-lism. The cellular specificity and mechanism of action of the enzyme carrying out the cleavage are research avenues that should be followed up to clarify what is cur-rently a rather open question.

REFERENCES

1. Hollander, D. 1973. Vitamin K_1 absorption by everted intestinal sacs of the rat. *Am J Physiol* 225:360–364.
2. Hollander, D. and E. Rim. 1976. Factors affecting the absorption of vitamin K-1 in vitro. *Gut* 17:450–455.
3. Hollander, D. and E. Rim. 1978. Effect of luminal constituents on vitamin K_1 absorption into thoracic duct lymph. *Am J Physiol* 234:E54–E59.
4. Hollander, D., E. Rim, and K.S. Muralidhara. 1977. Vitamin K_1 intestinal absorption in vivo: Influence of luminal contents on transport. *Am J Physiol* 232:E69–E74.
5. Shearer, M.J., A. McBurney, and P. Barkhan. 1974. Studies on the absorption and metab-olism of phylloquinone (vitamin K_1) in man. *Vitamins and Hormones* 32:513–542.
6. Suttie, J.W. 1995. The importance of menaquinones in human nutrition. *Annu Rev Nutr* 15:399–417.

7. Hollander, D. and E. Rim. 1976. Vitamin K_2 absorption by rat everted small intestinal sacs. *Am J Physiol* 231:415–419.

8. Hollander, D., K.S. Muralidhara, and E. Rim. 1976. Colonic absorption of bacterially synthesized vitamin K_2 in the rat. *Am J Physiol* 230:251–255.

9. Hollander, D., E. Rim, and P.E. Ruble. 1977. Vitamin K_2 colonic and ileal in vivo absorption: Bile, fatty acids, and pH effects on transport. *Am J Physiol* 233:E124–E129.

10. Ichihashi, T., Y. Takagishi, K. Uchida, and H. Yamada. 1992. Colonic absorption of menaquinone-4 and menaquinone-9 in rats. *J Nutr* 122:506–512.

11. Conly, J.M. and K.E. Stein. 1993. The absorption and bioactivity of bacterially synthesized menaquinones. *Clin Invest Med* 16:45–57.

12. Conly, J.M. and K. Stein. 1992. Quantitative and qualitative measurements of K vitamins in human intestinal contents. *Am J Gastroenterol* 87:311–316.

13. Hollander, D. and T.C. Truscott. 1974. Colonic absorption of vitamin K-3. *J Lab Clin Med* 83:648–656.

14. Hollander, D. and T.C. Truscott. 1974. Mechanism and site of vitamin K-3 small intestinal transport. *Am J Physiol* 226:1516–1522.

15. Gijsbers, B.L.M.G., K.-S.G. Jie, and C. Vermeer. 1996. Effect of food composition on vitamin K absorption in human volunteers. *Brit J Nutr* 76:223–229.

16. Garber, A.K., N.C. Binkley, D.C. Krueger, and J.W. Suttie. 1999. Comparison of phylloquinone bioavailability from food sources or a supplement in human subjects. *J Nutr* 129:1201–1203.

17. Booth, S.L., M.E. O'Brien-Morse, G.E. Dallal, K.W. Davidson, and C.M. Gundberg. 1999. Response of vitamin K status to different intakes and sources of phylloquinone-rich foods: Comparison of younger and older adults. *Am J Clin Nutr* 70:368–377.

18. Booth, S.L., A.H. Lichtenstein, and G.E. Dallal. 2002. Phylloquinone absorption from phylloquinone-fortified oil is greater than from a vegetable in younger and older men and women. *J Nutr* 132:2609–2612.

19. Dolnikowski, G.G., Z. Sun, M.A. Grusak, J.W. Peterson, and S.L. Booth. 2002. HPLC and GC/MS determination of deuterated vitamin K (phylloquinone) in human serum after ingestion of deuterium-labeled broccoli. *J Nutr Biochem* 13:168–174.

20. Erkkila, A.T., A.H. Lichtenstein, G.G. Dolnikowski, M.A. Grusak, S.M. Jalbert, K.A. Aquino, J.W. Peterson, and S.L. Booth. 2004. Plasma transport of vitamin K in men using deuterium-labeled collard greens. *Metabolism* 53:215–221.

21. Kurilich, A.C., S.J. Britz, B.A. Clevidence, and J.A. Novotny. 2003. Isotopic labeling and LC-APCI-MS quantification for investigating absorption of carotenoids and phylloquinone from kale (*Brassica oleracea*). *J Agric Food Chem* 51:4877–4883.

22. Jones, K.S., L.J.C. Bluck, and W.A. Coward. 2006. Analysis of isotope ratios in vitamin K_1 (phylloquinone) from human plasma by gas chromatography/mass spectrometry. *Rapid Commun Mass Spectrom* 20:1894–1898.

23. Jones, K.S., L.J.C. Bluck, L.Y. Wang, and W.A. Coward. 2008. A stable isotope method for the simultaneous measurement of vitamin K_1 (phylloquinone) kinetics and absorption. *Eur J Clin Nutr* 62:1273–1281.

24. van Beek, E., C. Lowik, G. van der Pluijm, and S. Papapoulos. 1999. The role of geranylgeranylation in bone resorption and its suppression by bisphosphonates in fetal bone explants in vitro: A clue to the mechanism of action of nitrogen-containing bisphosphonates. *J Bone Min Res* 14:722–729.

25. Schurgers, L.J. and C. Vermeer. 2000. Determination of phylloquinone and menaquinones in food. *Haemostasis* 30:298–307.

26. Lamon-Fava, S., J.A. Sadowski, K.W. Davidson, M.E. O'Brien, J.R. McNamara, and E.J. Schaefer. 1998. Plasma lipoproteins as carriers of phylloquinone (vitamin K_1) in humans. *Am J Clin Nutr* 67:1226–1231.

27. Kohlmeier, M., J. Saupe, H.J. Drossel, and M.J. Shearer. 1995. Variation of phylloquinone (vitamin K_1) concentrations in hemodialysis patients. *Thromb Haemostas* 74:1252–1254.

28. Sadowski, J.A., S.J. Hood, G.E. Dallal, and P.J. Garry. 1989. Phylloquinone in plasma from elderly and young adults: Factors influencing its concentration. *Am J Clin Nutr* 50:100–108.

29. Saupe, J., M.J. Shearer, and M. Kohlmeier. 1993. Phylloquinone transport and its influence on gamma-carboxyglutamate residues of osteocalcin in patients on maintenance hemodialysis. *Am J Clin Nutr* 58:204–208.

30. Yan, L., B. Zhou, S. Nigdikar, X. Wang, J. Bennett, and A. Prentice. 2005. Effect of apolipoprotein E genotype on vitamin K status in healthy older adults from China and the UK. *Brit J Nutr* 94:956–961.

31. Niemeier, A., M. Kassem, K. Toedter, D. Wendt, W. Ruether, U. Beissegel, and J. Heeren. 2005. Expression of LRP1 by human osteoblasts: A mechanism for the delivery of lipoproteins and vitamin K_1 to bone. *J Bone Miner Res* 20:283–293.

32. Newman, P., F. Bonello, A.S. Wierzbicki, P. Lumb, G.F. Savidge, and M.J. Shearer. 2002. The uptake of lipoprotein-borne phylloquinone (vitamin K_1) by osteoblasts and osteoblast-like cells: Role of heparan sulfate proteoglycans and apolipoprotein E. *J Bone Miner Res* 17:426–433.

33. Schurgers, L.J. and C. Vermeer. 2002. Differential lipoprotein transport pathways of K-vitamins in healthy subjects. *Biochim Biophys Acta* 1570:27–32.

34. Schurgers, L.J., K.J.F. Teunissen, K. Hamulyak, M.H.J. Knapen, H. Vik, and C. Vermeer. 2007. Vitamin K-containing dietary supplements: Comparison of synthetic vitamin K_1 and natto-derived menaquinone-7. *Blood* 109:3279–3283.

35. Shearer, M.J., C.N. Mallinson, G.R. Webster, and P. Barkhan. 1972. Clearance from plasma and excretion in urine, faeces and bile of an intravenous dose of tritiated vitamin K_1 in man. *Brit J Haematol* 22:579–588.

36. Bjornsson, T.D., P.J. Meffin, S.E. Sweezey, and T.F. Blaschke. 1979. Effects of clofibrate and warfarin alone and in combination on the disposition of vitamin K_1. *J Pharmacol Exp Therap* 210:322–326.

37. Olson, R.E., J. Chao, D. Graham, M.W. Bates, and J.H. Lewis. 2002. Total body phylloquinone and its turnover in human subjects at two levels of vitamin K intake. *Brit J Nutr* 88:543–553.

38. Usui, Y., H. Tanimura, N. Nishimura, N. Kobayashi, T. Okanoue, and K. Ozawa. 1990. Vitamin K concentrations in the plasma and liver of surgical patients. *Am J Clin Nutr* 51:846–852.

39. Li, Z.-Q., F.-Y. He, C.J. Stehle, Z. Wang, S. Kar, F.M. Finn, and B.I. Carr. 2002. Vitamin K uptake in hepatocytes and hepatoma cells. *Life Sci* 70:2085–2100.

40. Suhara, Y., A. Murakimi, K. Nakagawa, Y. Mizuguchi, and T. Okano. 2006. Comparative uptake, metabolism, and utilization of menaquinone-4 and phylloquinone in human cultured cell lines. *Bioorg Med Chem* 14:6601–6607.

41. Hoshi, K., K. Nomura, Y. Sano, and Y. Koshihara. 1999. Nuclear vitamin K_2 binding protein in human osteoblasts. *Biochem Pharmacol* 58:1631–1638.

42. Conly, J.M. and R.T. Stein. 1992. The production of menaquinones (vitamin K_2) by intestinal bacteria and their role in maintaining coagulation homeostasis. *Prog Food Nutr Sci* 16:307–343.

43. Ramotar, K., J.M. Conly, H. Chubb, and T.J. Louie. 1984. Production and menaquinones by intestinal anaerobes. *J Infect Dis* 150:213–218.

44. Fernandez, F. and M.D. Collins. 1987. Vitamin K composition of anaerobic gut bacteria. *FEMS Microbiol* 41:175–180.

45. Conly, J.M. 1997. Assay of menaquinones in bacterial cultures, stool samples, and intestinal contents. *Meth Enzymol* 282:457–466.

46. Greer, F.R., L.L. Mummah-Schendel, S. Marshall, and J.W. Suttie. 1988. Vitamin K_1 (phylloquinone) and vitamin K_2 (menaquinone) status in newborns during the first week of life. *Pediatrics* 81:137–140.

47. Savage, D. and J. Lindenbaum. 1983. Clinical and experimental human vitamin K deficiency. In *Nutrition in Hematology*, ed. J. Lindenbaum, 271–320. New York: Churchill Livingstone.

48. Lipsky, J.J. 1988. Antibiotic-associated hypoprothrombinaemia. *J Antimicrob Chemother* 21:281–300.

49. Conly, J. and K. Stein. 1994. Reduction of vitamin K_2 concentrations in human liver associated with the use of broad spectrum antimicrobials. *Clin Invest Med* 17:531–539.

50. Ramotar, K., H. Chubb, E. Rayner, J. Conley, E.J. Bow, and T.J. Louie. 1985. Effect of empiric antimicrobial regimens on fecal flora and menaquinone (MK) profiles in neutropenic patients. *Microecol Ther* 15:311–312.

51. Suttie, J.W., C.G. Kindberg, J.L. Greger, and N.U. Bang. 1988. Effects of vitamin K (phylloquinone) restriction in the human. In *Current Advances in Vitamin K Research*, ed. J.W. Suttie, 465–476. New York: Elsevier Science Publishing Co.

52. Bechtold, H., K. Andrassy, E. Jahnchen, J. Koderisch, H. Koderisch, L.S. Weilemann, H-G. Sonntag, and E. Ritz. 1984. Evidence for impaired hepatic vitamin K_1 metabolism in patients treated with N-methyl-thiotetrazole cephalosporins. *Thromb Haemostas* 51:358–361.

53. Creedon, K.A. and J.W. Suttie. 1986. Effect of N-methyl-thiotetrazole on vitamin K epoxide reductase. *Thrombosis Res* 44:147–153.

54. Cohen, H., S.D. Scott, I.J. Mackie, M. Shearer, R. Bax, S.J. Karran, and S.J. Machin. 1988. The development of hypoprothrombinaemia following antibiotic therapy in malnourished patients with low serum vitamin K_1 levels. *Brit J Haematol* 68:63–66.

55. Shearer, M.J., H. Bechtold, K. Andrassy, J. Koderisch, P.T. McCarthy, D. Trenk, E. Jahnchen, and E. Ritz. 1988. Mechanism of cephalosporin-induced hypoprothrombinemia: Relation to cephalosporin side chain, vitamin K metabolism, and vitamin K status. *J Clin Pharmacol* 28:88–95.

56. Reedstrom, C.K. and J.W. Suttie. 1995. Comparative distribution, metabolism, and utilization of phylloquinone and menaquinone-9 in rat liver. *Proc Soc Exp Biol Med* 209:403–409.

57. Harrington, D.J., R. Soper, C. Edwards, G.F. Savidge, S.J. Hodges, and M.J. Shearer. 2005. Determination of the urinary aglycone metabolites of vitamin K by HPLC with redox-mode electrochemical detection. *J Lipid Res* 46:1053–1060.

58. Taylor, J.D., G.J. Millar, L.B. Jaques, and J.W.T. Spinks. 1956. The distribution of administered vitamin K_1-^{14}C in rats. *Can J Biochem Physiol* 34:1143–1152.

59. Thierry, M.J., M.A. Hermodson, and J.W. Suttie. 1970. Vitamin K and warfarin distribution and metabolism in the warfarin-resistant rat. *Am J Physiol* 219:854–859.

60. Kindberg, C.G. and J.W. Suttie. 1989. Effect of various intakes of phylloquinone on signs of vitamin K deficiency and serum and liver phylloquinone concentrations in the rat. *J Nutr* 119:175–180.

61. Konishi, T., S. Baba, and H. Sone. 1973. Whole-body autoradiographic study of vitamin K distribution in rat. *Chem Pharm Bull* 21:220–224.

62. Duello, T.J. and J.T. Matschiner. 1972. Characterization of vitamin K from human liver. *J Nutr* 102:331–335.

63. Thijssen, H.H.W. and M.J. Drittij-Reijnders. 1994. Vitamin K distribution in rat tissues: Dietary phylloquinone is a source of tissue menaquinone-4. *Brit J Nutr* 72:415–425.

64. Kayata, S., C. Kindberg, F.R. Greer, and J.W. Suttie. 1989. Vitamin K_1 and K_2 in infant human liver. *J Pediatr Gastroenterol Nutr* 8:304–307.

65. Shearer, M.J., P.T. McCarthy, O.E. Crampton, and M.B. Mattock. 1988. The assessment of human vitamin K status from tissue measurements. In *Current Advances in Vitamin K Research*, ed. J.W. Suttie, 437–452. New York: Elsevier Science Publishing Co.

66. Will, B.H. and J.W. Suttie. 1992. Comparative metabolism of phylloquinone and menaquinone-9 in rat liver. *J Nutr* 122:953–958.

67. Denisova, N.A. and S.L. Booth. 2005. Vitamin K and sphingolipid metabolism: Evidence to date. *Nutr Rev* 63:111–121.

68. Lev, M. and A.F. Milford. 1971. Vitamin K stimulation of sphingolipid synthesis. *Biochem Biophys Res Commun* 45:358–362.

69. Sundaram, K.S. and M. Lev. 1988. Warfarin administration reduces synthesis of sulfatides and other sphingolipids in mouse brain. *J Lipid Res* 29:1475–1479.

70. Sundaram, K.S. and M. Lev. 1990. Regulation of sulfotransferase activity by vitamin K in mouse brain. *Arch Biochem Biophys* 277:109–113.

71. Sundaram, K.S., J.A. Engelke, A.L. Foley, J.W. Suttie, and M. Lev. 1996. Vitamin K status influences brain sulfatide metabolism in young mice and rats. *J Nutr* 126:2746–2751.

72. Carrie, I., J. Portoukalian, R. Vicaretti, J. Rochford, S. Potvin, and G. Ferland. 2004. Menaquinone-4 concentration is correlated with sphingolipid concentrations in rat brain. *J Nutr* 134:167–172.

73. Liu, P., W.-P. Li, and R.G.W. Machleidt. 1999. Identification of caveolin-2 in lipoprotein particles secreted by exocrine cells. *Nat Cell Biol* 1:369–375.

74. Thomas, D.D.H., K.J. Krzykowski, J.A. Engelke, and G.E. Groblewski. 2004. Exocrine pancreatic secretion of phospholipid, menaquinone-4, and caveolin-2 in vivo. *Biochem Biophys Res Commun* 319:974–979.

75. Green, J.P., E. Sondergaard, and H. Dam. 1956. Intracellular distribution of vitamin K in beef liver. *Biochim Biophys Acta* 19:182–183.

76. Bell, R.G. and J.T. Matschiner. 1969. Intracellular distribution of vitamin K in the rat. *Biochim Biophys Acta* 184:597–603.

77. Thierry, M.J. and J.W. Suttie. 1971. Effect of warfarin and the chloro analog of vitamin K on phylloquinone metabolism. *Arch Biochem Biophys* 147:430–435.

78. Nyquist, S.E., J.T. Matschiner, and D.J.J. Morre. 1971. Distribution of vitamin K among rat liver cell fractions. *Biochim Biophys Acta* 244:645–649.

79. Knauer, T.E., C.M. Siegfried, and J.T. Matschiner. 1976. Vitamin K requirement and the concentration of vitamin K in rat liver. *J Nutr* 106:1747–1756.

80. Kight, C.E., C.K. Reedstrom, and J.W. Suttie. 1995. Identification, isolation, and partial purification of a cytosolic binding protein for vitamin K from rat liver. *FASEB J* 9:A725.

81. Martius, C. and H.O. Esser. 1958. Uber die konstitution des im tierkorper aus methyl naphthochinon gebildenten K-vitamines. *Biochem Z* 331:1–9.

82. Martius, C. 1961. The metabolic relationships between the different K vitamins and the synthesis of the ubiquinones. *Am J Clin Nutr* 9:97–103.

83. Dialameh, G.H., K.G. Yekundi, and R.E. Olson. 1970. Enzymatic alkylation of menaquinone-o to menaquinones by microsomes from chick liver. *Biochim Biophys Acta* 223:332–338.

84. Taggart, W.V. and J.T. Matschiner. 1969. Metabolism of menadione-6,7-^{3}H in the rat. *Biochemistry* 8:1141–1146.

85. Billeter, M. and C. Martius. 1960. Uber die unwandlung von plyllochinon (vitamin K_2) in vitamin $K_{2(20)}$ in tierkorper. *Biochem Z* 333:430–439.

86. Billeter, M., W. Bollinger, and C. Martius. 1964. Untersuchungen uber die unwandlung von verfutterten K-vitaminen durch austausch der seitenkette und die rolle der darmbakterien hierbei. *Biochem Z* 340:290–303.

87. Will, B.H., Y. Usui, and J.W. Suttie. 1992. Comparative metabolism and requirement of vitamin K in chicks and rats. *J Nutr* 122:2354–2360.

88. Guillaumont, M., H. Weiser, L. Sann, B. Vignal, M. Leclercq, and A. Frederich. 1992. Hepatic concentration of vitamin K active compounds after application of phylloquinone to chickens on a vitamin K deficient or adequate diet. *Int J Vitam Nutr Res* 62:15–20.

89. Thijssen, H.H.W. and M.J. Drittij-Reijnders. 1996. Vitamin K status in human tissues: Tissue-specific accumulation of phylloquinone and menaquinone-4. *Brit J Nutr* 75:121–127.

90. Thijssen, H.H.W., M.J. Drittij-Reijnders, and M.A.J.G. Fischer. 1996. Phylloquinone and menaquinone-4 distribution in rats: Synthesis rather than uptake determines menaquinone-4 organ concentrations. *J Nutr* 126:537–543.

91. Davidson, R.T., A.L. Foley, J.A. Engelke, and J.W. Suttie. 1998. Conversion of dietary phylloquinone to tissue menaquinone-4 in rats is not dependent on gut bacteria. *J Nutr* 128:220–223.

92. Ronden, J.E., H.H.W. Thijssen, and C. Vermeer. 1998. Tissue distribution of K-vitamers under different nutritional regimens in the rat. *Biochim Biophys Acta* 1379:16–22.

93. Sato, T., R. Ozaki, S. Kamo, Y. Hara, S. Konishi, Y. Isobe, S. Saitoh, and H. Harada. 2003. The biological activity and tissue distribution of 2',3'-dihydrophylloquinone in rats. *Biochim Biophys Acta* 1622:145–150.

94. Thijssen, H.H.W., L.M.T. Vervoort, L.J. Schurgers, and M.J. Shearer. 2006. Menadione is a metabolite of oral vitamin K. *Brit J Nutr* 95:260–266.

95. Booth, S.L., J.W. Peterson, D. Smith, M.K. Shea, J. Chamberland, and N. Crivello. 2008. Age and dietary form of vitamin K affect menaquinone-4 concentrations in male Fischer 344 rats. *J Nutr* 138:492–496.

96. Okano, T., Y. Shimomura, M. Yamane, Y. Suhara, M. Kamao, M. Sugiura, and K. Nakagawa. 2008. Conversion of phylloquinone (vitamin K_1) into menaquinone-4 (vitamin K_2) in mice. Two possible routes for menaquinone-4 accumulation in cerebra of mice. *J Biol Chem* 283:11270–11279.

97. Matschiner, J.T., R.G. Bell, J.M. Amelotti, and T.E. Knauer. 1970. Isolation and characterization of a new metabolite of phylloquinone in the rat. *Biochim Biophys Acta* 201:309–315.

98. Bell, R.G., J.A. Sadowski, and J.T. Matschiner. 1972. Mechanism of action of warfarin: Warfarin and metabolism of vitamin K_1. *Biochemistry* 11:1959–1961.

99. Shearer, M.J., P. Barkhan, and G.R. Webster. 1970. Absorption and excretion of an oral dose of tritiated vitamin K_1 in man. *Brit J Haematol* 18:297–308.

100. Shearer, M.J., A. McBurney, A.M. Breckenridge, and P. Barkhan. 1977. Effect of warfarin on the metabolism of phylloquinone (vitamin K_1): Dose-response relationships in man. *Clin Sci Mol Med* 52:621–630.

101. Wiss, O. and H. Gloor. 1966. Absorption, distribution, storage and metabolites of vitamin K and related quinones. *Vitamins and Hormones* 24:575–586.

102. Tadano, K., T. Yuzuriha, T. Sato, T. Fujita, K. Shimada, K. Hashimoto, and T. Satoh. 1989. Identification of menaquinone-4 metabolites in the rat. *Pharmacobiodyn* 12:640–645.

103. Landes, N., M. Birringer, and R. Brigelius-Flohe. 2003. Homologous metabolic and gene activating routes for vitamins E and K. *Mol Aspects Med* 24:337–344.

104. Booth, S.L., A.H. Lichtenstein, M.E. O'Brien-Morse, N.M. McKeown, R.J. Wood, E.J. Saltzman, and C.M. Gundberg. 2001. Effects of a hydrogenated form of vitamin K on bone formation and resorption. *Am J Clin Nutr* 74:783–790.

105. Hoskin, F.C.G., J.W.T. Spinks, and L.B. Jaques. 1954. Urinary excretion products of menadione (vitamin K_3). *Can J Biochem Physiol* 32:240–250.

106. Solvonuk, P.F., L.B. Jaques, J.E. Leddy, L.W. Trevoy, and J.W.T. Spinks. 1952. Experiments with C^{14} menadione (vitamin K_3). *Proc Soc Exp Biol Med* 79:597–604.

107. Thompson, R.M., N. Gerber, R.A. Seibert, and D.M. Desiderio. 1972. Identification of 2-methyl-1,4-naphthohydroquinone monoglucuronide as a metabolite of 2-methyl-1, 4-naphthoquinone (menadione) in rat bile. *Res Commun Chem Path Pharmacol* 4:543–552.

108. Losito, R., C.A. Owen, and E.V. Flock. 1967. Metabolism of [C¹⁴] menadione. *Biochemistry* 6:62–68.

109. Losito, R., C.A. Owen, and E.V. Flock. 1968. Metabolic studies of vitamin K_1-^{14}C and menadione-^{14}C in the normal and hepatectomized rats. *Thrombos Diathes Heamorrh* 19:383–388.

110. Uchida, K. and T. Komeno. 1988. Relationships between dietary and intestinal vitamin K, clotting factor levels, plasma vitamin K and urinary Gla. In *Current Advances in Vitamin K Research*, ed. J.W. Suttie, 477–492. New York: Elsevier Science Publishing Co.

111. Usui, Y., N. Nishimura, N. Kobayashi, T. Okanoue, M. Kimoto, and K. Ozawa. 1989. Measurement of vitamin K in human liver by gradient elution high-performance liquid chromatography using platinum-black catalyst reduction and fluorimetric detection. *J Chromatogr* 489:291–301.

112. Harrington, D.J., S.L. Booth, D.J. Card, and M.J. Shearer. 2007. Excretion of the urinary 5C- and 7C-aglycone metabolites of vitamin K by young adults responds to changes in dietary phylloquinone and dihydrophylloquinone intakes. *J Nutr* 137:1763–1768.

7 Public Health Concerns Related to Vitamin K Status

7.1 VITAMIN K DEFICIENCIES

7.1.1 Hemorrhagic Disease of the Newborn

The classic example of human vitamin K deficiency is hemorrhagic disease of the newborn (HDN), now more appropriately called early vitamin K deficiency bleeding (VKDB), which occurs in healthy appearing neonates [1]. The disease has been sub-classified as early VKDB (within the first day of life), classic VKDB (within the first week), or late VKDB (second week to six months of age). The low vitamin K content of breast milk, low placental transfer of phylloquinone, low levels of clotting factors at birth, and a sterile gut all contribute to the disease. Classical VKDB presents as oozing of blood from the nose, intestine, cord, or broken skin sites, and in severe cases intracranial bleeding. Estimates of the incidence of VKDB vary considerably, but in the absence of prophylactic treatment might exceed 1% of infant births [2] with a high mortality rate from intracranial bleeding. Late VKDB has usually been considered rare (5 to 7 of every 100,000 live births in the absence of prophylaxis), but it is the cause of significant morbidity and mortality as intracranial hemorrhages occur in up to 60% of the affected infants [3]. This syndrome is seen predominantly in exclusively breastfed infants [4,5] or infants with severe intestinal malabsorption problems who may or may not have received vitamin K at birth [6]. A national study of the incidence of late VKDB in the Netherlands for all infants born in 2005 found a rate of 3.2 per 100,000 births [7], and all were breastfed. Infants that are breastfed and show biliary atresia-related cholestasis have been shown [8] to require substantial amounts of phylloquinone to maintain normal vitamin K-dependent clotting factor concentrations. Prevention of VKDB by oral or intramuscular administration of vitamin K immediately following birth is the standard practice in most countries. In the United States, this treatment is ensured by standard hospital guidelines, but severe cases of the disease have been reported following home deliveries where vitamin K was not administered [9]. Although oral administration of vitamin, which has not been widely used in the United States [10], appears to be as effective as parenteral administration to prevent early VKDB, recent increases in its use suggest that it may not be as effective for preventing late VKDB.

Reports in the early 1990s suggested that intramuscular injection of vitamin K to infants was associated with an increased incidence of certain childhood cancers. Golding [11] published the results of a large (16,000 infants) national cohort study in

Great Britain which was directed toward the relationship of various environmental and medical factors to the incidence of childhood cancers. Although vitamin K administration to newborn infants was not specifically addressed in the study protocol, it was concluded that it may have been a relevant factor. This study was then followed by a case controlled study of nearly 200 children with cancer, who were born at one of two hospitals, which differed in that vitamin K administration at birth was given orally at one and intramuscularly at the other [12]. This study suggested that the risk of cancer was doubled in infants receiving vitamin K intramuscularly and that oral administration of vitamin K should be the prophylaxis of choice. This conclusion was supported by a suggestion that the high plasma and presumably the high tissue concentration following IM administration was potentially carcinogenic [13]. There was no universal acceptance of the Golding report, and three other large epidemiological studies [14–16] published within a few years failed to confirm an association of IM vitamin K administration and cancer risk. The question of risk remained open, and four more large studies were published in the late 1900s [17–20]. Two of these found no relationship, one study found an increased risk for all cancers, and one an increased risk for a specific form of leukemia. Two comprehensive reviews of the available data have not found convincing evidence of childhood cancer risk associated with IM vitamin K [21,22], and a report from the United Kingdom childhood cancer study [23] concluded that there was no convincing evidence that neonatal vitamin K administration, by any route, influences the risk of children developing leukemia or any other cancer. This view is consistent with the current recommendation of the American Academy of Pediatrics [2] that "vitamin K (phylloquinone) should be given to all newborns as a single intramuscular dose of 0.5 to 1 mg." This firm recommendation for intramuscular administration does, however, not apply worldwide, and oral administration is recommended as preferable or an alternate treatment in some countries [24].

Although there does not appear to be a cancer risk associated with intramuscular injection, a great deal of coverage was given to the initial reports, and a switch to oral administration of vitamin K occurred in some countries and was associated with an increase in the incidence of late VKDB [25,26]. The low incidence of VKDB, independent of the method of vitamin K administration, has made it difficult to determine if there are real differences in the incidence of late VKDB between oral or IM administration, but cases of this disease are still reported in breastfed infants receiving oral therapy [7]. The most commonly used form of vitamin K for parenteral administration contains a nonionic detergent as a solubilizer and does not appear to be as highly bioavailable when given orally, but it has been shown [10,27] to be safe and effective. An alternate preparation containing a mixed micellar preparation to disperse the phylloquinone (see Chapter 2), which is not available in the United States, has been shown [28] to maintain infant plasma phylloquinone concentrations for the first two months of life as effectively as an IM injection when multiple doses are administered. As the infant formulas that are commercially available contain adequate amounts of vitamin K, the risk of late VKDB in breastfed infants receiving oral vitamin K appears to be limited to failure to follow the guidelines for multiple doses, lipid absorption problems, or cholestatic liver disease. An alternative to phylloquinone administration to breastfed newborns would be supplementation of the maternal diet [29,30]. Maternal milk phylloquinone concentrations are higher at the first day of lactation and decrease during the first month, are higher in foremilk than in hind milk, and are readily increased by dietary supplementation [4,30]. The data in Table 7.1 demonstrate that supplementation of the maternal diet with 5 µg/day of phylloquinone increased maternal plasma concentration about 30-fold and maternal milk concentration about 60-fold, while the plasma phylloquinone concentration of nursing infants was increased about 6-fold. This concentration of phylloquinone provides the nursing infant with nearly 10 µg/kg of body weight per day, which is substantially above the currently prescribed adequate intake. Although most healthy infants have normal prothrombin times, sensitive assays will detect PIVKA-II in a substantial fraction of infants not given prophylactic vitamin K [31,32]; and it has been shown [29] that maternal supplementation of vitamin K decreases the concentration of this sensitive marker in nursing infants.

Although the severe form of VKDB is present in early infancy, older infants with conjugated hyperbilirubinemia [33], chronic liver disease [34], or acute and intractable diarrhea [35] have been shown to require routine vitamin K supplementation to maintain normal vitamin K-dependent clotting factor levels. Some cases of late VKDB appear to be ideopathic and have been suggested to be due to a congenital increase in vitamin K requirement [36]. A prolonged prothrombin time is a common finding in sick preterm infants, and many of these cases are not the result of low vitamin K status but of other causes. Vitamin K status in premature infants has been assessed in a study [37] that found higher plasma phylloquinone concentration in premature infants because of a 1 mg IM injection and parenteral multivitamin administration, and it was concluded [38] that an IM

TABLE 7.1
Increase in Maternal Plasma and Milk Phylloquinone Concentration Following Dietary Supplementation

	Concentration of Plasma or Milk (ng/ml ± SD)		
	Before Birth	**2 Weeks**	**12 Weeks**
Maternal plasma			
Phylloquinone	0.3 ± 0.1	11.4 ± 4.7	10.7 ± 10.4
Placebo	0.3 ± 0.1	0.3 ± 0.2	0.4 ± 0.2
Maternal milk			
Phylloquinone	0.7 ± 0.4	76.5 ± 26.9	82.1 ± 40.0
Placebo	1.1 ± 0.8	1.2 ± 0.7	1.2 ± 0.4
Infant plasma			
Phylloquinone	–	2.3 ± 2.6	2.8 ± 3.1
Placebo	–	0.4 ± 0.3	0.3 ± 0.6

Note: Subjects (11/group) were given an oral 5 mg phylloquinone supplement or a placebo each day for 12 weeks. For details, see Reference [29].

injection of 0.5 mg of phylloquinone would be more than adequate for infants with a birth weight below 1,000 g.

7.1.2 ADULT HUMAN DEFICIENCIES

A vitamin K-responsive human hypoprothrombinemia (increased prothrombin time) is a rare finding as the adult human population normally consumes a diet containing an amount of vitamin K in excess of that needed to maintain normal hemostasis. Cases of an acquired vitamin K deficiency do, however, occur in the adult population and, though relatively rare, present a significant problem for some individuals. The potential problem areas and the basic factors needed to prevent a vitamin K deficiency have been reviewed [39] and are: (a) a normal diet containing the vitamin, (b) the presence of bile in the intestine, (c) a normal absorptive surface in the small intestine, and (d) a normal liver. Depression of the vitamin K-dependent coagulation factors has frequently been reported in malabsorption syndromes and in other gastrointestinal disorders, such as cystic fibrosis, sprue, celiac disease, ulcerative colitis, regional ileitis, ascaris infection, Crohn's disease, and short bowel syndrome [40–44]. It has usually been assumed that a general vitamin K deficiency in the population is not possible, but hypoprothrombinemia has been identified in patients undergoing prolonged intensive care [45]. A more recent study of adult patients with advanced cancer found [46] that about 75% had some degree of vitamin K deficiency as measured by circulating phylloquinone concentration or PIVKA-II assays. A relatively high percentage of older adult hospital-admitted populations have been reported [47–49] to have a hypoprothrombinemia that responds to administration of oral vitamin K. The basis for the apparent vitamin K deficiency in these studies was not determined, and was probably related to one or more of the factors listed above and to general malnutrition. Vitamin K status of the elderly is a particular concern [50], and animal studies have shown [51] that it is much easier to develop a vitamin K deficiency in older than younger rats. However, a comparison of biochemical indices for assessing the vitamin K nutritional status of younger and older adults [52] has demonstrated rather small differences, with the exception of a marked age-related increase in the urinary Gla/creatinine excretion ratio. The extent to which this was the result of a decreased muscle mass in the older population was not assessed.

Vitamin K-responsive hemorrhagic events have frequently been reported in patients receiving antibiotics and have been reviewed extensively [53,54]. These episodes have usually been assumed to be due to decreased menaquinone availability from the gut (see Chapter 6), but it is possible that in many cases they may represent low dietary intake alone and that the presumed effect on gut bacteria was not related to the observed hypoprothrombinemia. There is very little available data that would relate antibiotic administration to alterations in the numbers of menaquinone-producing bacteria in the gut, or to the amount of gut or fecal menaquinones. A study [55] of the administration of 10 different antibiotics for 10 days to subjects who were consuming an essentially vitamin K-free (<5 μg/day) diet did not indicate a clinically significant decrease in any of the vitamin K-dependent proteins. There was no prolongation of prothrombin time beyond the established upper normal limit, although at least one of the three subjects administered five of the antibiotics had a factor VII level that was below the range of the normal laboratory standard (75% to 132%) for at least one day. This response was also considered to be of no clinical significance. This study would suggest that the impact of antibiotic treatment, particularly when normal amounts of dietary vitamin K are consumed, might be less than often assumed. However, there are differences in the observed responses to different antibiotics, and some second- and third-generation cephalosporins have been implicated in a large number of hypoprothrombinemic episodes [56]. Studies of this response suggest that it is likely that these antibiotics were exerting a weak vitamin K-dependent carboxylase inhibition [57] or a coumarin-like response [58,59], which might be a more important factor in the developing hypoprothrombinemia than an influence on the gut bacterial population [60].

Experimental attempts to induce vitamin K deficiencies by dietary restriction utilizing as an endpoint a clinically significant increase in prothrombin time measurements have been rare and essentially unsuccessful. An often cited early study [61] investigated the vitamin K requirement of starved intravenously fed (5% glucose and vitamins) debilitated patients who were also given antibiotics in an attempt to decrease intestinal vitamin K synthesis. In these subjects, a significant degree of vitamin K-responsive hypoprothrombinemia was clearly established between 21 and 28 days. Some of the subjects were given small amounts of i.v. vitamin K, which resulted in short-term increases in prothrombin, factor VII, and factor X, but a minimum daily requirement value was not established. The very small intakes of vitamin K that are needed to maintain normal coagulation values are also indicated by the recent report [62] of a man who subjected himself to voluntary starvation (water only) for 44 days. His prothrombin time at the end of the starvation period was 14.7 seconds relative to a normal reference range of 12.5 to 14.5 seconds for the laboratory involved with the study. A number of more recent controlled studies utilizing diets containing approximately 10 µg/day or less of phylloquinone [55,63,64] have demonstrated alterations in procoagulant factors using more sensitive markers of vitamin K status, but a clinically significant decrease in prothrombin times was not seen.

7.2   CONTROL OF ANTICOAGULANT THERAPY

Anticoagulant agents are widely used for the acute treatment of venous and arterial thrombosis and for the long-term prevention of potentially recurring thrombotic events. Although injectable drugs such as heparin are used in the treatment of acute events, oral anticoagulants are widely used for patients needing long-term anticoagulation. Warfarin, which acts by an inhibition of the vitamin K epoxide reductase (see Chapter 4), is the most commonly used oral anticoagulant, while two other 4-hydroxycoumarins, acenocoumarol and phenprocoumon, are used to a small extent in North America, but more commonly in Europe. Oral anticoagulant treatment is used for the prevention and treatment of deep vein thrombosis, pulmonary embolism, atrial fibrillation, myocardial infarction, and hip and knee orthoplasty and surgery, and is therefore commonly administered. It is estimated that at any given time as high as 7% of the elderly are being prescribed these drugs [65]. Fetal warfarin syndrome is a severe embryopathy characterized by nasal hypoplasia, depression of the bridge of the nose, and stippling in uncalcified epiphyseal regions. The critical period of exposure appears to be between the sixth and ninth weeks of gestation [66]; but, as exposure at any stage of development may result in adverse effects, oral anti-coagulation utilizing warfarin or a similar compound is not prescribed for pregnant women. The ectopic calcification that is associated with the syndrome would suggest that a decrease in the amount of biologically active matrix Gla protein in the affected tissues is the underlying cause of the embryopathy.

Because of the narrow therapeutic range of these drugs, coumarin-based oral anticoagulants are potentially dangerous, and insufficient or excessive doses signifi-cantly increase the risk of thrombotic or bleeding events [67]. The anticoagulant effect of warfarin therapy is monitored by measurement of the prothrombin time (PT), a measure of combined procoagulant status rather than a true measure of prothrombin activity. As the thromboplastin reagents used in the assay vary widely in their sensi-tivity to depressed levels of various clotting factors, plasma from a warfarin-treated patient may yield very different values when tested with different thromboplastins. To overcome this problem the International Normalized Ratio (INR) is now used as a standardized method for reporting prothrombin time results. The INR allows interconversion of PT ratios (patient PT/mean normal PT) by use of an International Sensitivity Index (ISI) which corrects for differences in thromboplastin sensitivities. The goal of anticoagulant therapy is steady-state levels of vitamin K-dependent pro-coagulants, which are related to an INR that is somewhat dependent on the specific therapy but is often in the range of 2 to 3 [68]. This degree of stable anticoagulation does not result in an equal lowering of vitamin K-dependent clotting factors, but a decrease in the activity of prothrombin and factor X that is greater than that of fac-tors VII and IX (Table 7.2). The most common complication of anticoagulant ther-apy, bleeding, is directly related to the INR, with few bleeds at a stable INR of < 4.0 and a relatively high incidence with INRs of > 7.0. Maintaining patients within the stated therapeutic range is not easily accomplished, and a recent systematic review and meta-regression analysis [65] involving 67 studies and 50,000 patients indicated that patients were within the stated therapeutic range only 64% of the time. Oral anticoagulant therapy can be self-managed by patients using portable coagulometers [69]. A systematic review [70] of this procedure indicates that with careful selection of the patient population, ability to maintain a target INR is as good as or better than with conventional management. When overanticoagulation does occur, it can be brought back to the desired level by lowering the warfarin dose, or if severely out of range by subcutaneous or even slow i.v. infusion of phylloquinone.

The magnitude of the anticoagulant effect produced by a given dose of warfarin varies by as much as 20-fold between individuals, and patients who have just started on the therapy are closely monitored. The response to a given dose can also vary substantially in an individual patient over time. Drug interactions have been found to be responsible for some of this variation, and many commonly prescribed drugs [68,71] have been shown to alter displacement of warfarin from its plasma albumin carrier, induce the specific hepatic P450s that metabolize warfarin, interfere with warfarin clearance, or bind to warfarin in the gut. As the science of genomics has evolved, it has become clear that the genetic variability of the patient population also has a profound impact on the appropriate dose of warfarin. Clinically available warfarin is a racemic mixture of (R)-and (S)-warfarin, and (S)-warfarin is three to

TABLE 7.2
Influence of Long-Term Stable Warfarin Therapy on the Plasma Concentration of Vitamin K-Dependent Clotting Factors

Factor	% of Normal	
	Study 1 (mean ± SD)	Study 2 (median)
Prothrombin	35 ± 11	19
Factor VII	45 ± 14	33
Factor IX	49 ± 13	48
Factor X	16 ± 5	18

Note: Subjects in both studies were maintaining stable INR values for at least three months. For details, see: Study 1 [257]; Study 2 [258].

five times as effective as an inhibitor of the epoxide reductase. The major enzyme metabolizing the (S)-warfarin isomer is a specific cytochrome P450, CYP2C9 [72]. A meta-analysis of a number of studies [73] has indicated that variant alleles of this enzyme that decrease their ability to metabolize (S)-warfarin reduces the warfarin requirement by about 30%. Identification of the gene for the vitamin K epoxide reductase [74,75] led to the realization that haplotypes of this gene (VKORC1) were also associated with the dose of warfarin needed for effective anticoagulation of patients, and the genetic variability of VKOR1 has been found to be more important than the CYP2C9 in the INR response to warfarin [76].

Although thought so at one time, polymorphisms of the vitamin K-dependent carboxylase have been found to have little impact on warfarin dosage [77]. There are a large number of variants of the VKORC1 gene, which influence the warfarin dose needed for stable anticoagulation, and large differences in the genotypes of European, African American, and Asian populations [78–80]. These alterations can either increase or decrease the amount of the drug needed for effective treatment, and in extreme cases, a genetic alteration of the warfarin sensitivity of the epoxide reductase has been shown to result in an enzyme that is so resistant to warfarin that it is very difficult to achieve a desired therapeutic level [81]. Studies of the relationship between polymorphisms within the CYP2C9 and VKORC1 genes and the warfarin dose required for stable anticoagulation [82-85] suggest that 50% to 60% of the variation in amount of Warfarin needed for the INR targeted is related to these polymorphisms. This suggests that warfarin therapy is a practice where predictive genotyping might come into general use, and both the U.S. Food and Drug Administration [86] and the American College of Medical Genetics [87] have issued statements encouraging pharmacogenetic testing of CYP2C9 and VKORC1 alleles as an aid in determining the initial dosage of warfarin. A genetic variant of the CYP4F2 gene, which is involved in the degradation of the side chain of phylloquinone, has also been found [88] to alter the amount of warfarin needed to obtain the desired INR.

The widespread interest in this approach has led to efforts to validate pharmacogenetic algorithms used to calculate these dosages [89,90]. An extensive review of the large literature base related to the genetic factors that would lead to more appropriate initial doses of warfarin is now available [85]. This report and some more recent data [88] conclude that the extent to which various genetic or clinical factors contribute to the population variance in Warfarin maintenance doses is as follows: clinical factors, 20%; cytochrome P450 variants CYP2C9, 10% and CYP4F2, 2%; vitamin K epoxide reductase VKORC1, 25%; vitamin K-dependent carboxylase GGCX, 2%; and unknown factors, 41%.

Alterations of dietary vitamin K can be a significant factor in the stability of warfarin treatment. It has been reported [91] that patients who have low intakes of vitamin K, based on dietary records, have less stable control of their INR values and that changes in dietary intake can result in changes in anticoagulation status [92–96]. These studies and others [97,98] would suggest that meaningful changes in a patient's INR would require a shift of 100 to 150 µg of vitamin K in the diet. It has also been shown [99] that 25 µg of phylloquinone in the form of a multivitamin dietary supplement results in a subtherapeutic INR for those patients with a low dietary intake of vitamin K. Although the available data are not very extensive (see Chapter 6), it is likely that the bioavailability of the supplemental phylloquinone is two to five times that of the vitamin contained in a food matrix. This would indicate that 25 µg/day of a phylloquinone supplement would be the equivalent of doubling the vitamin K intake of most patients. Although advice to maintain normal dietary practices might be more appropriate, patients receiving anticoagulation therapy are often advised to restrict their intake of vitamin K-rich foods, mainly green leafy vegetables, which tend to put them in a situation where changes in their vitamin K intake are more likely to have an impact on the desired INR. This suggests that supplementation of the diet with 50 to 100 µg of phylloquinone would put patients in a situation where the warfarin dose would be increased but where changes in dietary vitamin K would be very unlikely to impact a stable INR history. Small studies of the utilization of this approach to stabilize patients within their target INR range have now been reported [100–102] and indicate that this approach might have benefit.

The goal of successful warfarin therapy includes the maintenance of a stable INR, and a large number of factors influence efforts to achieve this result [68,103]. The influence of drugs on the production of vitamin K in the gut does not seem to be as serious a problem as once thought [55], but antibiotics, particularly amoxicillin and doxycycline, have been reported [104] to increase the incidence of bleeding in patients receiving oral anticoagulants. As enteral nutrition products are supplemented with phylloquinone, their concurrent use with warfarin [105] also requires careful monitoring. In addition to numerous prescription drugs that can potentiate or counteract the action of warfarin [68], there are a large number of specialized foods, dietary supplements, botanicals, and nutraceuticals that have been claimed to influence standard anticoagulant therapy [106]. These include, but are not limited to, cranberry juice, green tea, high protein diets, seaweed, fiddlehead ferns, smoking, ginseng, royal jelly, and avocados. Much of the available data regarding these interactions is based on case reports [107], but there are two rather recent systematic reviews [71,108] and a special issue of *Thrombosis Research* containing the proceedings of a 2005 NIH Conference on Dietary Supplements, Coagulation, and Antithrombotic Therapies [109] that cover many of these potentially unwanted interactions in some detail.

Although warfarin and related inhibitors of the vitamin K epoxide reductase are relatively inexpensive and successful drugs for the control of thrombotic events, there are some downsides to their use. They have a rather short therapeutic range, monitoring is somewhat cumbersome, dosage differs substantially between patients, and there is an increased risk of bleeding complications. There has been a substantial effort by the pharmaceutical industry to develop oral anticoagulants that would be as effective as or better than warfarin as an inhibitor but would be easier to use and have a lower incidence of bleeding complications. These have focused on inhibitors of the propagation of the coagulation cascade, factor Xa or factor IXa, or on the inhibition of fibrin formation via thrombin inhibitors. Many of these drugs have been studied successfully in animal models, and some in clinical trials [110–114]. The most extensively studied direct oral thrombin inhibitor has been ximelagatran, which does not have antithrombin properties, but is a prodrug of melagatran, which is a direct active site inhibitor of thrombin. This drug did have promise as an effective anticoagulant in a number of trials but was removed from the market because of hepatoxicity. Efforts to produce an effective and safe drug of this type will undoubtedly continue.

7.3 VITAMIN K AND BONE HEALTH

7.3.1 RELATIONSHIP TO MARKERS OF VITAMIN K STATUS

As osteocalcin is present in relatively high concentrations in bone, a great deal of attention has been directed toward the concentration of osteocalcin in plasma and to the degree of vitamin K-dependent carboxylation of this protein as possible factors in bone health. Small amounts of this protein circulate in plasma at concentrations that are four- to fivefold higher in young children than in adults and reach the adult levels at puberty [115]. Assays of osteocalcin are usually performed with commercial antibody-based kits and, although they may all respond to changes in the same manner, the absolute values vary substantially in kits from different manufacturers [116]. As the protein is produced by mature osteoblasts, elevated plasma concentration has been commonly used as one of the markers for an increase in bone formation and turnover. Circulating osteocalcin in individuals within the normal population is not completely γ-carboxylated, and the extent of undercarboxylation has been studied extensively. Immunochemical assays for the des-γ-carboxylated forms have been developed [117], but most studies have defined under-γ-carboxylated osteocalcin (ucOC) as that fraction which does not adsorb to the form of calcium phosphate called hydroxyapatite under standardized conditions [118]. Depending on assay conditions and the specific epitopes detected by the assay kits utilized, the fraction of total circulating osteocalcin present as ucOC which has been reported in normal healthy populations has ranged from 30%–40% to <10%. This lack of uniformity in attempts to measure the fraction of total osteocalcin present as ucOC in a "normal" population has made it very difficult to compare much of the published data. At the present time it is also not known if all or only some of the three Gla residues in osteocalcin are required for their biological function, or how many of the three Gla residues are required to efficiently bind to the hydroxyapatite used in the assay.

Although fully carboxylated osteocalcin is often assumed to be a prerequisite to skeletal health, there is no clear evidence at the present time to support a link between an increase in the concentration of plasma ucOC and decreased mineralization. When γ-carboxylation of osteocalcin is effectively blocked in a rat model through the use of warfarin [119], a mineralization disorder characterized by complete fusion of the proximal tibia growth plate and cessation of longitudinal growth has been observed. These data have been interpreted to suggest that a skeletal vitamin K-dependent protein, probably osteocalcin, is involved in regulating bone mineralization, but they do not indicate that low vitamin K status would decrease mineralization. The opposite response seems to be more likely, as studies utilizing transgenic mice lacking the osteocalcin gene [120] have demonstrated that their phenotype is increased bone mineralization rather than decreased bone mass. A number of epidemiological studies have, however, shown [52,121–127] that populations with an increase in dietary vitamin K intake, and the increased plasma phylloquinone concentrations associated with it, are negatively related to the fraction of osteocalcin present as ucOC. These data have established that the normal dietary intake of vitamin K is not sufficient to maximally γ-carboxylate osteocalcin, and studies employing the supplementation of diets with vitamin K [64,128–131] have clearly demonstrated that increasing the amount of vitamin K ingested will decrease the ucOC fraction of osteocalcin. Although there is clearly a relationship between plasma phylloquinone concentrations and the extent of osteocalcin carboxylation, ethnic and apoE genotypes have also been shown to be involved [132]. It has, however, been shown [133] that supplementation with 1 mg phylloquinone per day (~10 times the current dietary reference intake (DRI)) is required to achieve maximal γ-carboxylation. Based on the available food composition data, this is an amount that would be very difficult to achieve with any type of "normal" diet.

There have been numerous studies attempting to link ucOC or other apparent markers of vitamin K insufficiency with bone health. These efforts have included a large number of epidemiological observations, including (1) that low vitamin K intake is associated with increased hip, spine, or femoral neck fracture risk [124,134–142]; (2) that lower serum vitamin K levels were associated with decreased bone mineral density [123,143,144]; (3) that undercarboxylated osteocalcin is a marker for hip fracture [117,145]; and (4) that undercarboxylated osteocalcin is correlated with low bone mass [127,146,147]. These reports vary considerably in number of subjects, study design, length of study, and methodology; details of many of them are available in recent reviews [148–152]. In a more recent 10-year study [153] of over 2,000 perimenopausal women with a wide range of vitamin K intakes, there was no association between vitamin K intake and alterations in bone mineral density or fracture risk. The possibility that vitamin K status might be related more to changes in the microarchitecture of bone than to bone mineral density has been raised [154], but a study assessing trabecular orientation by ultrasound has failed to find a strong relationship between vitamin K intake and this assay [155]. The positive associations found between increased vitamin K status and skeletal health in epidemiological studies do not necessarily imply causation. It is also possible that in regard to skeletal health, vitamin K might simply be a surrogate marker of a good healthy diet. As green vegetables are the major source of vitamin K in most diets, it is not surprising that assessment of the very large nutritional and disease risk databases such as the Framingham Offspring Cohort, the Nurses' Health Study, and the Health Professionals' Follow-Up Study have also found that increased dietary phylloquinone intake is a marker for a decrease in cardiovascular disease [156–158]. Although there have been numerous epidemiological studies that have attempted to assess the relationship between vitamin K status and bone health, it appears that long-term studies of vitamin K supplementation will be required to define this relationship.

7.3.2   WARFARIN THERAPY AND BONE HEALTH

The number of patients receiving warfarin or some other 4-hydroxycoumarin as an oral anticoagulant is large, and although treatment following orthopedic surgery may be short term, treatment following cardiovascular events is often very long. The dosages used substantially increase the ucOC fraction of circulating osteocalcin to a level that is much higher than would be observed in individuals consuming a low vitamin K diet. This induced vitamin K deficiency has raised concern about the influence of this very common treatment on skeletal health. The results of numerous studies are mixed. An increase in fracture rate within this patient population has been reported [159,160] in some but not in other studies [161–163], and no alteration in bone mineral density was observed in most of these studies [162–164]. A meta-analysis of nine studies with a total of 411 subjects [165] did, however, report an oral anticoagulant-related decrease in bone mineral density at the ultradistal radius but not at the lumbar spine or the femoral neck or trochanter. Although the possible impact of warfarin therapy on skeletal health has been studied widely, the available data differ substantially in the age and gender of the subjects, the length of therapy studied, and the sites used for fracture data and bone mineral density assessment.

The results of animal model studies of the influence of warfarin on bone health have also been somewhat mixed. A 28-day study of warfarin-treated adult rats [166] reported a decrease in bone strength, a reduction in cancellous bone volume, a decrease in rate of bone formation, and an increased rate of bone resorption. A somewhat longer (80 days) study utilizing younger (7 week) female rats found no impact of warfarin treatment on biomechanical properties of femur or vertebrae, bone mineral content or density, or on various measures of bone turnover [167]. A 30-month study of the impact of warfarin treatment (INR of 2.5) of adult male Rhesus monkeys has also found that there was no effect on bone mineral density or bone markers of skeletal turnover [168]. Although the available data are somewhat inconsistent, and the decrease in markers of vitamin K status following warfarin therapy are much more pronounced than would result from a low vitamin K diet, there does not appear to be sufficient evidence to support an indication of warfarin treatment as a risk factor for an increase in fracture rate.

7.3.3   DIETARY SUPPLEMENTATION OF VITAMIN K AND BONE HEALTH

Although the available data suggest that near maximal carboxylation of osteocalcin does not appear to be needed for normal bone mineralization, supplementation with one form of the vitamin, menaquinone-4, is a common therapy for osteoporosis in Japan and other Asian countries. The standard therapy is 45 mg of MK-4 (menatetrenone) per day, a pharmacological rather than a nutritional approach. There are a number of studies, mainly from Japan and with a relatively small number of subjects, that point to a reduction in the incidence of vertebral fractures and modest effects on bone mineral density from this therapy. These studies have been recently and comprehensively reviewed [169]. There has also been a systematic review and meta-analysis of seven randomized controlled MK-4 supplement trials [170–176] where hip and spine fracture of ~450 subjects, mainly elderly Japanese women, was an endpoint [177]. This analysis found an odds ratio favoring MK-4 of 0.40 (95% confidence interval, 0.25–0.65) for vertebral fractures and an odds ratio favoring MK-4 of 0.19 (95% confidence interval. 0.11–0.35) for all non-vertebral fractures. These decreases of fracture risk are as good as, or better than, the responses found for the impact of other drugs commonly prescribed for patients with osteoporosis. However, one of the trials [174] contributed about 50% of the weight of the analysis and in this trial the MK-4 supplemented group also received 1000 IU of ergocalciferol and 600 mg calcium daily for the two years of the study. As the subjects were shown to be vitamin D-deficient prior to the start of the study, the additional supplements may have impacted the results. There is also reference [178] to a report of a post-marketing research study of 2000 elderly osteoporotic Japanese subjects receiving the standard 45 mg per day dose of MK-4 and a calcium supplement compared to 2000 similar subjects receiving only the calcium supplement. The primary endpoint was new fracture rate, and during the first year of a three-year study, a beneficial effect of MK-4 was seen in only a small subpopulation of the subjects with multiple previous fractures. The results of the last two years of the study have not been reported.

There has also been an interest in using the ovariectomized rat as a model for assessing the possible influence of MK-4 on bone loss. A number of these studies have been reviewed recently [179], with the conclusion that MK-4 did reduce bone loss. There are, however, similar studies [180,181] that have not shown a positive response to MK-4 in this bone loss model. A study of bone mineral loss in gluco-corticoid-treated rats as measured by histomorphometric analysis [182] has found that MK-4 and a bis-phosphonate have similar efficacy reducing the glucocorticoid-induced decrease in periosteal bone formation and increase in endocortical bone erosion. Although MK-4 may not be as effective in preventing bone loss as once thought, it does have effects on cultured bone cells that are not seen with phylloquinone [183] and has apoptotic effects on malignant cell lines that are not seen with phylloquinone. Menaquinone-4 has been identified as a ligand for the steroid xenobiotic receptor in bone cells where it influences the expression of a number of osteoblastic markers [184–189], and various derivatives of geranylgeranyl, the side chain of MK4, have been found to have MK-4-like properties in cultured cell systems [190].

The major form of vitamin K in the diet is phylloquinone, and although phylloquinone supplementation has been shown repeatedly to decrease the concentration of circulating under-γ-carboxylated osteocalcin, there is very little data indicating that increased dietary intake of phylloquinone has any impact on skeletal health. The following four randomized controlled studies have been conducted, which suggest that any positive response to phylloquinone supplementation is limited:

1. The Braam et al. study [191]: This was a three-year study of 180 healthy 50- to 60-year-old postmenopausal women which compared the bone mineral density response of a placebo; a Ca, Zn, Mg and vitamin D supplement; and the mineral and vitamin D supplementation plus 1 mg of phylloquinone per day. There was a marginal reduction ($p <.05$) in the extent of the bone mineral density decrease of the femoral neck over the three-year period in the group with phylloquinone added to the mineral and vitamin D supplement, but no decrease in the loss of mineral from the lumbar spine. Mineral and vitamin D supplementation alone had no effect on the rate of bone mineral loss, and markers of bone turnover were not influenced by the treatments.

2. The Bolton-Smith et al. study [192]: This was a two-year study of 200 healthy postmenopausal women less than 60 years old which compared the bone mineral density response of a placebo, 200 μg phylloquinone per day, a Ca and vitamin D supplement, or the Ca and vitamin D supplement plus phylloquinone. In this two-year study, there was no significant difference in bone mineral density between any of the intervention groups at the end of the two years at any bone site. There was, however, an increase in bone mineral density of the ultradistal radius when compared to baseline values in the Ca and vitamin D plus phylloquinone group. This response was not seen in the other four bone sites measured.

3. The Booth et al. study [193]: This was a three-year study of 452 healthy 60- to 80-year-old men and women which compared the bone mineral density response of a group receiving a multivitamin preparation that contained a Ca and vitamin D supplement or the same preparation with 500 μg per day phylloquinone added. There were no differences in the change in bone mineral density at the femoral neck or lumbar spine.

4. The Binkley et al. study [194]: This was a one-year study of 381 healthy postmenopausal women which compared the bone mineral density response of a group given a Ca and vitamin D supplement only, or this supplement along with either 1 mg per day of phylloquinone or 45 mg of MK-4. There was no treatment effect on bone mineral density changes at the lumbar spine or proximal femur. Calconeal ultrasound parameters, a measure of bone quality, were also obtained and did not differ between the three groups. Standard markers of bone turnover were not influenced by treatment.

In all of these well-controlled trials, the phylloquinone supplementation raised the vitamin K intake of the treated subjects to a level that would be difficult to achieve in any normal diet, and other than the 200 μg/day supplementation, essentially impossible. In all of these studies, phylloquinone supplementation did increase the fraction of circulatory osteocalcin that was fully carboxylated, but the response of bone turnover markers was variable. A number of other smaller studies have found some influence of vitamin K supplementation on markers of bone turnover, but no consistent impact on alterations of bone mineral density [195–198]. There are also epidemiological studies of a possible relationship between the intake of MK-7, found uniquely in the fermented soybean product natto, and increased bone mineral density or decreased fracture rate [199,200]. Supplementation of the diet of ovariec-tomized rats with MK-7 [201] has also been reported to decrease bone mineral loss, and there are reports of the inhibition of osteoclastic bone resorption and stimulation of osteoblastic bone formation in vitro by MK-7 [202,203]. Whether or not this form of vitamin K has a unique ability to increase skeletal health in the human population will require some long-term, well-controlled studies.

7.4   VITAMIN K STATUS AND CALCIFICATION-RELATED DISEASES

7.4.1   RELATIONSHIP OF ECTOPIC CALCIFICATION TO MATRIX GLA PROTEIN

Although the relationship between decreases in the circulating levels of biologi-cally active osteocalcin and decreases in bone mineral density has been difficult to establish, the relationship between arterial vascular disease and matrix Gla protein appears to be more direct. Early studies of the matrix Gla protein "knockout" mouse indicated that these animals died from massive calcifications of the large arteries within eight weeks of birth [204], and a rapid calcification of the elastic lamellae of arteries and heart valves was soon demonstrated in a rat model where matrix Gla protein carboxylation was blocked [205] by warfarin administration. A subsequent study [206] utilizing warfarin-treated rats has suggested that MK-4 is much more effective than phylloquinone in reversing the arterial calcification seen in this model. There are also data [207] that have demonstrated that a combination of MK-4 and a bisphosphonate is capable of decreasing the extent of calcification that develops when inorganic phosphate is added to cultured bovine aortic smooth muscle cells. Matrix Gla protein (MGP) is expressed at a low level in healthy vascular tissue, but its expression is greatly upregulated in regions of ectopic arterial calcification. Calcification of vascular smooth muscle cells is a complex process associated with chondrocyte differentiation and cartilage formation and has been reviewed exten-sively [208–211]. The method by which γ-carboxylated MGP prevents soft tissue calcification is not yet clearly established [212,213], but is at least partially medi-ated through an interaction with cellular growth factors [214–217]. The major factor appears to be the ability of Gla-MGP, but not Glu-MGP, to inhibit vascular calcifi-cation by binding to and inhibiting bone morphogenetic protein-2 (BMP-2) which is a growth factor capable of triggering the transformation of a cell which renders it capable of depositing calcium. Studies of human vascular smooth muscle cells [218] have shown that treatment with warfarin decreases the ability of these cells to undergo calcification when the calcium concentration of the media is increased. In addition to carboxylation of the Gla domain of MGP, maximum inhibition of calci-fication is also dependent on phosphorylation of a number of serine residues. The complete MGP protein is not needed, and a short segment (residues 35–49) of MGP containing 3 Gla residues is capable of inhibiting the action of BMP-2 in transform-ing pro-myoblast cells into osteoblasts and subsequent calcification [219]. A number of actions other than those related to BMP-2 may be involved, as purified MGP has also been shown to inhibit the in vitro calcification of devitalized arteries and demineralized bone [211]. These animal studies have clearly shown an involvement

TABLE 7.3

Tissue Calcification Problems Possibly Associated with Matrix Gla Protein Function

Genetic diseases
   Keutel Syndrome
   Pseudoxanthoma elasticum
Public health concerns
   Cardiovascular calcification
   Warfarin-related tissue calcification
   Juvenile dermatomyositis
   Hand osteoarthritis
   Kidney stones

of MGP in the prevention of ectopic calcification and have generated a great deal of interest [220] in the possible relationship of vitamin K status to human diseases and public health concerns (Table 7.3).

7.4.2 GENETIC DISEASES

Keutel syndrome is a rare human autosomal recessive condition that leads to midfacial hypoplasia, abnormal diffuse cartilage calcification, hearing loss, peripheral pulmonary stenosis, and short tips of fingers. Although the disease has been recognized for some time, it has more recently been found to be associated with at least four mutations in the MGP gene [221,222] which alter the action of MGP.

A second, more common genetic disorder, pseudoxanthoma elasticum (PXE) has also been linked to the control of ectopic calcification by MGP [223]. It is an autosomal recessive disease characterized by the calcification of skin, eyes, and arterial blood vessels. The symptoms vary widely, but the predominant concern is often blindness resulting from damage to the elastic fibers of the eye. The mutations responsible for these changes do not directly involve the MGP gene, but are in the Abcc6 "multidrug Resistance Protein" (MRP6) gene [224–226]. A mouse model developed by the targeted ablation of the Abcc6 gene has been used to demonstrate that concentration of MGP in the serum of the knockout mouse is substantially reduced, and much of the MGP in tissues has been undercarboxylated [227]. It has also been shown that patients with PXE have statistically less circulating serum MGP [228] when compared to healthy nonrelatives. There is, however, a rather wide range of serum MGP in healthy controls, and the majority of the PXE patients would be within a normal range of serum MGP. The ratio of Gla-MGP/Glu-MGP is reduced in tissues obtained from patients with the disease [229], but the relationship between the genetic disorder and the decrease in MGP carboxylation has not been established. As the Abcc6 gene is an organic anion transported, it has been hypothesized that the low level of MGP carboxylation is related to a cellular inability to move vitamin K into the cells synthesizing MGP [230]. At this time there are very little data to support this view.

7.4.3 CARDIOVASCULAR CALCIFICATION

The relationship between serum MGP and coronary artery calcification in humans has been studied with somewhat variable results. It has been reported that, in patients suspected of coronary artery disease, the serum concentration of MGP was inversely correlated with the extent of coronary artery calcification measured by electron-beam computed tomography [231]. A large study using similar methods and subjects free of clinically apparent coronary heart disease found that serum MGP was positively associated with risk factors for atherosclerosis, but not with coronary artery calcification [232]. The initial attempts to relate circulating MGP with cardiovascular disease were conducted by the use of an antibody that detected both serum Gla-MGP and Glu-MGP [233]. A more recent study that utilized an antibody that is claimed to specifically measure under-γ-carboxylated MGP (ucMGP) has reported a much stronger relationship [234]. Compared to a reference healthy population, patients with angioplasty, aortic stenosis, calciphylaxis, or on hemodialysis had a substantially lowered concentration of serum ucMGP.

Attempts to relate polymorphisms of the MGP gene to vascular calcification or to the incidence of myocardial infarction [235] have not indicated any strong associations. However, studies [236–238] of the impact of genetic variants of the vitamin K epoxide reductase (VKOR) on arterial vascular diseases located a single nucleotide polymorphism which conferred almost twice the risk of stroke, coronary heart disease, and aortic dissection. The underlying basis for the response is not apparent and seems unlikely to be associated with a decreased γ-carboxylation of MGP as the plasma concentration of undercarboxylated osteocalcin and PIVKA-II were decreased rather than increased in subjects with this polymorphism. A similar study, but assessing a different polymorphism of VKOR, in a large population has reported an increase in calcification of the aortic far wall of nearly 20% in subjects carrying the polymorphism [239].

Whether or not a decreased intake of vitamin K is associated with an increase in vascular calcification has not been clearly defined. A study of the relationship between premature coronary calcification and phylloquinone intake [240] in a predominantly male 40- to 45-year-old population has found no relationship to a lower vitamin K intake. However, a much larger epidemiological study has shown an inverse relationship between dietary menaquinone and aortic calcification, myocardial infarction, and sudden cardiovascular death [241]. As the total mean vitamin K intake in this population was high (~275 µg/day) and the menaquinone intake represented only about 10% of the total, it is difficult at this time to assess the importance of this finding.

7.4.4 OTHER POSSIBLE INTERACTIONS INVOLVING MGP

The possible influence of the oral anticoagulant warfarin on arterial vascular disease has also been assessed. The extent of calcification of aortic values has been reported to be increased in patients who had received warfarin prior to undergoing aortic valve replacement [242], and coronary calcification has been found to be increased in subjects who were receiving standard oral anticoagulation for over a year [243–245].

Whether or not these responses were related to alterations in amount or degree of γ-carboxylation of MGP has not yet been determined. The incidence of vascular calcification is substantially increased in patients with chronic kidney disease [246,247], and the serum concentration of ucMGP, which may be a marker for active calcification, has been shown [248] to be significantly lowered in kidney dialysis patients. Another possible indication of the influence of MGP on human health is the finding that single nucleotide polymorphisms in the MGP gene have a substantial influence on the incidence of kidney stones [249]. An association of osteoarthritis of the hand and knee to low vitamin K status has also been reported [250], but a more recent clinical trial [251] failed to find an overall effect of vitamin K intake on radiographic hand osteoarthritis. It has also been found that the expression of MGP is increased in the damaged muscle tissues of patients with another disease characterized by cellular calcification, juvenile dermatomyositis [252].

7.5 CURRENT STATUS OF RESEARCH EFFORTS

The one clearly defined vitamin K-related deficiency, hemorrhagic disease of the healthy newborn, is an example of an extremely successful public health effort. When the advice for vitamin K supplementation at birth is followed, the incidence of the disease in the absence of complication is essentially nil. There remains the possibility that some infants delivered at home by midwives may not be treated. It is also likely that many of these same infants will be breastfed and that supplementation of the mother's diet would probably be a wise recommendation.

Stabilization of a target INR following warfarin therapy has been subject to a great deal of interest over the last 5 to 10 years, and there is no doubt that genetic typing of patients to calculate a starting dose would reduce the variation in response in the initial phase. There are, however, many drug and food interactions that make it difficult to maintain a stable INR, including short-term variations in vitamin K intake. In the last few years there have been reports that the daily supplementation of a standard amount of vitamin K can stabilize the INR by decreasing the daily variation in total vitamin K consumed in the diet. This approach appears to have promise but would probably require some studies with larger populations than are currently available to establish the most appropriate amount of supplementation. The pharmaceutical industry continues to develop oral drugs that would lower the procoagulant aspect of the normal hemostatic balance by direct inhibition of the involved proteases, and an effective and safe drug might be available in the future. It is likely that the cost of these drugs relative to the cost of warfarin monitoring practices will be one of the main factors involved in whether or not there will be a major change in the practice of oral anticoagulation.

The question of whether or not an increase in the intake of vitamin K would have a positive effect on the skeletal health of the population has been a very active research area over the last 15 to 20 years, and to a large extent it has shifted much of the efforts in vitamin K research from the laboratory to the epidemiologist. A great deal of effort has been directed toward measurements of the degree of γ-carboxylation of the circulating pool of osteocalcin with the assumption that, as with other vitamin K-dependent proteins, biological activity would be associated with this posttranslational modification of the protein. The value of the measurements of ucOC is, however, compromised by the great variation in values found in healthy populations. As the value ranges from <10% to >30% in what appear to be similar populations, it is difficult to interpret the data. The majority of studies have attempted to relate % ucOC or vitamin K intake to bone mineral density. There is, however, no known function of osteocalcin related to the calcification of bone, and the phenotype of the osteocalcin knockout mouse is a denser bone, not an osteoporotic bone. There have been four rather well-controlled, reasonably sized studies directed toward the impact of phylloquinone supplementation on measures of bone mineral density and bone turnover markers in adults. They have ranged from a supplement of from 200 μg to 1,000 μg of phylloquinone, and they have ranged from one to three years. The collective outcome of these studies does not support the view that increasing vitamin K intake sufficiently to substantially decrease ucOC will increase bone mineral density.

Although not conducted in large, randomized, blinded, placebo-controlled studies, there have been a number of small studies demonstrating that pharmacological doses of MK-4 do decrease fracture rate, although these same studies do not show a consistent increase in bone mineral density. This has led to the hypothesis that the positive impact of MK-4 is related to alterations in bone geometry or "bone mineral quality" rather than to an improvement in bone mineral density [253,254]. The available data to support this hypothesis is not yet conclusive, but as MK-4 has been shown to have metabolic impacts on bone cells, metabolism not shared by phylloquinone, this is a possibility. It also appears that the MK-4 studies were carried out for the most part in Japan with patients diagnosed as osteoporotic, while the more recent phylloquinone supplementation trials in Europe or the United States utilized subjects whose skeletal health was such that they would not have been treated with drugs to prevent osteoporotic fractures. The currently available data would not appear to support the widespread use of vitamin K supplements in an effort to improve the skeletal health of the population, although research in this area will continue in an attempt to more clearly define the role of the vitamin as it relates to bone. Recent reports [255,256] of the identification of osteocalcin as a bone-derived hormone that plays an important role in glucose intolerance and insulin resistance may redefine the metabolic role of this protein.

At the present time, much of the interest in the public health aspect of vitamin K status has shifted to the possibility that alterations in vitamin K intake could be a major factor in regulating those factors responsible for calcification of cells not predisposed to this pathway. It does appear that studies in cell culture systems have established that MGP, in its Gla-MGP state, can protect vascular smooth muscle cells from calcifying, which would be expected from the initial observation that the null MGP mouse dies from arterial calcification. It is likely that more epidemiological studies will soon be available. Two large epidemiological studies have indicated that high phylloquinone intake may be a marker for low coronary heart disease risk in women [156], but that other dietary and lifestyle patterns associated with phylloquinone intake rather than the nutrient itself might account for this association. Low phylloquinone intake by men [157] was not found to be an independent risk factor for cardiovascular diseases but was also a marker for other risk factors. As with the possible impact of increased vitamin K intake on bone health, large controlled supplementation studies will probably be required to determine if this is an approach that would benefit a large segment of the population.

REFERENCES

1. Lane, P.A. and W.E. Hathaway. 1985. Vitamin K in infancy. *J Pediatrics* 106:351–359.
2. Vitamin K ad Hoc Task Force, American Association of Pediatrics. 1993. Controversies concerning vitamin K and the newborn. *Pediatrics* 91:1001–1003.
3. Buck, M.L. 2001. Vitamin K for the prevention of bleeding in newborns. *Pediatr Pharmacotherapy* 7.
4. von Kries, R., M. Shearer, P.T. McCarthy, M. Haug, G. Harzer, and U. Gobel. 1987. Vitamin K_1 content of maternal milk: Influence of the stage of lactation, lipid composition, and vitamin K_1 supplements given to the mother. *Pediatr Res* 22:513–517.
5. Greer, F.R. 1995. The importance of vitamin K as a nutrient during the first year of life. *Nutrition Res* 15:289–310.
6. Zengin, E., N. Sarper, G. Turker, F. Corapcioglu, and V. Etus. 2006. Late haemorrhagic disease of the newborn. *Ann Trop Paediatr* 26:225–231.
7. Ijland, M.M., R.R. Pereira, and E.A. Cornelissen. 2008. Incidence of late vitamin K deficiency bleeding in newborns in the Netherlands in 2005: Evaluation of the current guideline. *Eur J Pediatr* 167:165–169.
8. van Hasselt, P.M., T.J. de Koning, N. Kvist, E. de Vries, C.R. Lundin, R. Berger, J.L. Kipen, R.H. Houwen, M.H. Jorgensen, and H.J. Verkade. 2008. Prevention of vitamin K deficiency bleeding in breastfed infants: Lessons from the Dutch and Danish biliary atresia registries. *Pediatrics* 121:e857–e863.
9. Hubbard, D. and J.D. Tobias. 2006. Intracerebral hemorrhage due to hemorrhagic disease of the newborn and failure to administer vitamin K at birth. *South Med J* 99:1216–1220.
10. Clark, F.I. and E.J. James. 1995. Twenty-seven years of experience with oral vitamin K_1 therapy in neonates. *J Pediatr* 127:301–304.
11. Golding, J., M. Paterson, and L.J. Kinien. 1990. Factors associated with childhood cancer in a national cohort study. *Br J Cancer* 62:304–308.
12. Golding, J., R. Greenwood, K. Birmingham, and M. Mott. 1992. Childhood cancer, intramuscular vitamin K, and pethidine given during labour. *Br Med J* 305:341–346.
13. Israels, L.G., E. Friesen, A.H. Jansen, and E.D. Israels. 1987. Vitamin K_1 increases sister chromatid exchange in vitro in human leukocytes and in vivo in fetal sheep cells: A possible role for "vitamin K deficiency" in the fetus. *Pediatr Res* 22:405–408.
14. Ekelund, H., O. Finnstrom, J. Gunnarskog, B. Kallen, and Y. Larsson. 1993. Administration of vitamin K to newborn infants and childhood cancer. *Biochem Mol J* 307:89–91.
15. Klebanoff, M.A., J.S. Read, J.L. Mills, and P.H. Shiono. 1993. The risk of childhood cancer after neonatal exposure to vitamin K. *New Engl J Med* 329:905–908.
16. Olsen, J.H., H. Hertz, K. Blinkenberg, and H. Verder. 1994. Vitamin K regimens and incidence of childhood cancer in Denmark. *Brit Med J* 308:895–896.
17. McKinney, P.A., E. Juszczak, E. Findlay, and K. Smith. 1998. Case-control study of childhood leukaemia and cancer in Scotland: Findings for neonatal intramuscular vitamin K. *Brit Med J* 316:173–177.
18. Parker, L., M. Cole, A.W. Craft, and E.N. Hey. 1998. Neonatal vitamin K administration and childhood cancer in the north of England: Retrospective case-control study. *Brit Med J* 316:189–193.

19. Passmore, S.J., C. Draper, P. Brownbill, and M. Kroll. 1998. Case-control studies of relation between childhood cancer and neonatal vitamin K administration. *Brit Med J* 316:178–184.
20. Passmore, S.J., G. Draper, P. Brownbill, and M. Kroll. 1998. Ecological studies of relation between hospital policies on neonatal vitamin K administration and subsequent occurrence of childhood cancer. *Brit Med J* 316:184–189.
21. Roman, E., N.T. Fear, P. Ansell, D. Bull, G. Draper, P. McKinney, J. Michaelis, S.J. Passmore, and R. von Kries. 2002. Vitamin K and childhood cancer: Analysis of individual patient data from six case-control studies. *Brit J Cancer* 86:63–69.
22. Ross, J.A. and S.M. Davies. 2000. Vitamin K prophylaxis and childhood cancer. *Med Pediatr Oncol*, 34:434–437.
23. Fear, N.T., E. Roman, P. Ansell, J. Simpson, N. Day, and O.B. Eden. 2003. Vitamin K and childhood cancer: A report from the United Kingdom Childhood Cancer Study. *Brit J Cancer* 89:1228–1231.
24. Clarke, P., S.J. Mitchell, S. Sundaram, V. Sharma, R. Wynn, and M. Shearer. 2005. Vitamin K status of preterm infants with a prolonged prothrombin time. *Acta Paediatr* 194:1822–1833.
25. Humpl, T., K. Bruhl, R. Brzezinska, G. Hagner, W. Coerdt, and M.J. Shearer. 1999. Fatal late vitamin K-deficiency bleeding after oral vitamin K prophylaxis secondary to unrecognized bile duct paucity. *J Pediatr Gastroenterol* 29:594–597.
26. Cornelissen, M., R. von Kries, P. Loughnan, and G. Schubiger. 1997. Prevention of vitamin K deficiency bleeding: Efficacy of different multiple oral dose schedules of vitamin K. *Eur J Pediatr* 156:126–130.
27. O'Connor, M.E. and J.E. Addiego. 1986. Use of oral vitamin K_1 to prevent hemorrhagic disease of the newborn infant. *J Pediatr* 108:616–619.
28. Greer, F.R., S.P. Marshall, R.R. Severson, D.A. Smith, M.J. Shearer, D.G. Pace, and P.H. Joubert. 1998. A new mixed micellar preparation for oral vitamin K prophylaxis: Randomised controlled comparison with an intramuscular formulation in breast fed infants. *Arch Dis Child* 79:300–305.
29. Greer, F.R., S.P. Marshall, A.L. Foley, and J.W. Suttie. 1997. Improving the vitamin K status of breastfeeding infants with maternal vitamin K supplements. *Pediatrics* 99:88–92.
30. Greer, F.R., S. Marshall, J. Cherry, and J.W. Suttie. 1991. Vitamin K status of lactating mothers, human milk, and breastfeeding infants. *Pediatrics* 88:751–756.
31. von Kries, R., S. Kreppel, A. Becker, R. Tangermann, and U. Gobel. 1987. A carboxy-prothrombin activity after oral prophylactic vitamin K. *Arch Dis Child* 62:938–940.
32. von Kries, R., M.J. Shearer, J. Widdershoven, K. Motohara, G. Umbach, and U. Gobel. 1992. Des-gamma-carboxyprothrombin (PIVKA II) and plasma vitamin K_1 in newborns and their mothers. *Thromb Haemostas* 68:383–387.
33. Pereira, S.P., M.J. Shearer, R. Williams, and G. Mieli-Vergani. 2007. Intestinal absorption of mixed micellar phylloquinone (vitamin K_1) is unreliable in infants with conjugated hyperbilirubinaemia: Implications for oral prophylaxis of vitamin K deficiency bleeding. *Arch Dis Child Fetal Neonatal Ed* 88:F113–F118.
34. Mager, D.R., P.L. McGee, K.N. Furuya, and E.A. Roberts. 2006. Prevalence of vitamin K deficiency in children with mild to moderate chronic liver disease. *J Pediatr Gastroenterol Nutr* 42:71–76.
35. Bay, A., A.F. Oner, V. Celebi, and A. Uner. 2006. Evaluation of vitamin K deficiency in children with acute and intractable diarrhea. *Adv Therapy* 23:469–474.
36. von Kries, R., J. Funda, M. Shearer, and U. Gobel. 1992. Late hemorrhagic disease of newborn: A case with increased vitamin K requirement. *Acta Paediatr* 81:728–730.
37. Kumar, D., F.R. Greer, D.M. Super, J.W. Suttie, and J.J. Moore. 2001. Vitamin K status of premature infants: Implications for current recommendations. *Pediatrics* 108:1117–1122.

38. Costakos, D.T., F.R. Greer, L.A. Love, L.R. Dahlen, and J.W. Suttie. 2003. Vitamin K prophylaxis for premature infants: 1 mg vs. 0.5 mg. *Am J Perinatol* 20:485–490.
39. O'Reilly, R.A. 1976. Vitamin K and the oral anticoagulant drugs. *Annu Rev Med* 27:245–261.
40. Krasinski, S.D., R.M. Russell, B.C. Furie, S.F. Kruger, P.F. Jacques, and B. Furie. 1985. The prevalence of vitamin K deficiency in chronic gastrointestinal disorders. *Am J Clin Nutr* 41:639–643.
41. Duggan, P., M. O'Brien, M. Kiely, J. McCarthy, F. Shanahan, and K.D. Cashman. 2004. Vitamin K status in patients with Crohn's disease and relationship to bone turnover. *Am J Gastroenterol* 99:2178–2185.
42. Cavallaro, R., P. Iovino, F. Castiglione, A. Palumbo, M. Marino, S. Di Bella, F. Sabbatini, F. Labanca, R. Tortora, G. Mazzacca, and C. Ciacci. 2004. Prevalence and clinical associations of prolonged prothrombin time in adult untreated coeliac disease. *Eur J Gastroenterol Hepatol* 16:219–223.
43. Rashid, M., P. Durie, M. Andrew, D. Kalnins, J. Shin, M. Corey, E. Tullis, and P.B. Pencharz. 1999. Prevalence of vitamin K deficiency in cystic fibrosis. *Am J Clin Nutr* 70:378–382.
44. Petersen, L.C., S. Valentin, and U. Hedner. 1995. Regulation of the extrinsic pathway system in health and disease: The role of factor VIIa and tissue factor pathway inhibitor. *Thrombosis Res* 79:1–47.
45. Ham, J.M. 1971. Hypoprothrombinemia in patients undergoing prolonged intensive care. *Med J Australia* 2:716–718.
46. Harrington, D.J., H. Western, C. Seton-Jones, S. Rangarajan, T. Beynon, and M.J. Shearer. 2008. A study of the prevalence of vitamin K deficiency in patients with cancer referred to a hospital palliative care team and its association with abnormal haemostasis. *J Clin Pathol* 61:537–540.
47. Hazell, K. and K.H. Baloch. 1970. Vitamin K deficiency in the elderly. *Gerontol Clin* 12:10–17.
48. Alperin, J.B. 1987. Coagulopathy caused by vitamin K deficiency in critically ill, hospitalized patients. *JAMA* 258:1916–1919.
49. O'Shaughnessy, D., C. Allen, T. Woodcock, K. Pearce, J. Harvey, and M. Shearer. 2003. Echis time, under-carboxylated prothrombin and vitamin K status in intensive care patients. *Clin Lab Haem* 25:397–404.
50. Booth, S.L. 2007. Vitamin K status in the elderly. *Curr Opinion Clin Nutr Metab Care* 10:20–23.
51. Doisy, E.A. Nutritional hypoprothrombinemia and metabolism of vitamin K. 1961. *Fed Proc* 20:989–994.
52. Sokoll, L.J. and J.A. Sadowski. 1996. Comparison of biochemical indexes for assessing vitamin K nutritional status in a healthy adult population. *Am J Clin Nutr* 63:566–573.
53. Shevchuk, Y.M. and J.M. Conly. 1990. Antibiotic-associated hypoprothrombinemia: A review of prospective studies, 1966–1988. *Rev Infect Dis* 12:1109–1126.
54. Savage, D. and J. Lindenbaum. 1983: Clinical and experimental human vitamin K deficiency. In *Nutrition in Hematology*, ed. J. Lindenbaum, 271–320. New York: Churchill Livingstone.
55. Allison, P.M., L.L. Mummah-Schendel, C.B. Kindberg, C.S. Harms, N.U. Bang, and J.W. Suttie. 1987. Effects of a vitamin K-deficient diet and antibiotics in normal human volunteers. *J Lab Clin Med* 110:180–188.
56. Weitekamp, M.R. and R.C. Aber. 1983. Prolonged bleeding times and bleeding diathesis associated with moxalactam administration. *JAMA* 249:69–71.
57. Lipsky, J.J. 1984. Mechanism of the inhibition of the gamma-carboxylation of glutamic acid by N-methylthiotetrazole-containing antibiotics. *Proc Natl Acad Sci USA* 81:2893–2897.

58. Suttie, J.W., J.A. Engelke, and J. McTigue. 1986. Effect of N-methyl-thiotetrazole on rat liver microsomal vitamin K-dependent carboxylation. *Biochem Pharmacol* 35:2429–2433.

59. Creedon, K.A. and J.W. Suttie. 1986. Effect of N-methyl-thiotetrazole on vitamin K epoxide reductase. *Thrombosis Res* 44:147–153.

60. Lipsky, J.J. 1988. Antibiotic-associated hypoprothrombinaemia. *J Antimicrob Chemother* 21:281–300.

61. Frick, P.G., G. Riedler, and H. Brogli. 1967. Dose response and minimal daily requirement for vitamin K in man. *J Appl Physiol* 23:387–389.

62. Jackson, J.M., D. Blaine, J. Powell-Tuck, M. Korbonitis, A. Carey, and M. Elia. 2006. Macro- and micronutrient losses and nutritional status resulting from 44 days of total fasting in a non-obese man. *Nutrition* 22:889–897.

63. Booth, S.L., M.E. O'Brien-Morse, G.E. Dallal, K.W. Davidson, and C.M. Gundberg. 1999. Response of vitamin K status to different intakes and sources of phylloquinone-rich foods: Comparison of younger and older adults. *Am J Clin Nutr* 70:368–377.

64. Sokoll, L.J., S.L. Booth, M.E. O'Brien, K.W. Davidson, K.I. Tsaioun, and J.A. Sadowski. 1997. Changes in serum osteocalcin, plasma phylloquinone, and urinary gamma-carboxyglutamic acid in response to altered intakes of dietary phylloquinone in human subjects. *Am J Clin Nutr* 65:779–784.

65. van Walraven, C., A. Jennings, N. Oake, D. Fergusson, and A.J. Forster. 2006. Effect of study setting on anticoagulation control. *Chest* 129:1155–1166.

66. Hall, J.G., R.M. Pauli, and K.M. Wilson. 1980. Maternal and fetal sequelae of anticoagulation during pregnancy. *Am J Med* 68:122–140.

67. Ansell, J., J. Hirsh, L. Poller, H. Bussey, A. Jacobson, and E.M. Hylek. 2004. The pharmacology and management of the vitamin K antagonists. *Chest* 126:204S–233S.

68. Williams, E.C. and J.W. Suttie. 1998. Vitamin K antagonists. In *Cardiovascular Thrombosis: Thrombocardiology and Thromboneurology*, ed. M. Verstraete, V. Fuster, and E.J. Topol, 285–300. Philadelphia: Lippincott-Raven Publishers.

69. Bauman, M.E., K.L. Black, M.P. Massicotte, M.L. Bauman, S. Kuhle, S. Howlett-Clyne, G.S. Cembrowski, and L. Bajzar. 2008. Accuracy of the CoaguChek XS for point-of-care international normalized ratio (INR) measurement in children requiring warfarin. *Thromb Haemost* 99:1097–1103.

70. Christensen, T.D., S.P. Johnsen, V.E. Hjortdal, and J.M. Hasenkam. 2007. Self-management of oral anticoagulant therapy: A systematic review and meta-analysis. *Int J Cardiol* 118:54–61.

71. Holbrook, A.M., J.A. Pereira, R. Labris, H. McDonald, J.D. Douketis, M. Crowther, and P.S. Wells. 2005. Systematic overview of warfarin and its drug and food interactions. *Arch Intern Med* 165:1095–1106.

72. Takahashi, H. and H. Echizen. 2003. Pharmacogenetics of CYP2C9 and interindividual variability in anticoagulant response to warfarin. *Pharmacogenomics J* 3:202–214.

73. Sanderson, S., J. Emery, and J. Higgins. 2005. CYP2C9 gene variants, drug dose, and bleeding risk in warfarin-treated patients: A HuGEnetTM systematic review and meta-analysis. *Genet Med* 7:97–104.

74. Rost, S., A. Frogin, V. Ivaskevicius, E. Conzelmann, K. Hortnagel, H.-J. Pelz, K. Lappegard, E. Seifried, I. Scharrer, E.G.D. Tuddenham, C.R. Muller, T.M. Strom, and J. Oldlenburg. 2004. Mutations in VKORC1 cause warfarin resistance and multiple coagulation factor deficiency type 2. *Nature* 427:537–541.

75. Li, T., C.-Y. Chang, D.-Y. Jin, P.-J. Lin, A. Khvorova, and D.W. Stafford. 2004. Identification of the gene for vitamin K epoxide reductase. *Nature* 427:541–544.

76. Schwarz, U.I., M.D. Ritchie, Y. Bradford, C. Li, S.M. Dudek, A. Frye-Anderson, R.B. Kim, D.M. Roden, and C.M. Stein. 2008. Genetic determinants of response to warfarin during initial anticoagulation. *N Engl J Med* 358:999–1008.

77. Rieder, M.J., A.P. Reiner, and A.F. Rettie. 2007. Gamma-glutamyl carboxylase (GGCX) tagSNPs have limited utility for predicting warfarin maintenance dose. *J Thromb Haemost* 5:2227–2234.

78. Li, T., L.A. Lange, X. Li, I. Susswain, B. Bryant, R. Malone, E.M. Lange, T-Y. Huang, D.W. Stafford, and J.P. Evans. 2006. Polymorphisms in the VKORC1 gene are strongly associated with warfarin dosage requirements in patients receiving anticoagulation. *J Med Genet* 43:740–744.

79. Geisen, C., M. Watzka, K. Sittinger, M. Stefens, L. Daugela, E. Seifried, M.C. R, T.F. Wienker, and J. Oldenburg. 2005. VKORC1 haplotypes and their impact on the inter-individual and inter-ethnical variability of oral anticoagulation. *Thromb Haemost* 94:773–779.

80. Rieder, M.J., A.P. Reiner, B.F. Gage, D.A. Nickerson, C.S. Eby, H.L. McLeod, D.K. Blough, K.E. Thummel, D.L. Veenstra, and A.E. Rettie. 2005. Effect of VKORC1 haplotypes on transcriptional regulation and warfarin dose. *New Engl J Med* 352:2285–2293.

81. O'Reilly, R.A. and P.M. Aggeler. 1965. Coumarin anticoagulant drugs: Hereditary resistance in man. *Fed Proc* 24:1266–1273.

82. Sato, Y., R. Nakamura, M. Satoh, K. Fujishita, S. Mori, S. Ishida, T. Yamaguchi, K. Inoue, T. Nagao, and Y. Ohno. 2005. Thyroid hormone targets matrix Gla protein gene associated with vascular smooth muscle calcification. *Circulation Res* 97:550–557.

83. Vecsler, M., R. Loebstein, S. Almog, D. Kurnik, B. Goldman, H. Halkin, and E. Gak. 2006. Combined genetic profiles of components and regulators of the vitamin K-dependent gamma-carboxylation system affect individual sensitivity to warfarin. *Thromb Haemost* 95:205–211.

84. Caldwell, M.D., R.L. Berg, K.Q. Zhang, I. Glurich, J.R. Schmelzer, S.H. Yale, H.J. Vidaillet, and J.K. Burmester. 2007. Evaluation of genetic factors for warfarin dose prediction. *Clin Med Res* 5:8–16.

85. Au, N. and A.E. Rettie. 2008. Pharmacogenomics of 4-hydroxycoumarin anticoagulants. *Drug Metab Rev* 40:355–375.

86. Thompson, C.A. 2007. FDA encourages genetics-aided warfarin dosing. *Am J Health Syst Pharm* 64:1994–1996.

87. Flockhart, D.A., D. O'Kane, M.S. Williams, M.S. Watson, D.A. Flockhart, B.F. Gage, R. Gandolfi, R.M. King, E. Lyon, R. Nussbaum, D. O'Kane, K. Schulman, D. Veenstra, M.S. Williams, and M.S. Watson. 2008. Pharmacogenetic testing of CYP2C9 and VKORC1 alleles for warfarin. *Genet Med* 10:139–150.

88. Caldwell, M.D., T. Awad, J.A. Johnson, B.F. Gage, M. Falkowski, P. Gardina, J. Hubbard, Y. Turpaz, T.Y. Langaee, C. Eby, C.R. King, A. Brower, J.R. Schmelzer, I. Glurich, H.J. Vidaillet, S.H. Yale, K.Q. Zhang, R.L. Berg, and J.K. Burmester. 2008. CYP4F2 genetic variant alters required warfarin dose. *Blood* 111:4106–4112.

89. Gage, B.F., C. Eby, J. Johnson, E. Deych, M.J. Rieder, P. Ridker, P. Milligan, G. Grice, P. Lenzini, A. Rettie, C. Aquilante, L. Grosso, S. Marsh, L.T.L. Farnett, D. Voora, D. Veenstra, R. Glynn, A. Barrett, and H. McLeod. 2008. Use of pharmacogenetic and clinical factors to predict the therapeutic dose of warfarin. *Clin Pharmacol Ther* 84:326–331.

90. Anderson, J.L., B.D. Horne, S.M. Stevens, A.S. Grove, S. Barton, N.Z. P, S.F. Kahn, H.T. May, K.M. Samuelson, J.B. Muhlestein, and J.F. Carlquist. 2007. Randomized trial of genotype-guided versus standard warfarin dosing in patients initiating oral anticoagulation. *Circulation* 116:2563–2570.

91. Sconce, E., T. Khan, J.B. Mason, F. Noble, H. Wynne, and F. Kamali. 2005. Patients with unstable control have a poorer dietary intake of vitamin K compared to patients with stable control of anticoagulation. *Thromb Haemostas* 93:872–875.

92. Schurgers, L.J., M.J. Shearer, K. Hamulyak, E. Stocklin, and C. Vermeer. 2004. Effect of vitamin K intake on the stability of oral anticoagulant treatment: Dose-response relationships in healthy subjects. *Blood* 104:2682–2689.

93. Franco, V., C.A. Polanczyk, N. Clausell, and L.E. Rohde. 2004. Role of dietary vitamin K intake in chronic oral anticoagulation: Prospective evidence from observational and randomized protocols. *Am J Med* 116:651–656.

94. das Dores, S.M.C., S.L. Booth, L.A. Martini, V. Hugo de Carvalho Gouvea, F. Humberto de Abreu Maffei, A.O. Campana, and S.A. Rupp de Paiva. 2007. Relationship between diet and anticoagulant response to warfarin: A factor analysis. *Eur J Nutr* 46:147–154.

95. Watson, A.J.M., M. Pegg, and J.R.B. Green. 1984. Enteral feeds may antagonise warfarin. *Brit Med J* 288:557.

96. Couris, R., G.R. Tataronis, W. McCloskey, L. Oertel, G. Dallal, J. Dwyer, and J.B. Blumberg. 2006. Dietary vitamin K variability affects international normalized ratio (INR) coagulation indices. *Int J Vitam Nutr Res* 76:65–74.

97. Bovill, E.G., M. Fung, and M. Cushman. 2004. Vitamin K and oral anticoagulation: Thought for food. *Am J Med* 116:711–713.

98. Johnson, M.A. 2005. Influence of vitamin K on anticoagulant therapy depends on vitamin K status and the source and chemical forms of vitamin K. *Nutr Rev* 63:91–97.

99. Kurnik, D., R. Loebstein, H. Rabinovitz, N. Austerweil, H. Halkin, and S. Almog. 2004. Over-the-counter vitamin K_1-containing multivitamin supplements disrupt warfarin anticoagulation in vitamin K_1-depleted patients. *Thromb Haemostas* 92:1018–1024.

100. Sconce, E., P. Avery, H. Wynne, and F. Kamali. 2007. Vitamin K supplementation can improve stability of anticoagulation for patients with unexplained variability in response to warfarin. *Blood* 109:2419–2423.

101. Ford, S.K., C.P. Misita, B.B. Shilliday, R.M. Malone, C.G. Moore, and S. Moll. 2007. Prospective study of supplemental vitamin K therapy in patients on oral anticoagulants with unstable international normalized ratios. *J Thromb Thrombolysis* 24:23–27.

102. Reese, A.M., L.E. Farnett, R.M. Lyons, B. Patel, L. Morgan, and H.I. Bussey. 2005. Low-dose vitamin K to augment anticoagulation control. *Pharmacotherapy* 25:1746–1751.

103. Siguret, V., E. Pautas, and I. Gouin-Thibault. 2008. Warfarin therapy: Influence of pharmacogenetic and environmental factors on the anticoagulant response to warfarin. In *Vitamin K*, ed. G. Litwack, 247–265. New York: Academic Press.

104. Penning-van Beest, F.J.A., J. Koerselman, and R.M. Herings. 2008. Risk of major bleeding during concomitant use of antibiotic drugs and coumarin anticoagulants. *J Thromb Haemost* 6:284–290.

105. Dickerson, R.N., W.M. Garmon, D.A. Kuhl, G. Minard, and R.O. Brown. 2008. Vitamin K-dependent warfarin resistance after concurrent administration of warfarin and continuous enteral nutrition. *Pharmacotherapy* 28:308–313.

106. Nutescu, E.A. 2006. Warfarin and its interactions with foods, herbs and other dietary supplements. *Expert Opin Drug Saf* 5:433–451.

107. Wittkowsky, A.K. 2008. Dietary supplements, herbs and oral anticoagulants: The nature of the evidence. *J Thromb Thrombolysis* 25:72–77.

108. Wittkowsky, A.K. 2005. A systematic review and inventory of supplement effects on warfarin and other anticoagulants. *Thrombosis Res* 117:81–86.

109. Marder, V.J., T.L. Ortel, A. Grollman, and A.A.K. Hasan (eds.). 2005. Special Issue: Papers from the NIH Conference on Dietary Supplements, Coagulation, and Antithrombotic Therapies. *Thrombosis Research* 117.

110. Bates, S.M. and J.I. Weitz. 2006. The status of new anticoagulants. *Brit J Nutr* 134:3–19.

111. Hirsh, J., M. O'Donnell, and J.I. Weitz. 2005. New anticoagulants. *Blood* 105:453–463.

112. Bauer, K.A. 2006. New anticoagulants: Anti IIa vs Anti Xa — Is one better? *J Thromb Thrombolysis* 21:67–72.

113. Stangier, J., K. Rathgen, H. Stahle, D. Gansser, and W. Roth. 2007. The pharmacokinetics, pharmacodynamics and tolerability of dabigatran extexilate, a new oral direct thrombin inhibitor, in healthy male subjects. *Br J Clin Pharmacol* 64:292–303.

114. Piccini, J.P., M.R. Patel, K.W. Mahaffey, K.A. Fox, and R.M. Califf. 2008. Rivaroxaban, an oral direct factor Xa inhibitor. *Expert Opin Investig Drugs* 17:925–937.

115. Gundberg, C.M., J.B. Lian, and P.M. Gallop. 1983. Measurements of gamma-carboxyglutamate and circulating osteocalcin in normal children and adults. *Clin Chim Acta* 128:1–8.

116. Masters, P.W., R.G. Jones, D.A. Purves, E.H. Cooper, and J.M. Cooney. 1994. Commercial assays for serum osteocalcin give clinically discordant results. *Clin Chem* 40:358–363.

117. Vergnaud, P., P. Garnero, P.J. Meunier, G. Breart, K. Kamilhagi, and P.D. Delmas. 1997. Undercarboxylated osteocalcin measured with a specific immunoassay predicts hip fracture in elderly women: The EPIDOS study. *J Clin Endocrinol Metab* 82:719–724.

118. Gundberg, C.M., S.D. Nieman, S. Abrams, and H. Rosen. 1998. Vitamin K status and bone health: An analysis of methods for determination of undercarboxylated osteocalcin. *J Clin Endocrinol Metab* 83:3258–3266.

119. Price, P.A., M.K. Williamson, T. Haba, R.B. Dell, and W.S.S. Jee. 1982. Excessive mineralization with growth plate closure in rats on chronic warfarin treatment. *Proc Natl Acad Sci USA* 79:7734–7738.

120. Ducy, P., C. Desbois, B. Boyce, G. Pinero, B. Story, C. Dunstan, E. Smith, J. Bonadio, S. Goldstein, C.M. Gundberg, A. Bradley, and G. Karsenty. 1996. Increased bone formation in osteocalcin-deficient mice. *Nature* 382:448–452.

121. McKeown, N.M., P.F. Jacques, C.M. Gundberg, J.W. Peterson, K.L. Tucker, D.P. Kiel, P.W.F. Wilson, and S.L. Booth. 2002. Dietary and nondietary determinants of vitamin K biochemical measures in men and women. *J Nutr* 132:1329–1334.

122. Collins, A., K.D. Cashman, and M. Kiely. 2006. Phylloquinone (vitamin K_1) intakes and serum undercarboxylated osteocalcin levels in Irish postmenopausal women. *Brit J Nutr* 95:982–988.

123. Booth, S.L., K.E. Broe, J.W. Peterson, D.M. Cheng, B. Dawson-Hughes, C.M. Gundberg, L.A. Cupples, P.W.F. Wilson, and D.P. Kiel. 2004. Associations between vitamin K biochemical measures and bone mineral density in men and women. *J Clin Endocrinol Metab* 89:4904–4909.

124. Kohlmeier, M., J. Saupe, M.J. Shearer, K. Schaefer, and G. Asmus. 1997. Bone health of adult hemodialysis patients is related to vitamin K status. *Kidney Int* 51:1218–1221.

125. Tsugawa, N., M. Shiraki, Y. Suhara, M. Kamao, K. Tanaka, and T. Okano. 2006. Vitamin K status of healthy Japanese women: Age-related vitamin K requirement for gamma-carboxylation of osteocalcin. *Am J Clin Nutr* 83:380–386.

126. Nimptsch, K., S. Hailer, S. Rohrmann, K. Gedrich, G. Wolfram, and J. Linseisen. 2007. Determinants and correlates of serum undercarboxylated osteocalcin. *Ann Nutr Metab* 51:563–570.

127. O'Connor, E.O., C. Molgaard, K.F. Michaelsen, J. Jakobsen, C.J.E. Lamberg-Allardt, and K.D. Cashman, 2007. Serum percentage undercarboxylated osteocalcin, a sensitive measure of vitamin K status, and its relationship to bone health indices in Danish girls. *Brit J Nutrition* 97:661–666.

128. Binkley, N.C., D.C. Krueger, J.A. Engelke, A.L. Foley, and J.W. Suttie. 2000. Vitamin K supplementation reduces serum concentrations of under-gamma-carboxylated osteocalcin in healthy young and elderly adults. *Am J Clin Nutr* 72:1523–1528.

129. Bugel, S., A.D. Sorensen, O. Heis, M. Kristensen, C. Vermeer, J. Jakobsen, A. Flynn, C. Molgaard, and K.D. Cashman. 2007. Effect of phylloquinone supplementation on biochemical markers of vitamin K status and bone turnover in postmenopausal women. *Brit J Nutr* 97:373–380.

130. Sokoll, L.J., S.L. Booth, K.W. Davidson, G.E. Dallal, and J.A. Sadowski. 1998. Diurnal variation in total and undercarboxylated osteocalcin: Influence of increased dietary phylloquinone. *Calcif Tissue Int* 62:447–452.

131. Douglas, A.S., S.P. Robins, J.D. Hutchison, R.W. Porter, A. Stewart, and D.M. Reid. 1995. Carboxylation of osteocalcin in post-menopausal osteoporotic women following vitamin K and D supplementation. *Bone* 17:15–20.

132. Beavan, S.R., A. Prentice, D.M. Stirling, B. Dibba, L. Yan, D.J. Harrington, and M.J. Shearer. 2005. Ethnic differences in osteocalcin gamma-carboxylation, plasma phylloquinone (vitamin K_1) and apolipoprotein E genotype. *Eur J Clin Nutr* 59:72–81.

133. Binkley, N.C., D.C. Krueger, T.N. Kawahara, J.A. Engelke, R.J. Chappell, and J.W. Suttie. 2002. A high phylloquinone intake is required to achieve maximal osteocalcin gamma-carboxylation. *Am J Clin Nutr* 76:1055–1060.

134. Booth, S.L., K.L. Tucker, H. Chen, M.T. Hannan, D.R. Gagnon, L.A. Cupples, P.W.F. Wilson, J. Ordovas, E.J. Schaefer, B. Dawson-Hughes, and D.P. Kiel. 2000. Dietary vitamin intakes are associated with hip fracture but not with bone mineral density in elderly men and women. *Am J Clin Nutr* 71:1201–1208.

135. Feskanich, D., P. Weber, W.C. Willett, H. Rockett, S.L. Booth, and G.A. Colditz. 1999. Vitamin K intake and hip fractures in women: A prospective study. *Am J Clin Nutr* 69:74–79.

136. Hodges, S.J., K. Akesson, P. Vergnaud, K.J. Obrant, and P.D. Delmas. 1993. Circulating levels of vitamin K_1 and K_2 decreased in elderly women with hip fracture. *J Bone Miner Res* 8:1241–1245.

137. Hart, J.P., M.J. Shearer, L. Klenerman, A. Catterall, J. Reeve, P.N. Sambrook, R.A. Dodds, and J. Chayen. 1985. Electrochemical detection of depressed circulating levels of vitamin K_1 in osteoporosis. *J Clin Endocrinol Metab* 60:1268–1269.

138. Hodges, S.J., M.J. Pilkington, T.C.B. Stamp, A. Catterall, M.J. Shearer, L. Bitensky, and J. Chayen. 1991. Depressed levels of circulating menaquinones in patients with osteoporotic fractures of the spine and femoral neck. *Bone* 12:387–389.

139. Szulc, P., M.-C. Chapuy, P.J. Meunier, and P.D. Delmas. 1993. Serum undercarboxylated osteocalcin is a marker of the risk of hip fracture in elderly women. *J Clin Invest* 91:1769–1774.

140. Tsugawa, N., M. Shiraki, Y. Suhara, M. Kamao, R. Ozaki, K. Tanaka, and T. Okano. 2008. Low plasma phylloquinone concentration is associated with high incidence of vertebral fracture in Japanese women. *J Bone Miner Metab* 26:79–85.

141. Kawana, K., M. Takahashi, H. Hoshino, and K. Kushida. 2001. Circulating levels of vitamin K_1, menaquinone-4, and menaquinone-7 in healthy elderly Japanese women and patients with vertebral fractures and patients with hip fractures. *Endocr Res* 27:337–343.

142. Yaegashi, Y., T. Onoda, T. Tanno, T. Kuribayashi, K. Sakata, and H. Orimo. 2008. Association of hip fracture incidence and intake of calcium, magnesium, vitamin D, and vitamin K. *Eur J Epidemiol* 23:219–225.

143. Kanai, T., T. Takagi, K. Masuhiro, M. Nakamura, M. Iwata, and F. Saji. 1997. Serum vitamin K level and bone mineral density in postmenopausal women. *Int J Gynecol Obstet* 56:25–30.

144. Macdonald, H.M., F.E. McGuigan, S.A. Lanham-New, W.D. Fraser, S.H. Ralston, and D.M. Reid. 2008. Vitamin K_1 intake is associated with higher bone mineral density and reduced bone resorption in ealy postmenopausal Scottish women: No evidence of gene-nutrient interaction with apolipoprotein E polymorphisms. *Am J Clin Nutr* 87:1513–1520.

145. Szulc, P., M.C. Chapuy, P.J. Meunier, and P.D. Delmas. 1996. Serum undercarboxylated osteocalcin is a marker of the risk of hip fracture: A three year follow-up study. *Bone* 18:487–488.

146. Szulc, P., M.E. Arlot, M.C. Chapuy, F. Duboeuf, P.J. Meunier, and P.D. Delmas. 1994. Serum undercarboxylated osteocalcin correlates with hip bone mineral density in elderly women. *J Bone Miner Res* 9:1591–1595.

147. van Summeren, M.J.H., S.C.C.M. van Coeverden, L.J. Schurgers, L.A.J. L.M. Braam, F. Noirt, C.S.P.M. Uiterwaal, W. Kuis, and C. Vermeer. 2008. Vitamin K status is associated with childhood bone mineral content. *Brit J Nutr* 100:852–858.

148. Weber, P. 2001. Vitamin K and bone health. *Nutrition* 17:880–887.

149. Vermeer, C., M.J. Shearer, A. Zittermann, C. Bolton-Smith, P. Szulc, S. Hodges, P. Walter, W. Rambeck, E. Stocklin, and P. Weber. 2004. Beyond deficiency: Potential benefits of increased intakes of vitamin K for bone and vascular health. *Eur J Nutr* 43:325–335.

150. Cashman, K.D. 2005. Vitamin K status may be an important determinant of childhood bone health. *Nutr Rev* 63:284–289.

151. Bugel, S. 2008. Vitamin K and bone health in adult humans. In *Vitamin K*, ed. G. Litwack, 393–416. New York: Academic Press.

152. Heiss, C., L.M. Hoesel, U. Wehr, S. Wenisch, I. Drosse, V. Alt, C. Meyer, U. Horas, M. Schieker, and R. Schnettler. 2008. Diagnosis of osteoporosis with vitamin K as a new biochemical marker. In *Vitamin K*, ed. G. Litwack, 417–434. New York: Academic Press.

153. Rejnmark, L., P. Vestergaard, P. Charles, A.P. Hermann, C. Brot, P. Eiken, and L. Mosekilde. 2006. No effect of vitamin K_1 intake on bone mineral density and fracture risk in perimenopausal women. *Osteoporosis Int* 17:1122–1132.

154. Liu, G. and M. Peacock. 1998. Age-related changes in serum undercarboxylated osteocalcin and its relationships with bone density, bone quality, and hip fracture. *Calcif Tissue Int* 62:286–289.

155. McLean, R.R., S.L. Booth, D.P. Kiel, K.E. Broe, D.R. Gagnon, K.L. Tucker, L.A. Cupples, and M.T. Hannan. 2006. Association of dietary and biochemical measures of vitamin K with quantitative ultrasound of the heel in men and women. *Osteoporosis Int* 17:600–607.

156. Erkkila, A., S.L. Booth, F.B. Hu, P.F. Jacques, J.E. Manson, K.M. Rexrode, M.J. Stampfer, and A.H. Lichtenstein. 2005. Phylloquinone intake as a marker for coronary heart disease risk but not stroke in women. *Eur J Clin Nutr* 59:196–204.

157. Erkkila, A.T., S.L. Booth, F.B. Hu, P.F. Jacques, and A.H. Lichtenstein. 2007. Phylloquinone intake and risk of cardiovascular diseases in men. *Nutr Metab Cardiovasc Dis* 17:58–62.

158. Braam, L., N. McKeown, P. Jacques, A. Lichtenstein, C. Vermeer, P. Wilson, and S. Booth. 2004. Dietary phylloquinone intake as a potential marker for a heart-healthy dietary pattern in the Framingham Offspring Cohort. *J Am Dietet Assoc* 104:1410–1414.

159. Caraballo, P.J. 1999. Long-term use of oral anticoagulants and the risk of fracture. *Arch Intern Med* 159:1750–1756.

160. Gage, B.F., E. Birman-Deych, M.J. Radford, D.S. Nilasena, and E.F. Binder. 2006. Risk of osteoporotic fracture in elderly patients taking warfarin. *Arch Intern Med* 166:241–246.

161. Mamdani, M., R.E.G. Upshur, G. Anderson, B.R. Bartle, and A. Laupacis. 2003. Warfarin therapy and risk of hip fracture among elderly patients. *Pharmacotherapy* 23:1–4.

162. Jamal, S.A., W.S. Browner, D.C. Bauer, and S.R. Cummings. 1998. Warfarin use and risk for osteoporosis in elderly women. *Ann Int Med* 128:829–832.

163. Chang, L.L., C.W. Shinoff, S.K. Ewing, S.R. Cummings, and D.C. Bauer. 2006. Warfarin use and risk of osteoporosis in elderly men: A prospective study. *J Bone Miner Res* 21(suppl 1):S277.

164. Rosen, H.N., L.A. Maitland, J.W. Suttie, W.J. Manning, R.J. Glynn, and S.L. Greenspan. 1993. Vitamin K and maintenance of skeletal integrity in adults. *Am J Med* 94:62–68.

165. Caraballo, P.J., S.E. Gabriel, M.R. Castro, E.J. Atkinson, and L.J.I. Melton. 1999. Changes in bone density after exposure to oral anticoagulants: A meta-analysis. *Osteoporosis Int* 9:441–448.

166. Simon, R.R., S.M. Beaudin, M. Johnston, K.J. Walton, and S.G. Shaughnessy. 2002. Long-term treatment with sodium warfarin results in decreased femoral bone strength and cancellous bone volume in rats. *Thrombosis Res* 105:353–358.

167. Haffa, A., D. Krueger, J. Bruner, J. Engelke, C.M. Gundberg, M. Akhter, and N. Binkley. 2000. Diet- or warfarin-induced vitamin K insufficiency elevates circulating undercarboxylated osteocalcin without altering skeletal status in growing female rats. *J Bone Miner Res* 15:872–878.

168. Binkley, N., D. Krueger, J. Engelke, and J. Suttie. 2007. Vitamin K deficiency from long-term warfarin anticoagulation does not alter skeletal status in male rhesus monkeys. *J Bone Miner Res* 22:695–700.

169. Iwamoto, J., T. Takeda, and Y. Sato. 2006. Menatetrenone (vitamin K_2) and bone quality in the treatment of postmenopausal osteoporosis. *Nutr Rev* 64:509–517.

170. Ishida, Y. and S. Kawai. 2004. Comparative efficacy of hormone replacement therapy, etidronate, calcitonin, alfacalcidol, and vitamin K in postmenopausal women with osteoporosis: The Yamaguchi osteoporosis prevention study. *Am J Med* 117:549–555.

171. Sasaki, N., E. Kusano, H. Takahashi, Y. Ando, K. Yano, E. Tsuda, and Y. Asano. 2005. Vitamin K_2 inhibits glucocorticoid-induced bone loss partly by preventing the reduction of osteoprotegerin (OPG). *J Bone Miner Metab* 23:41–47.

172. Sato, Y., Y. Honda, H. Kuno, and K. Oizumi. 1998. Menatetrenone ameliorates osteopenia in disuse-affected limbs of vitamin D- and K-deficient stroke patients. *Bone* 23:291–296.

173. Sato, Y., Y. Honda, M. Kaji, T. Asoh, K. Hosokawa, I. Kondo, and K. Satoh. 2002. Amelioration of osteoporosis by menatetrenone in elderly female Parkinson's disease in patients with vitamin D. *Bone* 31:114–118.

174. Sato, Y., T. Kanoko, K. Satoh, and J. Iwamoto. 2005. Menatetrenone and vitamin D_2 with calcium supplements prevent nonvertebral fracture in elderly women with Alzheimer's disease. *Bone* 36:61–68.

175. Shiraki, M., Y. Shiraki, C. Aoki, and M. Miura. 2000. Vitamin K_2 (menatetrenone) effectively prevents fractures and sustains lumbar bone mineral density in osteoporosis. *J Bone Miner Res* 15:515–521.

176. Iwamoto, J., T. Takeda, and S. Ichimura. 2001. Effect of menatetrenone on bone mineral density and incidence of vertebral fractures in postmenopausal women with osteoporosis: A comparison with the effect of etidronate. *J Orthop Sci* 6:487–492.

177. Cockayne, S., J. Adamson, S. Lanham-New, M.J. Shearer, S. Gilbody, and D.J. Torgerson. 2006. Vitamin K and the prevention of fractures. *Arch Intern Med* 166:1256–1261.

178. Tamura, T., S.L. Morgan, and H. Takimoto. 2007. Vitamin K and the prevention of fractures. *Arch Intern Med* 167:94.

179. Iwamoto, J., T. Takeda, and Y. Sato. 2006. Effects of vitamin K_2 on the development of osteopenia in rats as the models of osteoporosis. *Yonsei Med J* 47:157–166.

180. Binkley, N., D. Krueger, J. Engelke, T. Crenshaw, and J. Suttie. 2002. Vitamin K supplementation does not affect ovariectomy-induced bone loss in rats. *Bone* 30:897–900.

181. Otomo, H., A. Sakai, S. Ikeda, S. Tanaka, M. Ito, R.J. Phipps, and T. Nakamura. 2004. Regulation of mineral-to-matrix ratio of lumbar trabecular bone in ovariectomized rats treated with risedronate in combination with or without vitamin K_2. *J Bone Miner Metab* 22:404–414.

182. Iwamoto, J., H. Matsumoto, T. Takeda, Y. Sato, X. Liu, and J.K. Yeh. 2008. Effects of vitamin K(2) and risedronate on bone formation and resorption, osteocyte lacunar system, and porosity in the cortical bone of glucocorticoid-treated rats. *Calcif Tissue Int* 83:121–128.

183. Binkley, N.C. and J.W. Suttie. 1995. Vitamin K nutrition and osteoporosis. *J Nutr* 125:1812–1821.

184. Tabb, N.M., A. Sun, C. Zhou, F. Grun, J. Errandi, K. Romero, H. Pham, S. Inoue, S. Mallick, M. Lin, B.M. Forman, and B. Blumberg. 2003. Vitamin K2 regulation of bone homeostasis is mediated by the steroid and xenobiotic receptor SXR. *J Biol Chem* 278:43919–43927.

185. Ichikawa, T., K. Horie-Inoue, K. Ikeda, B. Blumberg, and S. Inoue. 2006. Steroid and xenobiotic receptor SXR mediates vitamin K_2-activated transcription of extracellular matrix-related genes and collagen accumulation in osteoblastic cells. *J Biol Chem* 281:16927–16934.

186. Igarashi, M., Y. Yogiashi, M. Mihara, I. Takada, H. Kitagawa, and S. Kato. 2006. Vitamin K stimulates osteoblastgenesis through PXR/SXR-mediated Msx2 induction. 21(Suppl 1):S381.

187. Horie-Inoue, K. and S. Inoue. 2008. Steroid and xenobiotic receptor mediates a novel vitamin K(2) signaling pathway in osteoblastic cells. *J Bone Miner Metab* 26:9–12.

188. Igarashi, M., Y. Yogiashi, M. Mihara, I. Takada, H. Kitagawa, and S. Kato. 2007. Vitamin K induces osteoblast differentiation through pregnane X receptor-mediated transcriptional control of the Msx2 gene. *Mol Cell Biol* 27:7947–7954.

189. Ichikawa, T., K. Horie-Inoue, K. Ikda, B. Blumberg, and S. Inoue. 2007. Vitamin K_2 induces phosphorylation of protein kinase A and expression of novel target genes in osteoblastic cells. *J Mol Endocrinol* 39:239–247.

190. Nanke, Y., S. Kotake, T. Ninomiya, T. Furuya, H. Ozawa, and N. Kamatani. 2005. Geranylgeranylacetone inhibits formation and function of human osteoclasts and prevents bone loss in tail-suspended rats and ovariectomized rats. *Calcif Tissue Int* 77:376–385.

191. Braam, L.A.J.L.M., M.H.J. Knapen, P. Geusens, F. Brouns, K. Hamulyak, M.J.W. Gerichhausen, and C. Vermeer. 2003. Vitamin K_1 supplementation retards bone loss in postmenopausal women between 50 and 60 years of age. *Calcif Tissue Int* 73:21–26.

192. Bolton-Smith, C., M.E.T. McMurdo, C.R. Paterson, P.A. Mole, J.M. Harvey, S.T. Fenton, C.J. Prynne, G.D. Mishra, and M.J. Shearer. 2007. Two-year randomized controlled trial of vitamin K_1 (phylloquinone) and vitamin D_3 plus calcium on the bone health of older women. *J Bone Miner Res* 22:509–519.

193. Booth, S.L., G. Dallal, M.K. Shea, C. Gundberg, J.W. Peterson, and B. Dawson-Hughes. 2008. Effect of vitamin K supplementation on bone loss in elderly men and women. *J Clin Endocrinol Metab* 93:1217–1223.

194. Binkley, N., J. Harke, D. Krueger, J. Engelke, N. Vallarta-Ast, D. Gemar, M. Checovich, R. Chappell, and J. Suttie. 2008. Vitamin K treatment reduces undercarboxylated osteocalcin but does not alter bone turnover, density, geometry in healthy postmenopausal North American women. *J Bone Miner Res* 2008 Dec 29. [Epub ahead of print] PMID: 19113922 [PubMed—as supplied by publisher].

195. Braam, L.A.J.L.M., M.H.J. Knapen, P. Geusens, F. Brouns, and C. Vermeer. 2003. Factors affecting bone loss in female endurance athletes. *Am J Sports Med* 31:889–895.

196. Martini, L.A., S.L. Booth, E.J. Saltzman, M. Rosario Dias de Oliveira Latorre, and R.J. Wood. 2006. Dietary phylloquinone depletion and repletion in postmenopausal women: effects on bone and mineral metabolism. *Osteoporosis Int* 17:929–935.

197. Kruger, M.C., C.L. Booth, J. Coad, L.M. Schollum, B. Kuhn-Sherlock, and M.J. Shearer. 2006. Effect of calcium fortified milk supplementation with or without vitamin K on biochemical markers of bone turnover in premenopausal women. *Nutrition* 22:1120–1128.

198. Nicolaidou, P., I. Stavrinadis, I. Loukou, A. Papadopoulou, H. Georgouli, K. Duouros, K.N. Priftis, D. DGourgiotis, Y.G. Matsinos, and S. Doudounakis. 2006. The effect of vitamin K supplementation on biochemical markers of bone formation in children and adolescents with cystic fibrosis. *Eur J Pediatr* 165:540–545.

199. Kaneki, M., S.J. Hedges, T. Hosoi, S. Fujiwara, A. Lyons, S.J. Crean, N. Ishida, M. Nakagawa, M. Takechi, Y. Sano, Y. Mizuno, S. Hoshino, M. Miyao, S. Inoue, K. Horiki, M. Shiraki, Y. Ouchi, and H. Orimo. 2001. Japanese fermented soybean food as the major determinant of the large geographic difference in circulating levels of vitamin K_2: Possible implications for hip-fracture risk. *Nutrition* 17:315–321.

200. Ikeda, Y., M. Iki, A. Morita, E.E. Kajita, S. Kagamimori, Y. Kagawa, and H. Yoneshima. 2006. Intake of fermented soybeans, natto, is associated with reduced bone loss in postmenopausal women: Japanese population-based osteoporosis (JPOS) study. *J Nutr* 136:1323–1328.

201. Yamaguchi, M., H. Taguchi, Y.H. Gao, A. Igarashi, and Y. Tsukamoto. 1999. Effect of vitamin K_2 (menaquinone-7) in fermented soybean (natto) on bone loss in ovariectomized rats. *J Bone Miner Metab* 17:23–29.

202. Yamaguchi, M. and Z.J. Ma. 2001. Inhibitory effect of menaquinone-7 (vitamin K_2) on osteoclast-like cell formation and osteoclastic bone resorption in rat bone tissues in vitro. *Mol Cell Biochem* 228:39–47.

203. Yamaguchi, M., E. Sugimoto, and S. Hachiya. 2001. Stimulatory effect of menaquinone-7 (vitamin K_2) on osteoblastic bone formation in vitro. *Mol Cell Biochem* 223:131–137.

204. Luo, G., P. Ducy, M.D. McKee, G.J. Pinero, E. Loyer, R.R. Behringer, and G. Karsenty. 1997. Spontaneous calcification of arteries and cartilage in mice lacking matrix Gla protein. *Nature* 386:78–81.

205. Price, P.A., S.A. Faus, and M.K. Williamson. 1998. Warfarin causes rapid calcification of the elastic lamellae in rat arteries and heart valves. *Arterioscler Thromb Vasc Biol* 18:1400–1407.

206. Spronk, H.M.H., B.A.M. Soute, L.J. Schurgers, H.H.W. Thijssen, J.G.R. De Mey, and C. Vermeer. 2003. Tissue-specific utilization of menaquinone-4 results in the prevention of arterial calcification in warfarin-treated rats. *J Vasc Res* 40:531–537.

207. Saito, E., H. Wachi, F. Sato, H. Sugitani, and Y. Seyama. 2007. Treatment with vitamin K(2) combined with bisphosphonates synergistically inhibits calcification in cultured smooth muscle cells. *J Atheroscler Thromb* 14:317–324.

208. El-Maadawy, S., M.T. Kaartinen, T. Schinke, M. Murshed, G. Karsenty, and M.D. McKee. 2003. Cartilage formation and calcification in arteries of mice lacking matrix Gla protein. *Connective Tissue Res* 44 (Suppl):272–278.

209. Berkner, K.L. and K.W. Runge. 2005. The physiology of vitamin K nutriture and vitamin K-dependent protein function in atherosclerosis. *J Thromb Haemostas* 2:2118–2132.

210. Hofbauer, L.C., C.C. Brueck, C.M. Shanahan, M. Schoppet, and H. Dobnig. 2007. Vascular calcification and osteoporosis: From clinical observation towards molecular understanding. *Osteoporosis Int* 18:251–259.

211. El-Abbadi, M. and C.M. Giachelli. 2007. Mechanisms of vascular calcification. *Adv Chronic Kidney Dis* 14:54–66.

212. Shearer, M.J. 2000. Role of vitamin K and Gla proteins in the pathophysiology of osteoporosis and vascular calcification. *Current Opinion Clin Nutr Metab Care* 3:433–438.

213. Price, P.A., S.A. Faus, and M.K. Williamson. 2000. Warfarin-induced artery calcification is accelerated by growth and vitamin D. *Arterioscler Thromb Vasc Biol* 20:317–327.

214. Cola, C., M. Almeida, D. Li, F. Romeo, and J.L. Mehta. 2004. Regulatory role of endothelium in the expression of genes affecting arterial calcification. *Biochem Biophys Res Commun* 320:424–427.

215. Yao, Y., A.F. Zebboudj, E. Shao, M. Perez, and K. Bostrom. 2006. Regulation of bone morphogenetic protein-4 by matrix Gla protein in vascular endothelial cells involves activin-like kinase receptor 1. *J Biol Chem* 28:33921–33930.

216. Zebboudj, A.F., M. Imura, and K. Bostrom. 2002. Matrix Gla protein, a regulatory protein for bone morphogenetic protein-2. *J Biol Chem* 277:4388–4394.

217. Bostrom, K., A.F. Zebboudj, Y. Yao, T.S. Lin, and A. Torres. 2004. Matrix Gla protein stimulates VEGF expression through increased transforming growth factor-beta1 activity in endothelial cells. *J Biol Chem* 279:52904–52913.

218. Schurgers, L.J., H.M.H. Spronk, J.N. Skepper, T.M. Hackeng, C.M. Shanahan, C. Vermeer, P.L. Weissberg, and D. Proudfoot. 2007. Post-translational modifications regulate matrix Gla protein function: Importance for inhibition of vascular smooth muscle cell calcification. *J Thromb Haemostas* 5:2503–2511.

219. Wallin, R., L.J. Schurgers, and N. Wajih. 2008. Effects of the blood coagulation vitamin K as an inhibitor of arterial calcification. *Thromb Res* 122:411–417.

220. Cranenburg, E.C.M., L.J. Schurgers, and C. Vermeer. 2007. Vitamin K: The coagulation vitamin that became omnipotent. *Thromb Haemost* 98:120–125.

221. Hur, D.J., G.V. Raymond, S.G. Kahler, D.L. Riegert-Johnson, B.A. Cohen, and S.A. Boyadjiev. 2005. A novel MGP mutation in a consanguineous family: Review of the clinical and molecular characteristics of Keutel syndrome. *Am J Med Genet* 135A:36–40.

222. Munroe, P.B., R.O. Olgunturk, J.-P. Fryns, L. Van Maldergem, F. Ziereisen, B. Yuksel, R.M. Gardiner, and E. Chung. 1999. Mutations in the gene encoding the human matrix Gla protein cause Keutel syndrome (Letter). *Nature Genet* 21:142–144.

223. Gheduzzi, D., F. Boraldi, G. Annovi, C.P. Devincenzi, L.J. Schurgers, C. Vermeer, D. Quaglino, and I. Pasquali Ronchetti. 2007. Matrix Gla protein is involved in elastic fiber calcification in the dermis of pseudoxanthoma elasticum patients. *Lab Invest* 87:998–1008.

224. Le Saux, O., Z. Urban, C. Tschuch, K. Csiszar, B. Bacchelli, D. Quaglino, I. Pasquali-Ronchetti, F.M. Pope, A. Richards, S. Terry, L. Bercovitch, A. de Paepe, and C.D. Boyd. 2000. Mutations in a gene encoding an ABC transporter cause pseudoxanthoma elasticum. *Nat Genet* 25:223–227.

225. Bergen, A.A., A.S. Plomp, E.J. Schuurman, S. Terry, M. Breuning, H. Dauwerse, J. Swart, M. Kool, S. van Soest, F. Baas, J.B. Ten Brink, and P.T. de Jong. 2000. Mutations in ABCC6 cause pseudoxanthoma elasticum. *Nat Genet* 25:228–231.

226. Ringpfeil, F., M.G. Lebwohl, A.M. Christiano, and J. Uitto. 2000. Pseudoxanthoma elasticum: mutations in the MRP6 gene encoding a transmembrane ATP-binding cassette (ABC) transporter. *Proc Natl Acad Sci USA* 97:6001–6006.

227. Li, Q., Q. Jiang, L.J. Schurgers, and J. Uitto. 2007. Pseudoxanthoma elasticum: Reduced gamma-glutamyl carboxylation of matrix Gla protein in a mouse model (abcc6-/-). *Biochem Biophys Res Commun* 364:208–213.

228. Hendig, D., R. Zarbock, C. Szliska, K. Kleesiek, and C. Gotting. 2008. The local calcification inhibitor matrix Gla protein in pesudoxanthoma elasticum. *Clin Biochem* 41:407–412.

229. Troy, L.M., P.F. Jacques, M.T. Hannan, D.P. Kiel, A.H. Lichtenstein, E.T. Kennedy, and S.L. Booth. 2007. Dihydrophylloquinone intake is associated with low bone mineral density in men and women. *Am J Clin Nutr* 86:504–508.

230. Borst, P., K. van de Wetering, and R. Schlingemann. 2008. Does the absence of ABCC6 (multidrug resistance protein 6) in patients with pseudoxanthoma elasticum prevent the liver from providing sufficient vitamin K to the periphery? *Cell Cycle* 7:1575–1579.

231. Jono, S., Y. Ikari, C. Vermeer, P. Dissel, K. Hasegawa, A. Shioi, H. Taniwaki, A. Kizu, Y. Nishizawa, and S. Saito. 2004. Matrix Gla protein is associated with coronary artery calcification as assessed by electron-beam computed tomography. *Thromb Haemostas* 91:790–794.

232. O'Donnell, C.J., M.K. Shea, P.A. Price, D.R. Gagnon, P.W.F. Wilson, M.G. Larson, D.P. Kiel, U. Hoffmann, M. Ferencik, M.E. Clouse, M.K. Williamson, L.A. Cupples, B. Dawson-Hughes, and S.L. Booth. 2006. Matrix Gla protein is associated with risk factors for atherosclerosis but not with coronary artery calcification. *Arterioscler Thromb Vasc Biol* 26:2769–2774.

233. Schurgers, L.J., K.J.F. Teunissen, M.H.J. Knapen, M. Kwaijtaal, R. van Diest, A. Appels, C.P. Reutelingsperger, P.M. Cleutjens, and C. Vermeer. 2005. Novel conformation-specific antibodies against matrix gamma-carboxyglutamic acid (Gla) protein. Undercarboxylated matrix Gla protein as marker for vascular calcification. *Arterioscler Thromb Vasc Biol* 25:1629–1633.

234. Cranenburg, E.C.M., C. Vermeer, R. Koos, M.-L. Boumans, T.M. Hackeng, F.G. Bouwman, M. Kwaijtaal, V.M. Brandenburg, M. Ketteler, and L.J. Schurgers. 2008. The circulating inactive form of matrix Gla protein (ucMGP) as a biomarker for cardiovascular calcification. *J Vasc Res* 45:427–436.

235. Herrmann, S.-M., C. Whatling, E. Brand, V. Nicaud, J. Gariepy, A. Simon, A. Evans, J.-B. Ruidavets, D. Arveiler, G. Luc, L. Tiret, A. Henney, and F. Cambien. 2000. Polymorphisms of the human matrix Gla protein (MGP) gene, vascular calcification, and myocardial infarction. *Arterioscler Thromb Vasc Biol* 20:2386–2393.

236. Spronk, H.M.H. 2006. Vitamin K epoxide reductase complex and vascular calcification. *Circulation* 113:1550–1552.

237. Wang, Y., W. Zhang, Y. Zhang, Y. Yang, L. Sun, S. Hu, J. Chen, C. Zhang, Y. Zheng, Y. Zhen, K. Sun, C. Fu, T. Yang, J. Wang, J. Sun, H. Wu, W.C. Glasgow, and R. Hui. 2006. VKORC1 haplotypes are associated with arterial vascular diseases (stroke, coronary heart disease, and aortic dissection). *Circulation* 113:1615–1621.

238. Lacut, K., C. Larramendy-Gozalo, G. Le Gal, J. Duchemin, B. Mercier, L. Gourhant, D. Mottier, L. Becquemont, E. Oger, and C. Verstuyft. 2007. Vitamin K epoxide reductase genetic polymorphism is associated with venous thromboembolism: Results from the EDITH Study. *J Thromb Haemost* 5:2020–2024.

239. Teichert, M., L.E. Visser, R.H.N. van Schaik, A. Hofman, A.G. Uitterlinden, P.A.M. De Smet, J.C.M. Witteman, and B.H.C. Stricker. 2008. Vitamin K epoxide reductase comlex subunit 1 (VKORC1) polymorphism and aortic calcification. The Rotterdam Study. *Arterioscler Thromb Vasc Biol* 28:771–776.

240. Villines, T.C., C. Hatzigeorgiou, I.M. Feuerstein, P.G. O'Malley, and A.J. Taylor. 2005. Vitamin K_1 intake and coronary calcification. *Coronary Artery Disease* 16:199–203.

241. Geleijnse, J.M., C. Vermeer, D.E. Grobbee, L.J. Schurgers, M.H.J. Knapen, M. van der Meer, A. Hofman, and J.C.M. Witteman. 2004. Dietary intake of menaquinone is associated with a reduced risk of coronary heart disease: The Rotterdam study. *J Nutr* 134:3100–3105.

242. Schurgers, L.J., H. Aebert, C. Vermeer, B. Bultmann, and J. Janzen. 2004. Oral anticoagulant treatment: Friend or foe in cardiovascular disease? *Blood* 15:3231–3232.

243. Koos, R., A.H. Mahnken, G. Muhlenbruch, V. Brandenburg, B. Pflueger, J.E. Wildberger, and H.P. Kuhl. 2005. Relation of oral anticoagulation to cardiac valvular and coronary calcium assessed by multislice spiral computed tomography. *Am J Cardiol* 96:747–749.

244. Donovan, J.L. and P. Whittaker. 2006. Long-term warfarin therapy is associated with tissue calcification: Influence of treatment duration, age, and gender. *Circulation* 114(Suppl II):30.

245. Holden, R.M., A.S. Sanfilippo, W.M. Hopman, D. Zimmerman, J.S. Garland, and A.R. Morton. 2007. Warfarin and aortic valve calcification in hemodialysis patients. *J Nephrol* 20:417–422.

246. Holden, R.M. and S.L. Booth. 2007. Vascular calcification in chronic kidney disease: The role of vitamin K. *Nat Clin Pract Nephrol* 3:522–523.

247. van Summeren, M.J.H., J.M. Hameleers, L.J. Schurgers, A.P.G. Hoeks, C.S.P.M. Uiterwaal, T. Kruger, C. Vermeer, W. Kuis, and M.R. Lilien. 2008. Circulating calcification inhibitors and vascular properties in children after renal transplantation. *Pediatr Nephrol* 23:985–993.

248. Hermans, M.M., C. Vermeer, J.P. Kooman, V. Brandenburg, M. Ketteler, U. Gladziwa, P.L. Rensma, K.M. Leunissen, and L.J. Schurgers. 2007. Undercarboxylated matrix Gla protein levels are decreased in dialysis patients and related to parameters of calcium-phosphate metabolism and aortic augmentation index. *Blood Purif* 25:395–401.

249. Gao, B., T. Yasui, Y. Itoh, K. Tozawa, Y. Hayashi, and K. Kohri. 2007. A polymorphism of matrix Gla protein gene is associated with kidney stones. *J Urol* 177:2361–2365.

250. Neogi, T., S.L. Booth, Y.Q. Zhang, P.F. Jacques, R. Terkeltaub, P. Aliabadi, and D.T. Felson. 2006. Low vitamin K status is associated with osteoarthritis in the hand and knee. *Arthritis Rheumatism* 54:1255–1261.

251. Neogi, T., D.T. Felson, R. Sarno, and S.L. Booth.. 2008. Vitamin K in hand osteoarthritis: Results from a randomized clinical trial. *Ann Rheum Dis* 67:1570–1573.

252. van Summeren, M.J.H., W.G.M. Spliet, A. van Royen-Kerkhof, C. Vermeer, M. Lilien, W. Kuis, and L.J. Schurgers. 2008. Calcinosis in juvenile dermatomyositis: A possible role for the vitamin K-dependent protein matrix Gla protein. *Rheumatology* 47:267–271.

253. Knapen, M.H.J., L.J. Schurgers, and C. Vermeer. 2007. Vitamin K_2 supplementation improves hip bone geometry and bone strength indices in postmenopausal women. *Osteoporosis Int* 18:963–972.

254. Sugiyama, T., T. Takaki, K. Sakanaka, H. Sadamaru, K. Mori, Y. Kato, T. Taguchi, and T. Saito. 2007. Warfarin-induced impairment of cortical bone material quality and compensatory adaptation of cortical bone structure to mechanical stimuli. *J Endocrinol* 194:213–222.

255. Lee, N.K., H. Sowa, E. Hinoi, M. Ferron, J.D. Ahn, C. Confavreux, R. Dacquin, P.J. Mee, M.D. McKee, D.Y. Jung, Z.-Y. Zhang, J.K. Kim, F. Mauvais-Jarvis, P. Ducy, and G. Karsenty. 2007. Endocrine regulation of energy metabolism by the skeleton. *Cell* 130:456–469.

256. Ferron, M., E. Hinoi, G. Karsenty, and P. Ducy. 2008. Osteocalcin differentially regulates beta cell and adipocyte gene expression and affects the development of metabolic diseases in wild-type mice. *Proc Natl Acad Sci USA* 105:5266–5270.

257. Paul, B., A. Oxley, K. Brigham, T. Cox, and P.J. Hamilton. 1987. Factor II, VII, IX and X concentrations in patients receiving long term warfarin. *J Clin Pathol* 40:94–98.

258. Kumar, S., J.R.M. Haigh, G. Tate, M. Boothby, D.N. Joanes, J.A. Davies, B.E. Roberts, and M.P. Feely. 1990. Effect of warfarin on plasma concentrations of vitamin K dependent coagulation factors in patients with stable control and monitored compliance. *Brit J Haematol* 74:82–85.

8 Vitamin K Requirements, Toxicity, and Other Metabolic Interactions

8.1 DIETARY REFERENCE INTAKES FOR VITAMIN K

The first published Recommended Dietary Allowances (RDAs) for vitamins, proteins, minerals, and energy were issued by the National Research Council of the National Academy of Sciences in 1941. These values were used to establish various federal and state food and nutrition policies, and over time the responsibility for revision of guidelines was transferred to the Food and Nutrition Board of the Institute of Medicine (IOM). Until the 10th edition of the RDAs, there was no RDA for vitamin K; and, as with a number of other nutrients, it was assumed that a normal diet provided an "estimated safe and adequate daily dietary intake" of vitamin K. The 10th edition of the RDAs was completed in 1985, but after outside review was postponed for further consideration by a second panel and was published in 1989. Based on rather limited data, an RDA of approximately 1 µg of vitamin K per kilogram body weight (65 to 80 µg/day for adult males and 55 to 65 µg/day for adult females) was established. A somewhat different and unofficial recommendation, called a Recommended Dietary Intake, was published in 1987 [1] by a member of the original panel. This recommendation was 45 µg per day for adult males and 35 µg per day for adult females. The 10th edition of the RDAs was published in 1989, and in 1994 the Food and Nutrition Board, in cooperation with Health Canada, began a process that included Dietary Reference Intakes (DRIs) other than the RDA. Most importantly, an upper limit (UL) value and an estimated average requirement (EAR) were established. The EAR is not a recommended intake but is an intake used to determine the most widely used reference intake, the RDA, which was defined as the EAR plus two standard deviations. The RDA should, therefore, be an average intake that meets the nutritional needs of nearly all (97% to 98%) of the healthy population. Not all RDAs have been calculated from an EAR, but if the RDA is to be derived from the EAR, two factors are of critical importance: the amount and quality of the research data needed to establish an EAR, and the selection of an endpoint that will become the basis for the recommendation. Both of these factors have made it difficult to establish an RDA for vitamin K.

8.1.1 POSSIBLE ENDPOINTS TO ESTABLISH A VITAMIN K RDA

As the plasma concentration of phylloquinone, the major source of vitamin K in the diet, reflects intake over the last day or two rather than an average of a more extended period, this is not a measure that is of value as an indicator of vitamin K status. The only indicator of vitamin K status with a clearly defined clinical significance is the prothrombin time (PT), and alterations in the PT by changes in dietary intake of vitamin K alone are uncommon to nonexistent. This does not suggest that decreases in the plasma concentration of functional prothrombin which would be logical endpoints cannot be caused by low intakes of the vitamin, but that the PT assay is very insensitive to moderate changes in the concentration of functional prothrombin. An increase in the prothrombin time of 2 seconds would be needed to bring it out of the "normal" range, and as shown in Figure 8.1, this would require about 50% of the prothrombin pool to be inactive. This type of response is consistent with the observation [2] that none of the 33 subjects consuming a "vitamin K-free diet" (~5 µg/day) in a controlled clinical ward for 13 days developed a PT outside of the normal range. Most of these subjects were also receiving an antibiotic, and 10% of them did show a lowered, but not clinically significant, level of factor VII. The amount of functionally active prothrombin in plasma (presumably that fraction containing sufficient Gla residues to be activated) has also been measured. This can be done in a number of ways: by comparing the amount of thrombin generated from prothrombin through the normal prothrombinase (phospholipid, factor Xa, factor V) pathway to that generated by a snake venom protease (Ecarin), by measuring the fraction of prothrombin not adsorbed to $BaSO_4$, or by very sensitive immunoassays of PIVKA-II, the under-γ-carboxylated fraction of prothrombin (see Chapter 5). The sensitivity of each of these measures to detect a lower than normal concentration of functional prothrombin or an increase in a nonfunctional form varies widely (Table 8.1). The sensitivity of the immunochemical assays for PIVKA-II is such that very large increases of this nonfunctional form of vitamin K can be observed with no evidence of an alteration in the important physiological function of the prothrombin-driven plasma procoagulant pathway.

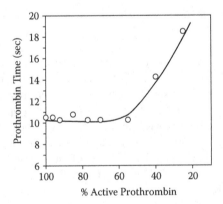

FIGURE 8.1 Effect of alterations of prothrombin concentration on prothrombin time. Normal human plasma was mixed with plasma from a warfarin-treated patient (25% of normal prothrombin) in varying amounts to produce a series of plasma samples containing 25% to 100% of the normal concentration of prothrombin. Standard clinical prothrombin times were then determined.

TABLE 8.1

Sensitivity of Assays for the Activity of Normal and Nonfunctional Prothrombin

Assay	Plasma Prothrombin			
	100% of Normal	90% of Normal	Δ	% Change
Prothrombin time (seconds)	10–11	10–11	0	0
Prothrombin concentration (%)[a]	100	90	10	10
Active/total prothrombin (ratio)[b]	0.95	0.70	0.25	26
PIVKA-II by barium salt method (units)[c]	1.12	7.70	6.58	587
PIVKA-II by antibody assay (units)[d]	0.05	1.01	0.96	1,920

Note: Assays used were: [a] chromogenic assay for prothrombin [111]; [b] S/E ratio as described in [2]; [c] Ecarin activation of prothrombin not absorbable by barium salt [112]; or [d] specific antibody for des-γ-carboxyprothrombin [113].

Source: Modified from Suttie [110], the various assays were performed on normal plasma or normal plasma diluted with plasma from a warfarin-treated patient to contain 90% of normal prothrombin.

There are a number of Gla-containing proteins other than the vitamin K-dependent clotting factors, and when these proteins are subjected to turnover and degradation to amino acids, the Gla residues are not subjected to further metabolism, but are excreted in the urine [3]. As the vitamin K-dependent proteins are presumably at a steady-state concentration in an adult, the amount of Gla excreted should be a measure of the synthesis of these proteins, and a drop in Gla excretion would be an indication of a lack of optimal intakes of vitamin K. There are data indicating that modifications of phylloquinone intake over ranges that are within the normal variation of the population intake do have an influence on urinary Gla excretion. In a study [4] in which young adult males consuming a normal diet (~80 μg phylloquinone/day) reduced their intake by 50% by eliminating high vitamin K foods from their diet, urinary Gla excretion was decreased by 22% after 17 days. Excretion of Gla was returned to the initial levels by supplementation of either 50 or 500 μg of phylloquinone per day. Both age and gender appear to influence the excretion of Gla, and a study of 260 subjects [5] has clearly shown that the urinary Gla/creatinine ratio is significantly higher in females and that Gla excretion in both males and females increases substantially with age. In a well-controlled study [6] in which subjects were housed in a metabolic ward and fed a diet containing 80 μg phylloquinone per day for 4 days and then a vitamin K-deficient diet (10 μg phylloquinone/day) for 13 days, Gla excretion dropped about 10% in the young (20- to 40-year-old) subjects, but remained unchanged in the older (60- to 80-year-old) subjects. At the present time there are no data that link a change in Gla excretion to specific proteins or to explain the basis for the influence of age and gender on Gla excretion.

Because of the large amount of interest that has developed regarding the possible role of vitamin K in maintaining skeletal health (see Chapter 7), the bone protein osteocalcin has been seen as a regulatory factor in maintaining skeletal health, and the extent to which circulating osteocalcin is fully γ-carboxylated has become a major issue. The majority of the available data have not focused on the amount of circulating fully carboxylated osteocalcin (OC), but rather on the extent to which plasma osteocalcin is fully γ-carboxylated and the data expressed as percent undercarboxylated osteocalcin (ucOC). Most of the available data related to this value have been obtained by the use of an antibody that reacts with both carboxylated and undercarboxylated osteocalcin, and ucOC has been defined as that fraction of the total which does not bind to hydroxyapatite [7]. The percent ucOC of the circulating osteocalcin in apparently healthy and vitamin K-sufficient subjects in a large number of studies has ranged from less than 10% to 40%–45% [8–12]. These differences have made it difficult to compare various studies and are most probably due to the differences in epitope specificity in the antibodies used in various commercial assay kits. Osteocalcin is rather sensitive to the action of proteases, and in the case of studies with high "normal ucOC values" small peptides that would not bind to hydroxyapatite are probably being included in the fraction called ucOC. Regardless of the stated percent ucOC values, numerous studies have shown that supplementation with vitamin K will substantially decrease the percent ucOC, although in many of the reported studies the resulting percent ucOC is still high. In a two-week dose response study [13] in which young healthy males and females consuming approximately 100 µg of dietary phylloquinone per day were supplemented with from 250 µg to 2,000 µg of phylloquione per day, it was found that 1000 µg per day was needed to reduce ucOC from 7% to 2% (the presumed lower limit of the assay).

8.1.2 ESTABLISHMENT OF THE CURRENT DRI FOR VITAMIN K

There are, therefore, a number of possible endpoints that could have been used to define the appropriate vitamin K intake (Table 8.2), but other than the maximization of γ-carboxylation of osteocalcin, there are no dose response studies utilizing an adequate range of intakes that would allow the calculation of an estimated average requirement (EAR) and subsequently an RDA based on these markers. Reports that decreases in bone or vascular health (see Chapter 7) might be related to alterations in vitamin K status have also failed to provide the data needed to establish an RDA based on a public health concern. There are ample data to establish that very few, if any, individuals consume sufficient vitamin K to maximally γ-carboxylate their circulating osteocalcin. As there appears to be no clinical significance of this apparent deficiency, and as supplementation with about 1 mg per day of phylloquinone is needed to achieve this response, this index of adequacy was not used to set a reference value. As sufficient data to determine an EAR were not available, the RDI currently in use and published in 2001 [14] is the adequate intake (AI) for different age groups shown in Tables 8.3 and 8.4. This value is defined as "the recommended average daily intake level based on observed or experimentally determined

TABLE 8.2

Estimated Daily Intake of Vitamin K to Assure Various Endpoints

Endpoint	µg/day
1. Normal prothrombin time	<10
2. Normal urinary Gla	~75
3. Absence of nonfunctional prothrombin[a]	~80
4. Absence of PIVKA-II[b]	~100
5. Fully carboxylated osteocalcin	>1000

Note: Very little dose response data that could be used to set an intake for endpoints 2 to 4 (see Reference [15]) are available. The daily intakes indicated are based on available data but, other than endpoint 5, it is not possible to indicate the possible error of the value.

[a] Assay based on snake venom and physiological activation.

[b] Assay based on specific antibody.

TABLE 8.3

Adequate Intakes of Vitamin K, 19 Years and Older[a]

AI for Men (µg/day of vitamin K)	
19–30 years	120
31–50 years	120
51–70 years	120
>70 years	120
AI for Women[b] (µg/day of vitamin K)	
19–30 years	90
31–50 years	90
51–70 years	90
>70 years	90

[a] Values from 2001 Dietary Reference Intakes [14].

[b] No alteration of intake for pregnancy or lactation.

approximations or estimates of nutrient intake by a group or groups of apparently healthy people that are assumed to be adequate."

Based on the data currently available and the framework used to establish the DRIs, the use of an AI seems appropriate for the following reasons. A clinically significant deficiency of vitamin K is extremely rare (see Chapter 7) and usually results from severe malabsorption syndromes. There are a number of determinants of vitamin K status in humans [15], and there are data demonstrating that decreases in vitamin K intake can produce alterations in some sensitive indicators. There is insufficient dose response data to establish an EAR from these

TABLE 8.4

Adequate Intake of Vitamin K, Birth through 12 Months[a]

AI for Infants (µg/day of vitamin K)	
0–6 months	2.0
7–12 months	2.5
AI for Children (µg/day of vitamin K)	
1–3 years	30
4–8 years	55
AI for Boys	
9–13 years	60
14–18 years	75
AI for Girls (µg/day of vitamin K)	
9–13 years	60
14–18 years[b]	75

[a] Values from 2001 Dietary Reference Intakes [14].
[b] No alteration of intake for pregnancy or lactation.

data, and there are no known health consequences associated with these possible endpoints. There may be sufficient data to establish an EAR based on fully carboxylated circulating osteocalcin, but the RDA resulting from this value would require substantial supplementation of the entire population with vitamin K. At the present time there are no data to support such a large universal supplementation. The current adult DRI for vitamin K is, therefore, an adequate intake based on the median intake of vitamin K available from the National Health and Nutrition Examination Survey III (NHANES III) data. The AI for children is also based on the NHANES III data, and the AI for 0- to 6-month-old infants is based on the amount of vitamin K in human milk with the assumption that the infants have received 0.5 to 1.0 mg of phylloquinone intramuscularly or 2.0 mg orally within 6 hours of birth. The AI for infants from 7 months to 1 year is based on extrapolation from the younger infants.

8.2 VITAMIN K REQUIREMENT OF DOMESTIC AND COMPANION ANIMALS

The determination of the vitamin K requirement for various species has been difficult and is extremely variable because of the varying degrees to which each species utilizes the large amount of vitamin K synthesized by intestinal bacteria and the degree to which different species practice coprophagy. A spontaneous deficiency of vitamin K was first noted in chicks [16], and poultry consuming a low vitamin K diet are much more likely to develop symptoms of a dietary deficiency than any other species. This response has usually been assumed to be due to the rapid transit rate of nutrients through the relatively short intestinal tract of the chick or to limited synthesis of menaquinones in this species. There are, however, data that would suggest that there are other factors that might influence the differences in vitamin K requirements between various species. A study [17] of the response of various vitamin-related physiological and biochemical measures in the rat and the chick when they are fed the same concentration in their diet is shown in Table 8.5. These data demonstrate that the consumption of the same diet by rats and chicks results in very similar serum and liver concentrations of total phylloquinone (phylloquinone and phylloquinone-2,3-epoxide) but substantial increases in prothrombin time and decreases in prothrombin concentration in chicks. The elevation of phylloquinone epoxide in the chick suggests that the hepatic vitamin K-epoxide reductase in chicks is not able to effectively recycle this product of the action of the vitamin K-dependent carboxylase. As it appears (see Chapter 4) that the epoxide reductase also furnishes the reduced form of phylloquinone needed to drive the carboxylase, the nearly 10-fold higher V_{max} of the vitamin K-epoxide reductase from rat liver would suggest that the decreased activity of this enzyme in the chick could be a major factor in the high vitamin K requirement in this species. There are undoubtedly a large number of variations in the metabolism of different species that would influence their requirement for vitamin K, but there is very little information that has been used to explain the rather large differences between species.

TABLE 8.5
Response of Rats and Chicks to the Consumption of Diets Containing 500 µg Phylloquinone/kg

Vitamin K-Related Response	Rat	Chick
Prothrombin time (sec)	10.7 (10.4-11.4)	36.4 (29.4-45.7)
Prothrombin conc (% normal rat plasma)	87 ± 2	22 ± 2
Serum phylloquinone (nmol/L)	36 ± 5	24 ± 3
Serum phylloquinone-2,3-epoxide (nmol/L)	2 ± 1	16 ± 3
% Total serum phylloquinone as epoxide	5	40
Liver phylloquione (nmol/kg wet wt)	37 ± 3	24 ± 5
Liver phylloquinone-2,3-epoxide (nmol/kg wet wt)	1 ± 1	13 ± 2
% Total liver phylloquinone as epoxide	3	48
Liver vitamin K-dependent carboxylase		
K_m (µmol/L)	99 ± 7	308 ± 85
V_{max} ($^{14}CO_2$ fixation)	26 ± 1	14 ± 2
Liver vitamin K-epoxide reductase		
K_m (µmol/L)	78 ± 4	48 ± 13
V_{max} (phylloquinone/min g prot)	280 ± 2	26 ± 2

Note: Both 250 g male rats and 4- to 5-week-old Leghorn chicks (8/group) were fed the same vitamin K-deficient (<5 µg phylloquinone/kg) diet for 3 days and then fed the same vitamin K-deficient diet with 500 µg phylloquinone added/kg diet for 8 days before measurements were made (see Reference [17] for details).

Ruminal microorganisms synthesize large amounts of vitamin K, and ruminants do not appear to need a source of vitamin in the diet. Deficiencies have, however, been produced in most monogastric species. Estimations of vitamin K requirements of various species from different laboratories are difficult to compare. The majority of these data are old, different forms of the vitamin were used, and different methods were employed to establish the requirement. Some of these studies did utilize dose response data to determine the amount of vitamin K required to obtain maximal clotting activity over an extended period of time. Other studies, particularly some of the earliest attempts to establish requirements, utilized a curative assay in which vitamin K-deficient, hypoprothrombinemic animals were administered vitamin K over varying periods of time to reestablish a "normal" clotting factor level. Phylloquinone has been the form of vitamin K added to defined diets for small animals used in nutritional studies, although other less expensive forms of vitamin K are usually used in practical rations. Menadione has been widely used and is usually considered to be from 20% to 40% as effective as phylloquinone on a molar basis, but this conversion factor depends a great deal on the type of assay that is used. It is rather ineffective in a curative assay where the rate of its alkylation to biologically active menaquinone-4 is probably the rate-limiting factor, but on a weight basis menadione often shows activity nearly equal to phylloquinone in a long-term preventive assay. Commercial poultry and livestock rations usually utilize water-soluble forms of menadione (see Chapter 2) such as menadione sodium bisulfite (MSB), menadione sodium bisulfite complex (MSBC), menadione dimethyl pyrimidinal bisulfite (MPB), or menadione nicotinamide bisulfite (MNB), as they are much cheaper than phylloquinone. When added to poultry rations, these forms of vitamin K have an activity which, on a molar basis, is near that of phylloquinone, although MSBC appears to be a better source than MSB. The newer forms of menadione such as MPB [18–21] and NMB [22,23] are somewhat more active than MSBC. Increasing the vitamin K content of rations for growing chicks above that needed to maintain normal prothrombin times has been reported to increase bone ash content in one study [24] but not in another [25].

Detailed reviews of the vitamin K requirements of various species are available [26–28]. The available data, which are often limited, indicate that the requirement for most species falls in a range of 2 to 200 µg vitamin K per kilogram of body weight per day. The data in Table 8.6, which have been adopted from a table developed by Griminger [28], give an indication of the magnitude of the vitamin K requirement for various species. It should be assumed that this requirement can be altered by age, sex, or strain of animal, and that any condition influencing lipid absorption or conditions altering intestinal flora will have an influence on these values. A considerably higher level of dietary vitamin K has been recommended for most laboratory animals by the National Academy of Sciences Study of the Nutrient Requirements of Laboratory Animals [29]. Recommendations for most species are in the range of 3,000 µg vitamin K per kilogram of diet, but the rat requirement was set at 50 µg vitamin K per kilogram of diet.

Purified laboratory rodent diets have been utilized in a large number of studies directed at a wide range of nutritional problems, and they have undoubtedly

TABLE 8.6

Vitamin K Requirements of Various Species[a]

Species	Daily Intake (µg/kg per day)	Dietary Concentration (µg/kg diet)
Dog	1.25	60
Pig	5	50
Rhesus monkey	2	60
Rat, male	11–16	100–150
Chicken	80–120	530
Turkey poult	180–270	1,200

[a] Data have been summarized from a more extensive table [28] and are presented as the amount of vitamin needed to prevent the development of a deficiency. No correction for differences in potency of equal weights of different forms of the vitamin has been made.

been fortified with varying amounts and forms of vitamin K. Historically most have contained sufficient amounts of vitamin K, but rare instances of a vitamin K-responsive spontaneous hemorrhagic condition have been observed in rats fed these purified diets. Few, if any, of these incidences were reported in the literature, but were solved by increasing the amount of vitamin K in the diet. The issue was addressed in the early 1990s by the American Institute of Nutrition (now the American Society of Nutrition) by the appointment of an ad hoc committee charged with updating their recommendations for the composition of purified diets for laboratory rodents. The previous diet (AIN-76A) contained 500 µg menadione per kilogram, and the newer diet (AIN-93G) contains 750 µg phylloquinone per kilogram [30]. There have been no reports of spontaneous hemorrhagic events in rodents fed this diet. The establishment of a vitamin K requirement for rodents fed purified diets involves the same problem as that faced in setting an appropriate DRI for the human population. It depends on what endpoint to choose. The recommendation of 500 µg phylloquinone will certainly prevent bleeding, achieve a "normal" prothrombin time, and achieve near maximal plasma prothrombin concentrations. The activity of the hepatic vitamin K-dependent carboxylase as measured by the carboxylation of a synthetic peptide with $^{14}CO_2$ (peptide carboxylation) is known [31] to be increased in deficient rats, as is the amount of clotting factor precursors that accumulate in the microsomal fraction of deficient animals that can be measured [32] by $^{14}CO_2$ incorporation of the intracellular pool (protein carboxylation). The data shown in Figure 8.2 indicate that although the consumption of a diet containing 500 µg phylloquinone per kilogram by rats results in substantial changes from those seen in deficient animals in all markers assayed, increasing the amount of vitamin K in the diet will result in additional changes [33]. There are, however, no data to suggest that the rats consuming 1500 µg phylloquinone per kilogram are "healthier rats." The use of a recommendation of 500 µg per kilogram of phylloquinone therefore appears to be reasonable at the present time.

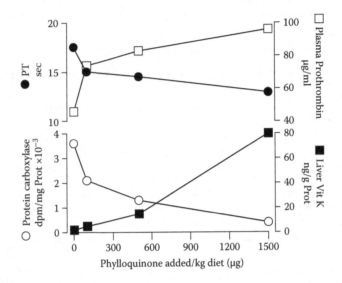

FIGURE 8.2   Response of various measures of vitamin K status of rats to a wide range of vitamin K intakes. Male 100-g rats were fed a vitamin K-deficient diet (9.5 µg/kg) or this diet with 100, 500, or 1,500 µg phylloquinone added for 24 days. At this time plasma was drawn for prothrombin times and prothrombin concentration assays, and liver microsomal preparations were obtained for vitamin K-dependent carboxylase assays (for details, see Reference [33]).

8.3   DIETARY AND PHYSIOLOGICAL FACTORS INFLUENCING VITAMIN K STATUS

Early attempts to determine the vitamin K requirement of laboratory animals demonstrated that female rats had higher plasma prothrombin concentrations than males and that they were more responsive to nutritional deficiencies than male rats. The increased concentration of prothrombin in female rats and the increase observed during pregnancy have been shown to be due to an increase in the rate of synthesis rather than a decreased degradation rate [34]. Castration of both sexes unifies that vitamin K response, and in the castrated rat, concentrations of prothrombin can be increased with estrogens and decreased with androgens [35]. There are some indications [36] from studies utilizing [3H]-phylloquinone that the estrogen effects are related to the amount of vitamin needed in the liver to maintain normal levels of prothrombin. The currently available evidence suggests that the influence of estrogens on rate of prothrombin synthesis is reflected in both a higher rate of synthesis and increased accumulation of prothrombin precursors in the microsomes [36,37]. Hypothysectomy has been reported [38] to prevent the estrogen stimulation of prothrombin synthesis in castrated female rats, and hypothyroidism in humans results in a decrease in both the rate of synthesis and destruction of the vitamin K-dependent clotting factors [39]. These hormonal effects on vitamin K-dependent proteins are apparently not related to any impact on vitamin K metabolism, but are associated with changes in the rate of synthesis of the proteins involved.

Although the extent to which humans can utilize menaquinones produced in the gut has been difficult to quantitate (see Chapter 6), early studies [40] of vitamin K action and requirements soon established the need to prevent coprophagy to produce a severe vitamin K deficiency in the rat. A series of studies into the nutritional impact of raising rats in a germ-free environment by Gustafsson [41] noted spontaneous hemorrhages in these rats, and subsequent studies utilizing a vitamin K-deficient diet ("vitamin free" casein, potato starch, salts, and vitamins) established the curative effect of vitamin K or intestinal organisms [42]. As the vitamin K requirement of the rat is greatly increased under germ-free conditions, coprophagy preventing cages [43,44] are routinely used in studies where a severe deficiency is required. A high incidence of spontaneous hemorrhage was also noted in rats fed irradiated beef as a protein source in a diet with an otherwise very low vitamin K content [45], which was traced to the degradative effect of the irradiation process on vitamin K [46]. The inclusion of mineral oil in the diet during early studies of vitamin K function was also shown to prevent its absorption [47], and mineral oil, as well as coprophagy prevention, has often been used in diets to ensure the development of a deficiency. Sulfa drugs such as sulfaquinoxaline have been shown to have a profound effect in increasing the vitamin K requirement of the chick [48], particularly when the source of vitamin K activity is menadione or menadione sodium bisulfite complex rather than phylloquinone. A number of other substances have been found to interfere with vitamin K action in ways that are not fully understood. Dietary butylated hydroxytoluene has been reported [49,50] to cause a hemorrhagic condition in rats that can be cured by vitamin K supplementation, and phenobarbital and diphenylhydantoin administration to pregnant women has been reported [51] to produce a vitamin K-responsive hemorrhage in the newborn.

Diets containing high levels of vitamin A have been reported for some time [26,40] to adversely influence vitamin K action. Hypervitaminosis A was found to result in hypoprothrombinemia in rats [52] in a manner that was not related to any influence of vitamin A on the intestinal flora [53]. Whether the antagonism by vitamin A is the result of a general effect on the absorption of nonpolar lipids or a specific antagonism of vitamin K is not known. More recently it has been shown that retinyl acetate and N-(4-hydroxyphenyl) retinamide could increase clotting times of rats fed a low vitamin K diet [54], but were not antagonists when the vitamin K content of the diets were increased. In this study, 13-cis-retinoic acid did not appear to antagonize the action of vitamin K. Retinoic acid has also been shown to increase osteocalcin secretion from osteoblastic cells in vitro [55] and to decrease the fraction of under-γ-carboxylated osteocalcin when the cells were incubated in the presence of warfarin. The details of the mechanism of action of these retinoid-vitamin K interactions are not known.

The possibility that vitamin E may antagonize the action of vitamin K has received more attention. The administration of d-α-tocopherol hydroquinone has been shown to produce a vitamin K-responsive hemorrhagic syndrome in the pregnant rat [56], and the addition of vitamin E to the diet of patients on coumarin anticoagulant therapy has been reported [57,58] to result in a hemorrhagic episode. These findings have suggested that this interaction may be of clinical significance, and it is possible that high vitamin E intakes may exacerbate a borderline vitamin K deficiency. The vitamin K-dependent carboxylase is competitively inhibited by vitamin E, and there are indications that the α-tocopherol quinone, rather than α-tocopherol [59,60] may be the causative agent and a possible mechanism for this interaction has been proposed [61]. The currently available information would suggest that the risk of serious complications is rare. A study of the influence of supplementation of adult men and women with 1,000 IU of RRR α-tocopherol for 12 weeks [62] has not shown any major response. A very sensitive measure of vitamin K deficiency, circulating PIVKA-II, was increased, but a more commonly used indicator of vitamin K status, under-γ-carboxylated osteocalcin, was not altered. It has also been reported [63] that supplementation of the diet of patients receiving chronic warfarin therapy with vitamin E did not alter their stabilized INR. This is, however, a rather insensitive measure of vitamin K status and additional studies of this interaction would be useful. In addition to the well-demonstrated ability of α-tocopherol quinone to inhibit the vitamin K-dependent carboxylase, a study [64] utilizing male rats has shown that increasing the intake of α-tocopherol resulted in decreased concentrations of phylloquinone and MK-4 in spleen, kidney, and brain, but not in plasma, liver, or testis. A second rat study [65] has indicated an adverse influence of vitamin E on absorption of phylloquinone. The mechanism for these responses is not yet known.

8.4 HAZARDS OF THE INGESTION OF LARGE AMOUNTS OF VITAMIN K

The Dietary Reference Intake used to define the intake of vitamin K that would be hazardous to the general population is "the tolerable upper intake level," the UL. It is defined as the highest level of daily nutrient intake that is likely to pose no risk of adverse health effects for almost all individuals. The current edition of the DRIs [14] found that no adverse effects associated with vitamin K consumption from food or supplements have been reported in humans or animals. Therefore, a quantitative risk assessment could not be performed, and a UL for vitamin K could not be derived. A more comprehensive earlier review of the literature relevant to the pharmacology and toxicology of vitamin K is available [66], and a National Research Council study [67] also failed to find evidence of vitamin K toxicity in animals.

For treatment of prolonged clotting times when hemorrhage is not a problem, pylloquinone can be given orally or parenterally. If given orally to patients with impaired biliary function, bile salts should also be administered. Phylloquinone is available as the pure compound, and an aqueous colloidal solution that can be given intramuscularly or intravenously, or a mixed micellar formulation that is more bioavailable when given orally. Vitamin K is used following an overdose of oral anticoagulants [68], and some adverse reactions have been noted following intravenous administration. An extensive review of the literature [69] relative to anaphylactoid reactions following administration suggests that these reactions can occur but that available data do not allow a calculation of the risk. Because of these concerns, slower acting intramuscular injections have often been recommended. A more recent study has, however, found that i.v. administration of vitamin K did not pose a clinically significant risk [70]. Effective therapy to reverse a prolonged prothrombin time requires synthesis of normal clotting factors, and a number of hours may be necessary before a substantial decrease in clotting times is apparent.

The relative safety of phylloquinone and, as far as is known, menaquinones does not hold for menadione or its water-soluble derivatives. These forms of vitamin K are safely used at low levels in domestic and companion animal rations to prevent the development of a deficiency but should not be used as a pharmacological treatment for a human hemorrhagic condition. Although once prescribed for treatment of the hemorrhagic disease of the newborn, these compounds are known to react with free sulfhydryl groups of various tissues and to cause hemolytic anemia, hyperbilirubinemia, and kernicterus. This marked increase in conjugated bilirubin is extremely toxic to the neonatal brain and has caused death in some instances [66]. Menadione and its water-soluble derivatives can also cause hepatic damage [71] which appears to be related to lipid peroxidation [72].

8.5   ADDITIONAL REPORTS OF BIOLOGICAL EFFECTS OF VITAMIN K

As is the case with many other nutrients, there are numerous reports of the impact of altered vitamin K status or the use of pharmacological amounts of vitamin K that are not directly related to known functions of the vitamin.

There have been studies suggesting that vitamin K status may influence glucose homeostasis. In rats fed a diet with a relatively low amount of phylloquinone (~150 µg/kg diet), it was found that glucose concentrations were higher and insulin response was delayed following intravenous glucose infusion when compared to rats consuming an additional 750 µg phylloquinone per kilogram diet [73]. These results were followed by small studies of human subjects indicating that a high dose of MK-4 (90 mg/day) for one week improved insulin response [74] and that subjects with higher dietary vitamin K intake had lower plasma glucose levels following glucose loading [75]. A recent large study utilizing data from nearly 3,000 subjects from the Framingham Offspring Study has also found that higher phylloquionone intake may be associated with greater insulin sensitivity and better glycemic status [76]. Data obtained from an elderly nondiabetic population that was supplemented with 500 µg phylloquinone/day for 36 months [77] has indicated that insulin resistance was reduced by supplementation in male subjects ($P = 0.01$) but not in female subjects. The possible relationship between vitamin K status and glucose homeostasis needs additional study before it is accepted, and the relationship between these data and the possible role of osteocalcin in the control of energy metabolism [78,79] will also need to be assessed.

Another possible public health related impact of alterations of vitamin K status relates to inflammation. DNA microarray techniques have been used to identify the increased expression of genes involved in acute inflammatory responses in rats fed a vitamin K-deficient diet [80] which were not seen in control or vitamin K-supplemented rats, and a second epidemiological study involving subjects from the Framingham Offspring Study has found an increase in a number of circulating inflammatory markers that were inversely associated with phylloquinone intake or plasma phylloquinone concentration [81]. At this time, there have been no supplementation trials involving human subjects to assess the influence of increased vitamin K intake on the inflammatory response.

Increases [82,83] in the circulating level of under-γ-carboxyprothrombin (PIVKA-II) (see Chapter 5) in individuals who are not vitamin K deficient have been used as a marker for hepatocellular carcinoma, and comparisons of this marker rather than serum α-fetoprotein as a diagnostic tool have indicated that it is more sensitive and specific in differentiating patients with hepatocellular carcinoma from those with cirrhosis and chronic hepatitis [84]. This malignancy is treated by surgery or radiofrequency ablation therapy, and the recurrence rate is relatively high. Vitamin K administration has also been used to treat this malignancy, and there are numerous reports of the ability of oral MK-4 treatment (usually 45 mg/day) to both lower recurrence rates and prolong the survival of patients with this disease [85–87]. Although the mode of action has not been completely elucidated [88,89], studies utilizing a number of different cultured cell lines and in animal models [90–92] clearly indicate an apoptotic response to MK-4 administration. Both MK-4 and menadione, but not phylloquinone, will generate superoxide when taken up by cells, and it is likely that this is involved in triggering the apoptotic response, although it is possible that the geranylgeranyl side chain of MK-4 acting as a ligand for an unidentified receptor may also be a factor [93–95].

The concentrations of vitamin K-dependent clotting factors are low in the human fetus and in newborns compared to older infants and adults. This is partially due to a low level of expression of these proteins prior to birth and, as indicated by increased PIVKA-II levels, partially to the low concentration of vitamin K in cord blood. The cellular impact of this relatively deficient state in neonates has been studied by looking at the response of various systems to alterations in vitamin K status. Sister chromatid exchange in cultured leukocytes, which is an index of mutagenic activity, increases as blood phylloquinone increases [96]. Increasing the phylloquinone concentration also amplifies the metabolism of benzo(α)pyrene in chick embryos or rat liver microsomal preparations [97,98], a response that would be expected to increase the mutagenic and carcinogenic potential of polycyclic hydrocarbons. The identification of Gas6 as a vitamin K-dependent protein which is a ligand for receptor tyrosine kinases has also led to theories [99,100] suggesting that there are possible benefits of low fetal vitamin K concentrations.

There are also published data that indicate responses in animal models that do not appear to be related to any known action of vitamin K-dependent proteins. Studies of calcium balance in ovariectomized rats [101] or in rats receiving varying amounts of calcium in their diet [102] have found that the addition of MK-4 to the diet, in amounts much higher than those needed to support known vitamin K functions, results in the improvement of calcium balance in rats fed normal amounts of calcium in the diet. The research interest in the possible role of vitamin K in skeletal health (Chapter 7) has led to other studies that might be related to calcium or phosphorus metabolism, and the supplementation of rat diets with very high amounts of either phylloquinone or MK-4 has been reported [103] to increase the activity of intestinal alkaline phosphatase. A recent study [104] has also demonstrated that increasing the phylloquinone content of the diet of female rats from weaning to 21 months of age increases the thickness of the equatorial/peripheral retina. Neither the basis for this change, nor the influence on sight, is currently known.

A wide range of cellular and organ preparations have been reported to respond in some manner to alterations in vitamin K concentrations. In most cases, the vitamin K levels involved would be considered pharmacological rather than nutritional. There are studies [105,106] demonstrating an attenuation of hypoxia-induced relaxation of rat carotid artery preparations by phylloquinone which would fall in this category. A DNA microarray approach has been used [107] to identify genes whose testicular expression in rats was affected by a vitamin K-deficient diet. Plasma and testis testosterone concentrations were decreased in the vitamin K-deficient rat, and the mRNA levels of Cyp11a, a rate-limiting enzyme in testosterone synthesis, were decreased. Interestingly, the expression of Cyp11a was related to the testicular concentration of MK-4, suggesting that vitamer produced from phylloquinone is a regulator of steroid production in this organ. A somewhat related study conducted in HepG2 cells [108] has suggested that estrogen metabolism can be modulated by the binding of MK-4 to 17β-hydroxysteroid dehydrogenase-4. Both of these studies support the view that the conversion of phylloquinone to MK-4 in selected tissues is related in some manner to metabolic control in their tissues.

Epidemiological studies have also pointed to possible relationships between vitamin K status and subsequent responses. A relatively large study followed 200 subjects from birth to 30 years of age [109] to assess various factors related to alcohol dependence. Only 20% of the subjects had received vitamin K at birth, and at age 30 only 5% of this group were assessed as being alcohol dependent, while the incidence of alcohol dependence in those not treated at birth was 18%. This study, as well as many others, needs substantially more data before responses attributed to vitamin K status can be verified. It is of interest that participants in this study, which started in the late 1960s, were administered menadione rather than phylloquinone and that brain tissue would have been subject to the possible pro-oxidant properties of menadione.

REFERENCES

1. Olson, J.A. 1987. Recommended dietary intakes (RDI) of vitamin K in humans. *Am J Clin Nutr* 45:687–692.
2. Allison, P.M., L.L. Mummah-Schendel, C.B. Kindberg, C.S. Harms, N.U. Bang, and J.W. Suttie. 1987. Effects of a vitamin K-deficient diet and antibiotics in normal human volunteers. *J Lab Clin Med* 110:180–188.
3. Shah, D.V., J.K. Tews, A.E. Harper, and J.W. Suttie. 1978. Metabolism and transport of gamma-carboxyglutamic acid. *Biochim Biophys Acta* 539:209–217.
4. Suttie, J.W., L.L. Mummah-Schendel, D.V. Shah, B.J. Lyle, and J.L. Greger. 1988. Vitamin K deficiency from dietary vitamin K restriction in humans. *Am J Clin Nutr* 47:475–480.
5. Sokoll, L.J. and J.A. Sadowski. 1996. Comparison of biochemical indexes for assessing vitamin K nutritional status in a healthy adult population. *Am J Clin Nutr* 63:566–573.
6. Ferland, G., J.A. Sadowski, and M.E. O'Brien. 1993. Dietary induced subclinical vitamin K deficiency in normal human subjects. *J Clin Invest* 91:1761–1768.

7. Gundberg, C.M., S.D. Nieman, S. Abrams, and H. Rosen. 1998. Vitamin K status and bone health: An analysis of methods for determination of undercarboxylated osteocalcin. *J Clin Endocrinol Metab* 83:3258–3266.

8. Sokoll, L.J., S.L. Booth, M.E. O'Brien, K.W. Davidson, K.I. Tsaioun, and J.A. Sadowski. 1997. Changes in serum osteocalcin, plasma phylloquinone, and urinary gamma-carboxyglutamic acid in response to altered intakes of dietary phylloquinone in human subjects. *Am J Clin Nutr* 65:779–784.

9. Binkley, N.C., D.C. Krueger, J.A. Engelke, A.L. Foley, and J.W. Suttie. 2000. Vitamin K supplementation reduces serum concentrations of under-gamma-carboxylated osteocalcin in healthy young and elderly adults. *Am J Clin Nutr* 72:1523–1528.

10. Szulc, P., M.C. Chapuy, P.J. Meunier, and P.D. Delmas. 1996. Serum undercarboxylated osteocalcin is a marker of the risk of hip fracture: A three year follow-up study. *Bone* 18:487–488.

11. O'Connor, E.O., C. Molgaard, K.F. Michaelsen, J. Jakobsen, C.J.E. Lamberg-Allardt, and K.D. Cashman. 2007. Serum percentage undercarboxylated osteocalcin, a sensitive measure of vitamin K status, and its relationship to bone health indices in Danish girls. *Brit J Nutrition* 97:661–666.

12. Kohlmeier, M., J. Saupe, M.J. Shearer, K. Schaefer, and G. Asmus. 1997. Bone health of adult hemodialysis patients is related to vitamin K status. *Kidney Int* 51:1218–1221.

13. Binkley, N.C., D.C. Krueger, T.N. Kawahara, J.A. Engelke, R.J. Chappell, and J.W. Suttie. 2002. A high phylloquinone intake is required to achieve maximal osteocalcin gamma-carboxylation. *Am J Clin Nutr* 76:1055–1060.

14. Food and Nutrition Board, Institute of Medicine (eds.). 2001. Dietary Reference Intakes: Vitamin A, Vitamin K, Arsenic, Boron, Chromium, Copper, Iodine, Iron, Manganese, Molybdenum, Nickel, Silicon, Vanadium, and Zinc. Washington, D.C.: National Academy Press.

15. Booth, S.L. and A.A. Rajabi. 2008. Determinants of vitamin K status in humans. In *Vitamin K*, ed. G. Litwack, 1–22. New York: Academic Press.

16. Dam, H. 1934. Haemorrhages in chicks reared on artificial diets: A new deficiency disease. *Nature* 133:909–910.

17. Will, B.H., Y. Usui, and J.W. Suttie. 1992. Comparative metabolism and requirement of vitamin K in chicks and rats. *J Nutr* 122:2354–2360.

18. Almquist, H.J. and A.A. Klose. 1939. The antihemorrhagic activity of certain naphthoquinones. *J Am Chem Soc* 61:1923–1924.

19. Griminger, P. 1966. Biological activity of the various vitamin K forms. *Vitamins and Hormones* 24:605–618.

20. Griminger, P. 1965. Relative vitamin K potency of two water-soluble menadione analogues. *Poultry Sci* 44:211–213.

21. Dua, P.N. and E.J. Day. 1966. Vitamin K activity of menadione dimethyl-pyrimidinol bisulfite in chicks. *Poultry Sci* 45:94–96.

22. Jin, S. and J.L. Sell. 2001. Dietary vitamin K_1 requirement and comparison of biopotency of different vitamin K sources for young turkeys. *Poultry Sci* 80:615–620.

23. Oduho, G.W., T.K. Chung, and D.H. Baker. 1993. Menadione nicotinamide bisulfite is a bioactive source of vitamin K and niacin activity for chicks. *J Nutr* 123:737–743.

24. Zhang, C.D., D. Li, F. Wang, and T. Dong. 2003. Effects of dietary vitamin K levels on bone quality in broilers. *Arch Anim Nutr* 57:197–206.

25. Jin, S., J.L. Sell, and J.S. Haynes. 1980. Effect of dietary vitamin K_1 on selected plasma characteristics and bone ash in young turkeys fed diets adequate or deficient in vitamin D_3. *Poult Sci* 80:607–614.

26. Doisy, E.A. and J.T. Matschiner. 1970. Biochemistry of vitamin K. In *Fat-Soluble Vitamins*, ed. R.A. Morton, 293–331. Oxford: Pergamon Press.

27. Scott, M.L. 1966. Vitamin K in animal nutrition. *Vitamins and Hormones* 24:633–647.

28. Griminger, P. 1971. Nutritional requirements for vitamin K-animal studies. In *Symposium Proceedings on the Biochemistry, Assay, and Nutritional Value of Vitamin K and Related Compounds*, 39–59. Chicago: Association of Vitamin Chemists.

29. National Academy of Sciences. 1978. *Nutrient Requirements of Laboratory Animals*, 3rd ed. Washington, D.C.: National Academy Press.

30. Reeves, P.G., F.H. Nielsen, and G.C. Fahey, Jr. 1993. AIN-93 purified diets for laboratory rodents: Final report of the American Institute of Nutrition ad hoc writing committee on the reformulation of the AIN-76A rodent diet. *J Nutr* 123:1939–1951.

31. Shah, D.V. and J.W. Suttie. 1978. Vitamin K-dependent carboxylase: Increased activity in a hypoprothrombinemia state. *Arch Biochem Biophys* 191:571–577.

32. Shah, D.V. and J.W. Suttie. 1983. Vitamin K-dependent carboxylase: Effect of endogenous microsomal protein precursors on the rate of exogenous substrate carboxylation. *Proc Soc Exp Biol Med* 173:148–152.

33. Kindberg, C.G. and J.W. Suttie. 1989. Effect of various intakes of phylloquinone on signs of vitamin K deficiency and serum and liver phylloquinone concentrations in the rat. *J Nutr* 119:175–180.

34. Matschiner, J.T. and R.G. Bell. 1973. Effect of sex and sex hormones on plasma prothrombin and vitamin K deficiency. *Proc Soc Exp Biol Med* 144:316–320.

35. Matschiner, J.T. and A.K. Willingham. 1974. Influence of sex hormones on vitamin K deficiency and epoxidation of vitamin K in the rat. *J Nutr* 104:660–665.

36. Siegfried, C.M., G.R. Knauer, and J.T. Matschiner. 1979. Evidence for increased formation of preprothrombin and the noninvolvement of vitamin K-dependent reactions in sex-linked hyperprothrombinemia in the rat. *Arch Biochem Biophys* 194:486–495.

37. Jolly, D.W., B.M. Kadis, and T.E. Nelson. 1977. Estrogen and prothrombin synthesis. The prothrombinogenic action of estrogen. *Biochem Biophys Res Commun* 74:41–49.

38. Nishino, Y. 1979. Hormonal control of prothrombin synthesis in rat liver microsomes, with special reference to the role of estradiol, testosterone and prolactin. *Arch Toxicol Suppl* 2:397–402.

39. van Oosterom, A.T., P. Kerkhoven, and J.J. Veltkamp. 1979. Metabolism of the coagulation factors of the prothrombin complex in hypothyroidism in man. *Thromb Haemostas* 41:273–285.

40. Doisy, E.A. 1961. Nutritional hypoprothrombinemia and metabolism of vitamin K. *Fed Proc* 20:989–994.

41. Gustafsson, B.F. 1959. Vitamin K deficiency in germfree rats. *Ann NY Acad Sci* 78:166–174.

42. Gustafsson, B.E., F.S. Daft, E.G. McDaniel, and J.C. Smith. 1962. Effects of vitamin K-active compounds and intestinal microorganisms in vitamin K-deficient germfree rats. *J Nutr* 78:461–468.

43. Barnes, R.H. and G. Fiala. 1959. Effects of the prevention of coprophagy in the rat. VI. Vitamin K. *J Nutr* 68:603–614.

44. Metta, V.C., L. Nash, and B.C. Johnson. 1961. A tubular coprophagy-preventing cage for the rat. *J Nutr* 74:473–476.

45. Metta, V.C., M.S. Mameesh, and B.C. Johnson. 1959. Vitamin K deficiency in rats induced by the feeding of irradiated beef. *J Nutr* 69:18–22.

46. Mameesh, M.S., V.C. Metta, P.B. Rama Rao, and B.C. Johnson. 1962. On the cause of vitamin K deficiency in male rats fed irradiated beef and the production of vitamin K deficiency using an amino acid synthetic diet. *J Nutr* 77:165–170.

47. Elliott, G.R., E.M. Odam, and M.G. Townsend. 1976. An assay procedure for the vitamin K_1 2,3-epoxide-reducing systems of rat liver involving high-performance liquid chromatography. *Biochem Soc Trans* 4:615–617.

48. Nelson, T.S. and L.C. Norris. 1961. Studies on the vitamin K requirement of the chick. II. Effect of sulfaquinoxaline on the quantitative requirements of the chick for vitamin K_1, menadione and menadione sodium bisulfite. *J Nutr* 73:135–142.

49. Suzuki, H., T. Nakao, and K. Hiraga. 1979. Vitamin K deficiency in male rats fed diets containing butylated hydroxytoluene (BHT). *Toxicol Appl Pharmacol* 50:261–266.

50. Takahashi, O. and K. Hiraga. 1979. Preventive effects of phylloquinone on hemorrhagic death induced by butylated hydroxytoluene in male rats. *J Nutr* 109:453–457.

51. Morrison, S.A. and M.P. Esnouf. 1973. The nature of the heterogeneity of prothrombin during dicoumarol therapy. *Nature New Biol* 242:92–94.

52. Matschiner, J.T. and E.A. Doisy, Jr. 1962. Role of vitamin A in induction of vitamin K deficiency in the rat. *Proc Soc Exp Biol Med* 109:139–142.

53. Wostmann, B.S. and P.L. Knight. 1965. Antagonism between vitamins A and K in the germfree rat. *J Nutr* 87:155–160.

54. McCarthy, D.J., C. Lindamood III, C.M. Gundberg, and D.L. Hill. 1989. Retinoid-induced hemorrhaging and bone toxicity in rats fed diets deficient in vitamin K. *Toxicol Appl Pharmacol* 97:300–310.

55. Szulc, P. and P.D. Delmas. 1996. Influence of vitamin D and retinoids on the gamma-carboxylation of osteocalcin in human osteosarcoma MG63 cells. *Bone* 19:615–620.

56. Rao, G.H. and K.E. Mason. 1975. Antisterility and antivitamin K activity of D-alpha-tocopheryl hydroquinone in the vitamin E-deficient female rat. *J Nutr* 105:495–498.

57. Corrigan, J.J. and F.I. Marcus. 1974. Coagulopathy associated with vitamin E ingestion. *J Am Med Assoc* 230:1300–1301.

58. Corrigan, J.J. and L.L. Ulfers. 1981. Effect of vitamin E on prothrombin levels in warfarin-induced vitamin K deficiency. *J Nutr* 34:1701–1705.

59. Olson, R.E. and J.P. Jones. 1979. The inhibition of vitamin K action by D-alpha-tocopherol and its derivatives. *Fed Proc* 38:710.

60. Uotila, L. 1988. Inhibition of vitamin K-dependent carboxylase by vitamin E and its derivatives. In *Current Advances in Vitamin K Research*, ed. J.W. Suttie, 59–64. New York: Elsevier Science Publishing Co.

61. Dowd, P. and Z.B. Zheng. 1995. On the mechanism of anticlotting action of vitamin E quinone. *Proc Natl Acad Sci USA* 92:8171–8175.

62. Booth, S.L., I. Golly, J.M. Sacheck, R. Roubenoff, G.E. Dallal, K. Hamada, and J.B. Blumberg. 2004. Effect of vitamin E supplementation on vitamin K status in adults with normal coagulation status. *Am J Clin Nutr* 80:143–148.

63. Kim, J.M. and R.H. White. 1996. Effect of vitamin E on the anticoagulant response to warfarin. *Am J Cardiol* 77:545–546.

64. Tovar, A., C.K. Ameho, J.B. Blumberg, J.W. Peterson, D. Smith, and S.L. Booth. 2006. Extrahepatic tissue concentrations of vitamin K are lower in rats fed a high vitamin E diet. *Nutr Metab* 3:29–34.

65. Alexander, C.D. and J.W. Suttie. 1999. The effects of vitamin E on vitamin K activity. *FASEB J* 13:A535.

66. Owen, C.A. 1971. Vitamin K group XI pharmacology and toxicology. In *The Vitamins*, 2nd ed., Vol. 3, ed. W.H. Sebrell and R.S. Harris, 492–509. New York: Academic Press.

67. National Research Council 1987. *Vitamin Tolerance of Animals*. Washington, D.C.: National Academy Press.

68. DeZee, K.J., W.T. Shimeall, K.M. Douglas, N.M. Shumway, and P.G. O'Malley. 2006. Treatment with excessive anticoagulation with phytonadione (vitamin K). *Arch Intern Med* 166:391–397.

69. Fiore, L.D., M.A. Scola, C.E. Cantillon, and M.T. Brophy. 2001. Anaphylactoid reactions to vitamin K. *J Thrombosis Thrombolysis* 11:175–183.

70. Bosse, G.M., M.N.S. Mallory, and G.J. Malone. 2002. The safety of intravenously administered vitamin K *Vet Human Toxicol* 44:174–176.

71. Badr, M., H. Yoshihara, F. Kauffman, and R. Thurman. 1987. Menadione causes selective toxicity to periportal regions of the liver lobule. *Toxicol Lett* 35:241–246.
72. Chiou, T.J., Y.T. Chou, and W.F. Tzeng. 1998. Menadione-induced cell degeneration is related to lipid peroxidation in human cancer cells. *Proc Natl Sci Counc Repub China B* 22:13–21.
73. Sakamoto, N., I. Wakabayashi, and K. Sakamoto. 1999. Low vitamin K intake effects on glucose tolerance in rats. *Int J Vit Nutr Res* 69:27–31.
74. Sakamoto, N., T. Nishiike, H. Iguchi, and K. Sakamoto. 2000. Possible effects of one week vitamin K (menaquinone-4) tablets intake on glucose tolerance in healthy young male volunteers with different descarboxy prothrombin levels. *Clin Nutr* 19:259–263.
75. Sakamoto, N., T. Nishiike, H. Iguchi, and K. Sakamoto. 1999. Relationship between acute insulin response and vitamin K intake in healthy young male volunteers. *Diab Nutr Metab* 12:37–41.
76. Yoshida, M., S.L. Booth, J.B. Meigs, E.J. Saltzman, and P.F. Jacques. 2008. Phylloquinone intake, insulin sensitivity, and glycemic status in men and women. *Am J Clin Nutr* 88:210–215.
77. Booth, S.L., G. Dallal, M.K. Shea, C. Gundberg, J.W. Peterson, and B. Dawson-Hughes. 2008. Effect of vitamin K supplementation on bone loss in elderly men and women. *J Clin Endocrin Metab* 93:1217–1223.
78. Lee, N.K., H. Sowa, E. Hinoi, M. Ferron, J.D. Ahn, C. Confavreux, R. Dacquin, P.J. Mee, M.D. McKee, D.Y. Jung, Z.-Y. Zhang, J.K. Kim, F. Mauvais-Jarvis, P. Ducy, and G. Karsenty. 2007. Endocrine regulation of energy metabolism by the skeleton. *Cell* 130:456–469.
79. Ferron, M., E. Hinoi, G. Karsenty, and P. Ducy. 2008. Osteocalcin differentially regulates beta cell and adipocyte gene expression and affects the development of metabolic diseases in wild-type mice. *Proc Natl Acad Sci USA* 105:5266–5270.
80. Ohsaki, Y., H. Shirakawa, K. Hiwatashi, Y. Furukawa, T. Mizutani, and M. Komai. 2006. Vitamin K suppresses lipopolysaccharide-induced inflammation in the rat. *Biosci Biotechnol Biochem* 70:926–932.
81. Shea, M.K., S.L. Booth, J.M. Massaro, P.F. Jacques, R.B. D'Agostino, Sr, B. Dawson-Hughes, J.M. Ordovas, C.J. O'Donnell, S. Kathiresan, J.F. Keany, Jr, R.S. Vasan, and E.J. Benjamin. 2008. Vitamin K and vitamin D status: Associations with inflammatory markers in the Framingham Offspring Study. *Am J Epidemiol* 167:313–320.
82. Hemker, H.C., A.D. Muller, and E.A. Loeliger. 1970. Two types of prothrombin in vitamin K deficiency. *Thrombos Diathes Haemorrh* 23:633–637.
83. Widdershoven, J., P. van Munster, R.A. De Abreu, H. Bosman, T. van Lith, M. van der Putten-van Meyel, K. Motohara, and I. Matsuda. 1987. Four methods compared for measuring des-carboxy-prothrombin (PIVKA-II). *Clin Chem* 33:2074–2078.
84. Marrero, J.A., G.L. Su, W. Wei, D. Emick, H.S. Conjeevaram, R.J. Fontana, and A.S. Lok. 2003. Des-gamma carboxyprothrombin can differentiate hepatocellular carcinoma from nonmalignant chronic liver disease in American patients. *Hepatology* 37:1114–1121.
85. Kakizaki, S., N. Sohara, K. Sato, H. Suzuki, M. Yanagisawa, H. Nakajima, H. Takagi, A. Naganuma, T. Otsuka, H. Takahashi, T. Hamada, and M. Mori. 2007. Preventive effects of vitamin K on recurrent disease in patients with hepatocellular carcinoma arising from hepatitis C viral infection. *J Gastroenterol Hepatol* 22:518–522.
86. Jackson, J.M., D. Blaine, J. Powell-Tuck, M. Korbonits, A. Carey, and M. Elia. 2006. Macro- and micronutrient losses and nutritional status resulting from 44 days of total fasting in a non-obese man. *Nutrition* 22:889–897.
87. Tamori, A., D. Habu, S. Shiomi, S. Kubo, and S. Nishiguchi. 2007. Potential role of vitamin K(2) as a chemopreventive agent against hepatocellular carcinoma. *Hepatol Res* 37(Suppl 2):S303–S307.

88. Kaneda, M., D. Zhang, R. Bhattacharjee, K. Nakahama, S. Aril, and I. Morita. 2008. Vitamin K_2 suppresses malignancy of HuH7 hepatoma cells via inhibition of connexin 43. *Cancer Lett* 263:53–60.

89. Sasaki, R., Y. Suzuki, Y. Yonezawa, Y. Ota, Y. Okamoto, Y. Demizu, P. Huang, H. Yoshida, K. Sugimura, and Y. Mizushina. 2008. DNA polymerase gamma inhibition by vitamin K_3 induces mitochondria-mediated cytotoxicity in human cancer cells. *Cancer Sci* 99:1040–1048.

90. Ozaki, I., H. Zhang, T. Mizut, Y. Ide, Y. Eguchi, T. Yasutake, T. Sakamaki, R.G. Pestell, and K. Yamamoto. 2007. Menatetrenone, a vitamin K_2 analogue, inhibits hepatocellular carcinoma cell growth by suppressing cyclin D_1 expression through inhibition of nuclear factor kB activation. *Clin Cancer Res* 13:2236–2245.

91. Tsujioka, T., Y. Miura, T. Otsuki, Y. Nishimura, F. Hyodoh, H. Wada, and T. Sugihara. 2006. The mechanisms of vitamin K_2-induced apoptosis of myeloma cells. *Haematologica* 91:613–619.

92. Ogawa, M., S. Nakai, A. Deguchi, T. Nonomura, T. Masaki, N. Uchida, H. Yoshiji, and S. Kuriyama. 2007. Vitamins K_2, K_3 and K_5 exert antitumor effects on established colorectal cancer in mice by inducing apoptotic death of tumor cells. *Int J Oncol* 31:323–331.

93. Shibayama-Imazu, T., I. Sonoda, S. Sakairi, T. Aiuchi, W.-W. Ann, S. Nakajo, H. Itabe, and K. Nakaya. 2006. Production of superoxide and dissipation of mitochondrial transmembrane potential by vitamin K_2 trigger apoptosis in human ovarian cancer TYK-nu cells. *Apoptosis* 11:1535–1543.

94. Lim, D., R.J. Morgan, Jr, S. Akman, K. Margolin, B.I. Carr, L. Leong, O. Odujinrin, and J.H. Doroshow. 2005. Phase I trial of menadiol diphosphate (vitamin K_3) in advanced malignancy. *Invest New Drugs* 23:235–239.

95. Sakagami, H., K. Hashimoto, F. Suzuki, M. Ishihara, H. Kikuchi, T. Katayama, and K. Satoh. 2008. Tumor-specificity and type of cell death induced by vitamin K_2 derivatives and prenylalcohols. *Anticancer Res* 28:151–158.

96. Israels, L.G., E. Friesen, A.H. Jansen, and E.D. Israels. 1987. Vitamin K_1 increases sister chromatid exchange in vitro in human leukocytes and in vivo in fetal sheep cells: A possible role for "vitamin K deficiency" in the fetus. *Pediatr Res* 22:405–408.

97. Israels, L.G., D.J. Ollmann, and E.D. Israels. 1985. Vitamin K_1 as a modulator of benzo(a)pyrene metabolism as measured by in vitro metabolite formation and in vivo DNA-adduct formation. *Int J Biochem* 17:1263–1266.

98. Dogra, S.C. and L.G. Israels. 1987. Vitamin K_1 amplification of benzo(a)pyrene metabolism in chick embryos. *Int J Biochem* 19:471–473.

99. Israels, L.G. and E.D. Israels. 1995. Observations on vitamin K deficiency in the fetus and newborn: Has nature made a mistake? *Sem Thromb* 21:357–363.

100. Saxena, S.P., E.D. Israels, and L.G. Israels. 2001. Novel vitamin K-dependent pathways regulating cell survival. *Apoptosis* 6:57–68.

101. Kobayashi, M., K. Hara, and Y. Akiyama. 2002. Effects of vitamin K_2 (menatetrenone) on calcium balance in ovariectomized rats. *Jpn J Pharmacol* 88:55–61.

102. Iwamoto, J., J.K. Yeh, T. Takeda, and Y. Sato. 2005. Comparative effects of vitamin K and vitamin D supplementation on calcium balance in young rats fed normal or low calcium diets. *J Nutr Sci Vitaminol* 51:211–215.

103. Sogabe, N., R. Maruyama, T. Hosoi, and M. Goseki-Sone. 2007. Enhancement effects of vitamin K_1 (phylloquinone) or vitamin K_2 (menaquinone-4) on intestinal alkaline phosphatase activity in rats. *J Nutr Sci Vitaminol* 53:219–224.

104. Carrie, I., G. Ferland, and M.S. Obin. 2003. Effects of long-term vitamin K (phylloquinone) intake on retina aging. *Nutr Neurosci* 6:351–359.

105. Tirapelli, C.R., F.E. Mingatto, and A.M. de Oliveira. 2002. Vitamin K_1 prevents the effect of hypoxia on phenylephrine-induced contraction in the carotid artery. *Pharmacology* 66:36–43.

106. Tirapelli, C.R., F.E. Mingatto, M.A. De Godoy, R. Ferreira, and A.M. De Oliveira. 2002. Vitamin K_1 attenuates hypoxia-induced relaxation of rat carotid artery. *Pharmacological Res* 46:483–490.
107. Shirakawa, H., Y. Ohsaki, Y. Minegishi, N. Takumi, K. Ohinata, Y. Furukawa, T. Mizutani, and M. Komai. 2006. Vitamin K deficiency reduces testosterone production in the testis through down-regulation of the Cyp11a a cholesterol side chain cleavage enzyme in rats. *Biochim Biophys Acta* 1760:1482–1488.
108. Otsuka, M., N. Kato, T. Ichimura, S. Abe, Y. Tanaka, H. Taniguchi, Y. Hoshida, M. Moriyama, Y. Wang, R.-X. Shao, D. Narayan, R. Muroyama, F. Kanai, T. Kawabe, T. Isobe, and M. Omata. 2005. Vitamin K_2 binds 17beta-hydroxysteroid dehydrogenase 4 and modulates estrogen metabolism. *Life Sci* 76:2473–2482.
109. Manzardo, A.M., E.C. Penick, J. Knop, E.J. Nickel, S. Hall, P. Jensen, C.C. Miller, and W.F. Gabrielli. 2005. Neonatal vitamin K might reduce vulnerability to alcohol dependence in Danish men. *J Stud Alcohol* 66:586–592.
110. Suttie, J.W. 1992. Vitamin K and human nutrition. *J Am Dietet Assoc* 92:585–590.
111. Shah, D.V., J.C. Swanson, and J.W. Suttie. 1984. Abnormal prothrombin in the vitamin K-deficient rat. *Thrombosis Res* 35:451–458.
112. Francis, J.L. 1988. A rapid and simple micromethod for the specific determination of descarboxylated prothrombin (PIVKA II). *Med Lab Sci* 45:69–73.
113. Motohara, K., Y. Kuroki, H. Kan, F. Endo, and I. Matsuda. 1985. Detection of vitamin K deficiency by use of an enzyme-linked immunosorbent assay for circulating abnormal prothrombin. *Pediatric Res* 19:354–357.

Index

Printed in the United States
by Baker & Taylor Publisher Services